The Advancing Frontier of Survival

Monographs on Population Aging

General editors
Bernard Jeune and James W. Vaupel

Vol. 1
Development of Oldest-Old Mortality, 1950-1990
Väinö Kannisto

Vol. 2
Exceptional Longivety: From Prehistory of the Present
Bernard Jeune and James W. Vaupel (Eds.)

Vol. 3
The Advancing Frontier of Survival:
Life Tables for Old Age
Väinö Kannisto

Vol. 4
Population Data at a Glance
James W. Vaupel, Wang Zhenglian, Kirill F. Andrew,
and Anatoli J. Yashin

Aging Research Unit
Centre for Health & Social Policy
Odense University Medical School

The Advancing Frontier of Survival

Life Tables for Old Age

Väinö Kannisto

Monographs on Population Aging, 3.

Odense University Press

The Advancing Frontier of Survival
© Väinö Kannisto and Odense University Press, 1996
Printed in Denmark by Special-Trykkeriet Viborg a-s
Cover illustration: Jens Bohr
ISBN 87-7838-185-1
ISSN 0909-119x

Odense University Press
55, Campusvej
DK-5230 Odense M
Tlf. +45 66 15 79 99   Fax. +45 66 15 81 26
E-mail: Press @ forlag.ou.dk

Contents

Acknowledgements 11

1. Introduction 12
2. The data 14
3. Probability of dying 20
4. Old age life tables 25
5. Changing mortality 36
6. Life expectancy at age 80 42
7. Other longevity parameters 50
8. Age shift in mortality 56
9. Slope of mortality 62
10. The road from 80 to 100 69
11. The centenarians 75
12. Gender and mortality 84
13. Stationary population 91
14. The changing survival curve 97
15. Realized living potential 102
16. Seven ways of looking at mortality change 108
17. Growing numbers of old people 117
18. The expanding frontier of survival 128
19. Conclusions 136

References 140

Annex 145
   by Väinö Kannisto, Zhenglian Wang, Kirill Andreev

Lists of tables and figures

Tables

1. Total data volume for 28 countries 19
2. Probability of dying by age and sex, by decade.
   Thirteen countries with good data 21
3. Probability of dying by age and sex, 1980-1990.
   Groups of countries with good data 23
4. Old age life table. Thirteen countries with good data, 1980-1990 26
5. Percent change in mortality between 1960-70 and 1980-90 38
6. Life expectancy at age 80, by country, aggregate and sex, each decade . 43
7. Ranking of countries according to life expectancy at 80 for both sexes,
   1950-60 and 1980-90, 19 countries with good data 44
8. Increase in life expectancy at age 80 from 1950-60 to 1980-90, years.
   19 countries with good data 47
9. Median, quartiles and inter-quartile range of age at death after 80
   in life table population. Thirteen countries with good data 50
10. Modal length of life 52
11. Age when life expectancy equals a given number of years.
    Low, medium and high mortality countries 55
12. Mean age shift in age groups from 1960-70 to 1980-90. By country . . . 60
13. Life table aging rate k in specified age intervals, by decade.
    Thirteen countries with good data 63
14. Life table aging rate k between ages 83 and 98 66
15. Probability of survival by age and sex and increase from 1960-70
    to 1980-90. Thirteen countries with good data; 5-year moving averages . 70
16. 5-year probabilities of survival by age and sex and increase between
    specified periods. Thirteen countries with good data 71
17. Persons reaching age 100 out of 1000 80-year-old 73
18. Survivors from age 80 to 100 in actual cohorts, per 1000 74
19. Proportion of centenarians in total population, 1960 and 1990 76
20. Sex ratio of centenarians. Thirteen countries with good data 77
21. Centenarian life table, 1980-90. Fourteen countries with good data 78

22.	Nordic centenarian life table, 1980-90, Denmark, Finland, Iceland, Norway, Sweden	79
23.	Life expectancy at age 100. Rates based on at least 100 person-years	82
24.	The road from 100 to 110 years. Thirteen countries with good data	84
25.	Gender indicators of mortality. Thirteen countries, 1980-1990	85
26.	Female advantage in life expectancy at 80 and female age delay	89
27.	Stationary oldest-old population. Thirteen countries, 1960-70 and 1980-90	92
28.	Stationary centenarian population. Thirteen countries, 1960-70 and 1980-90	93
29.	Age distribution of stationary population	95
30.	Years gained per 10,000 persons aged 80 through mortality decline between successive decades. Thirteen countries with good data	100
31.	Years gained per 10,000 persons aged 80 by mortality decline between 1950-60 and 1980-90. Low, medium and high mortality countries	101
32.	Realized living potential (percent) at ages 80-100 and years lived in each 5-year age interval per each person reaching age 80. Life tables 1980-90	103
33.	Mortality change indicators. Thirteen countries with good data from 1960-70 to 1980-90	110
34.	Growth of the oldest-old population. By country	118
35.	Proportion aged 80 and over in total population, percent	120
36.	Increase in the number of centenarians and contribution of mortality decline above age 80 to it, 1960-1990	126
37.	Contribution of mortality decline at ages 80 and over to population growth from 1960 to 1990, percent	127
38.	Probability of dying per 10,000 according to three scenarios	130
39.	Some demographic effects if the decline of oldest-old mortality in the last 20 years is repeated one, two or three more times. Thirteen countries with good data	132

Figures

1. Probability of dying by age and sex. Thirteen countries 1980-90 22
2. Probability of dying by age and sex. Countries with low, medium and high mortality, 1980-1990 24
3. Probability of dying by age and sex. Thirteen countries by decade 24
4. Life expectancy at age 80 according to official and Odense life tables .. 30
5. Percentage decline of mortality by age between successive decades. Thirteen countries with good data 37
6. Percent decline of mortality from 1960-70 to 1980-90 40
7. Life expectancy at age 80 in 1980-90 by sex. Nineteen countries with good data 45
8. Life expectancy at age 80 by sex and decade. Low, medium and high mortality countries 46
9. Correlation between life expectancy at age 80 in 1950-60 and its gain until 1980-90. Nineteen countries with good data 48
10. Long term development of life expectancy at 80 in Sweden, Finland and Norway 49
11. Length of life of 1000 persons who reached age 80. Thirteen countries with good data 53
12. Length of life of 1000 persons who reached age 80. Selected countries, 1980-90 54
13. Age when life expectancy equals 5 years. Low, medium and high mortality countries 56
14. Age shift in mortality from 1960-70 to specified periods. Thirteen countries 57
15. Age shift in mortality from 1960-70 to 1980-90 59
16. Comparison of age shift with increase in life expectancy at 80 from 1960-70 to 1980-90 61
17. Slope of mortality (k) in 5-year age intervals. Thirteen countries with good data 64
18. Correlation of life expectancy at age 80 and slope of mortality (k) between ages 83 and 98, twenty countries in 1980-90 67

19.	Correlation between change in life expectancy at age 80 and in slope of mortality (k) from 1960-70 to 1980-90. Twenty countries	68
20.	Increase from 1960-70 to 1980-90 in age-specific probability of survival. Thirteen countries with good data	70
21.	Percent surviving through specified age intervals. Thirteen countries with good data	72
22.	Probability of dying at ages 100 and over. 1980-90	80
23.	Survival curve of centenarians. Thirteen countries with good data	83
24.	Gender indicators of mortality. Thirteen countries with good data	86
25.	Female advantage in life expectancy and female age delay in mortality, 1980-90	90
26.	Proportionate age pyramid of the oldest-old. Thirteen countries with good data	91
27.	Proportionate age pyramid of centenarians. Thirteen countries with good data	94
28.	Age distribution of stationary population	96
29.	Survivors out of 100 persons aged 80	98
30.	Years of life gained per 100 persons aged 80	99
31.	Years lived at specified age intervals per each person reaching age 80	104
32.	Mortality change indicators. Thirteen countries. Change in mortality from 1960-70 to 1980-90	112
33.	Seven indicators of mortality change. Females. Thirteen countries from 1960-70 to 1980-90	116
34.	Annual growth rate of oldest-old population in ten countries involved in World War I	119
35.	Growth of the oldest-old population. Thirteen countries with good data.	122
36.	Growth factor of oldest-old population from 1960 to 1990 and contribution of mortality decline above age 80 to it. (in colour)	124
37.	Life and death at ages 80 and over. Female	135

Annex tables

1. Population aged 80 and over by age and sex, 1950-90, by country.
2. Decennial life tables by country.
3. Decennial life tables for aggregates.
4. Life expectancy at age 80 according to official life tables.
5. Mean values of q in age groups per 10.000.
6. Age shift of mortality from 1960-70 to 1980-90, by age. By country.
7. Survivors from age 80 to 100 in actual cohorts.
8. Probability of dying at ages 100 and over, pooled data for 14 countries.
9. Gender indicators of mortality by decade. Thirteen countries.
10. Stationary oldest-old population by country in 1980-90. Based on 10.000 persons (3500 male and 6500 female) annually reaching the age of 80 years.
11. Years lived at specified age intervals per each person reaching age 80. By country and decade.
12. Years lived at specified age intervals per each person reaching the interval. By country and decade.
13. Annual population growth (%) in countries involved and not involved in World War I.
14. Oldest-old population on 1 January 1960-1990.
15. Persons aged 80 and over, 1960-1990. Both sexes.
16. Population growth factor from 1960 to 1990.

Acknowledgements

I am greatly indebted to Professor James W. Vaupel who arranged to computerize my data and to extract from them ever since large numbers of statistical tables and graphs, and finally to have the work published. He and A. Roger Thatcher as well as Dr. Bernard Jeune have greatly helped me with their views, suggestions and comments. Thatcher who has generously given of his time to an intensive correspondence, also contributed the data on England and Wales to this study, and Jeune oversaw as editor its publication.

Many thanks are due to Mrs. Zhenglian Wang who has produced all the figures and many of the tables in this book, and to Kirill Andreev who with his thorough knowledge of the database has been very helpful. Wang and Andreev are my co-authors for the Annex. I thank Ms. Lis Bluhme for typing the text and many of the tables, Ms. Vaina Berntsen for assisting in the task and Ms. Klöjgaard for composing the final typescript.

I gratefully recognize the initial impetus and further encouragement given by Peter Laslett, Advisory Director, Cambridge Group, through the project on Maximal Length of Life which has invited interested colleagues to many useful meetings in Cambridge.

Finally, I wish to pay tribute to government statisticians past and present who have carefully tended the vital statistics of their respective countries and have been helpful to me in assembling the data.

Lisbon, December 1995

Väinö Kannisto

1. Introduction

The present book is intended to be an additional contribution to the description of the mortality of the oldest-old in the postwar era, begun with "Development of Oldest-Old Mortality, 1950-1990" by the same author. While the first publication was essentially a *time series study* of the momentous changes that took place in the mortality of old people in advanced countries, their timing and magnitude, their acceleration or deceleration or absence of either, in each of the 28 countries examined, the present one is a *life table analysis* of the same countries in the same period, less precise on timing and more sharply focused on age. Instead of annual fluctuations in 5-year or broader age groups, dealt with in the former, the present study examines mortality by single years of age. To do it successfully, the data are combined into 10-year periods in order to secure meaningful numbers of observations at ages where they are few. This has, in fact, allowed calculation of fairly robust death rates up to age 109 for an aggregate of several countries.

In the period 1950-1990, the developed countries experienced an unprecedented and entirely unexpected decline in old age mortality as documented on a broad front in the above-mentioned publication. Division of this period into four decades and preparation of life tables for each of them yields only a rough time series but provides a sharper view of the levels and changes in mortality by age. As data for the 1950s are unavailable for some countries and since the change from then up to 1960s was relatively small, the dimensions and nature of the changes that have so far occurred can perhaps best be seen when comparing the 1960-70 and 1980-90 life tables. This will be frequently done.

Both studies spring from the Kannisto-Thatcher Oldest-Old Database which is incorporated in the Odense Archive of Population Data on Aging. All the countries comprised in the database, 28 of which have been included in both these studies, are industrialized and can be considered in the global context to be low-mortality countries because the life expectancy at birth for both sexes combined in all of them is at least 69 and in most cases 75 years. This allows, however, significant differences in mortality levels, and the results will in some connections be presented separately for what are termed low, medium and high mortality groups of countries, so classified according to level of oldest-old mortality. It should be stressed that all of these are nevertheless advanced countries with relatively low death rates.

The geographic limitation of the database to essentially low-mortality countries was by no means planned but was reluctantly accepted for the reason that we have not found reliable data on age at death among the old in the national statistics of developing countries.

For the calculation of any kind of death rate, both the number of deaths and the size of the population at risk are needed. It may be surprising but it is nevertheless a fact that in most of the advanced countries of the world, including all the larger ones, the numbers of population at very high ages are not well known. Censuses regularly produce figures which at ages approaching or exceeding one hundred years are obviously overstated and, when examined over time, incompatible with data on deaths. This realization, together with the finding that the age information on death certificates was in many of the same countries quite accurate, prompted Paul VINCENT to pioneer his *method of extinct generations* (Vincent, 1951) in which the populations at risk are obtained by summing up the deaths in each cohort beginning with the oldest. Today, more than 40 years later, it is still the method of choice for the study of mortality at very high ages in all countries except the few which maintain reliable permanent population registers.

A third study which is currently under preparation, will use the same database to attempt to draw and define the trajectory of mortality as far up as is at present possible (Thatcher et al., forthcoming).

2. The data

2.1. Deaths

The database has been constructed in the first place from official national statistics giving annual numbers of deaths by sex and single years of age, beginning with the age of 80 years. In most countries, the single-year classification by age continues till the highest age recorded while in several others, the deaths at ages such as 100 and over are given in a lump sum which naturally impairs their usefulness. Often, however, this is done because the detailed age data are considered unreliable by the national office.

In about half of the countries of the database the age at death is cross-tabulated with the year of birth (cohort) and this information is used for arranging the data by cohort in order to make use of the extinct cohorts method. A problem rises when the cohort is not given and the deaths at a given age have to be allocated to the two alternative cohorts by an arbitrary rule. This was done at first in proportions observed in a neighbouring country but has later been done at a 50/50 split because the choice makes no appreciable difference in decennial life tables for either periods or cohorts. On the other hand, no arbitrary cohort allocation can lead to satisfactory results when calculating death rates by this method for one-year periods or for single cohorts. For this, double classification by age/cohort is needed and it is available for the following 15 countries: Belgium, Czechoslovakia, Denmark, Finland, France, West Germany, Hungary, Iceland, Italy, Japan, the Netherlands, Poland, Spain, Sweden and Switzerland. In Norway, the data were classified until 1976 by cohort only, thereafter by age only.

As mentioned, the data on deaths are in several countries limited by the fact that the single-year classification ends at age 99 or 100 after which the older deceased are given in a lump sum. This is the case for Canada, Czechoslovakia, Estonia, East Germany, Hungary, Latvia, Luxembourg and Scotland for the entire period, for West Germany until 1963, Australia until 1967, Belgium until 1973 and Singapore until 1988. The data for Spain are similarly limited since 1981 while Estonia removed the age restriction in 1990.

The official death counts have been accepted in the database virtually without correction. The deaths at ages 110 and over in England and Wales include only cases verified against a birth registration.

2.2. Exposed-to-risk

When a cohort is judged extinct, the numbers of deaths are summed up beginning with the oldest, to give the number of persons who reached each successive age. This ignores international migration which has been found to be negligible at high ages. The same procedure is applied even for countries which produce accurate migration data in their population registers, the reason being the methodological advantage of interlocking data on population and deaths.

For cohorts which are not yet extinct, the number of current survivors is needed in order to obtain the populations-at-risk. To determine these numbers, official population data have been compared with our own estimates made under the assumption that recent age-specific survival ratios in two or more successive cohorts have been equal or have changed linearly. Official population data are in these countries generally very reliable except at ages approaching or exceeding 100 years when they often become unreliable and even implausibly high. In such cases, the "own estimate" is accepted because, though not exact, it is consistent with information on deaths and generally plausible. With younger ages the "own estimates" become increasingly uncertain while the official figures gain in accuracy. Therefore, as a rule, a switch is made to the official figures at some such age as 95 or 90, often made easy by a convergence of the two series. However, for countries with reliable population register the official data are accepted as such.

This method of estimating survivors has been tested by applying it to past situations which can be verified by post-facto evidence and it has been found quite satisfactory.

2.3. Data quality

On the basis of rigorous quality tests, the data were classified into the following four categories:

A. Good quality (19 countries)

*	Austria	*	Iceland
	Belgium	*	Italy
	Czechoslovakia	*	Japan
*	Denmark		Luxembourg
*	England & Wales	*	Netherlands
*	Finland	*	Norway
*	France		Scotland
	Germany, East	*	Sweden
*	Germany, West	*	Switzerland
	Hungary		

Thirteen of the nineteen countries above, marked with an asterisk, have been combined into a hard core of best information because in them the age at death is known without an upper limit. This group of thirteen, though not uniform, shares a low level of mortality as well as the experience of a substantial recent decline in it. It will therefore be frequently used for measurement of various aspects of old age survival and their recent developments.

In the other six countries, the detailed classification ends at 99 or 100; in Belgium this was the case until 1973.

B. Acceptable quality (4 countries)

Australia
New Zealand, non-Maori
Portugal
Singapore, Chinese

The data for Australia and New Zealand carry traces of possible age overstatement which may now have come under control. All data presented in this study for New Zealand exclude the Maori. The Portuguese data have improved over time and have been in the last two decades quite reliable except at ages above 105. The series for Singapore is as yet too short for conclusive evaluation. Data for other races in Singapore are available but the numbers are too small for analysis.

C. Conditionally acceptable quality (5 countries)

    Estonia
    Ireland
    Latvia
    Poland
    Spain

These data give probably a roughly correct description of the mortality trend though at a level artificially lowered by age overstatement.

D. Weak quality (4 countries)

    Canada
    Chile
    New Zealand, Maori
    United States

Used with caution, these data may give approximate information on the size and development of the population below age 90 but estimation of mortality by the extinct cohort method would be too uncertain. The data for New Zealand Maori and United States non-white are the weakest due to large-scale age overstatement.

A report on data quality assessment is under preparation.

2.4. What does the database represent?

The "World Population Data Sheet" of the Population Reference Bureau Inc. (1994) lists 35 countries or territories in which the life expectancy at birth for both sexes combined is 75 years or more. These have a total population of 838 million which may be divided as follows:[1]

---

[1] United Kingdom and Germany are each counted as one entity; data for the U.S., Canada and Chile are entered in the database but were only exceptionally made use of in the study.

core thirteen	434 million
five others	71 "
covered in this study	505 million
United States	261 "
Canada	29 "
others	43 "
total	838 million

If, as we believe, old age mortality in the United States and Canada is comparable to that in the "thirteen" of the database, these latter represent well the low-mortality countries of the world. However, if - as has been claimed but not proven - old age mortality is lower in the U.S. than anywhere else, then the representativeness is of course greatly limited. Whichever case one chooses to believe, the database represents the cutting edge of the decline in old age mortality as far as it can be accurately measured. This holds true particularly of the core of thirteen, composed as it is of exactly the countries with the lowest proven levels of mortality among the oldest-old.

The combined population of the 28 countries included in the present study is according to the same source 590 million and the life expectancy in all of them is at least 70 years with the exception of Hungary and Latvia where it is 69.

The European countries of the database are further characterized by an advanced degree of aging. The fourteen countries in which according to the U.S. Bureau of the Census (1991) the proportion aged 75 and over is the highest in the world, includes eleven of the thirteen (without Iceland and Japan) plus Belgium, Greece and Luxembourg.

2.5. Data volume

The size of the population aged 80 and over in 1950-1990 is given by sex, age and country in Annex Table 1. The total volume of the data used in the present study amounted to 386 million person-years of observation of which 52 million ended in death as summarized in Table 1. The bulk of the information, 333 million person-years-at-risk (86.9 percent) refers to the 19 countries with good quality data, and 287 million (74.9 percent) to the core of thirteen countries with unrestricted age information in the 1960-90 period.

Table 1. TOTAL DATA VOLUME FOR 28 COUNTRIES.

Age, sex and period	Person-years placed at risk	Of these ended in death	Mean annual probability of dying
Both sexes:			
80 - 84	247 985 447	26 807 960	0.108
85 - 89	104 496 313	17 204 914	0.165
90 - 94	28 962 717	6 818 449	0.235
95 - 99	4 687 244	1 479 684	0.316
100 -	298 183	121 915	0.409
Total	386 429 904	52 432 922	**0.136**
Male	129 812 728	20 080 851	**0.155**
Female	256 617 176	32 352 071	**0.126**
1950 - 60	51 109 416	7 808 667	0.153
1960 - 70	76 480 754	11 261 282	0.147
1970 - 80	110 520 857	15 141 741	0.137
1980 - 90	148 318 877	18 221 232	0.123

The rapid attrition of the oldest-old population by death leads to a very uneven age distribution. Persons aged 90-94 are little more than one-tenth of those ten years younger but are almost 100 times as numerous as the centenarians. The analytically and scientifically important centenarian group is therefore only a tiny fraction of the total - yet, the nearly 300,000 life years which they began and of which nearly 122,000 ended in death, constitute probably a larger body of reliable evidence of survival after age 100 than has been assembled before.

In population terms, almost exactly one-third of the evidence pertains to the male but due to their higher mortality, they account for more than 38 percent of the deaths.

In the short historical period encompassed by the study, the oldest-old population grew vigorously. A part of the increase in Table 1 is due to inclusion of more countries in the course of the years. However, the greatest factor by far has been an increase in the number of persons surviving to high ages in the countries studied.

The mean annual probability of dying, though only a rough summary measure, reflects the steep increase of mortality by age, the greater vulnerability of men, and an unmistakable decline over time.

3. Probability of dying

The basic life table parameter q_x is in the present study obtained through follow-up of a closed group of persons as they move from one age to the next. The database gives for each country, sex and cohort the number of persons who reached the exact age x and the number of them who died without reaching the age x + 1. The proportion of the latter among the former or D_x/N_x indicates the probability q_x of dying at age x. The direct follow-up ensures strict correspondence between numerator and denominator which is a great advantage with the small numbers observed at high ages. It also allows easy measurement of chance variation.

The use of cohort histories is not predicated by a belief that cohort is the main or even an important factor in mortality but actually serves to eliminate the effect of the often uneven size of adjacent cohorts. The one-year observations of exposed-to-risk and the corresponding deaths are used as building blocks in the construction of period life tables with only the peculiarity that tables for two consecutive periods overlap in one calendar year. At high ages where observations are few, meaningful numbers can only be assembled by joining a number of calendar years together in which case the exact chronology becomes less important while the need for accuracy of age remains paramount.

The annual probability of dying may be converted into a central death rate m_x in which case it maintains its property of internal consistency while in an m_x calculated from the mean population, deaths are not necessarily included among the exposed-to-risk of the same age, with the result that rates may become volatile. An annual probability of dying is also convertible to force of mortality μ_x.

The probability of dying q_x and its complement $p_x = 1 - q_x$ will in some connections below be extended to wider age bands. For 5-year age groups, central values of q have been calculated as geometric means of single-age probabilities.

Table 2 gives a general account of the probability of dying in old age in today's low-mortality societies. Its thirteen component countries have experienced the recent remarkable progress in reduction of old age mortality. The table gives the results for each of the four post-war decades with an overlap in years ending in zero. The 1950-60 period includes the persons who reached age x during 1950-59 and follows them to age x + 1 which they would reach in 1951-1960. The survivors from 1959 to 1960 are then included in the risk population of age x + 1 in 1960-70 and successively at each age which they reach in that or the following decades. This procedure and this designation of overlapping time periods was already used by VINCENT (1951) and DEPOID (1973) in their pathbreaking work.

Table 2. **PROBABILITY OF DYING BY AGE AND SEX, BY DECADE.**
Thirteen countries with good data[1]). 3-year moving averages[2]).

Age	Male				Female			
	1950-60	1960-70	1970-80	1980-90	1950-60	1960-70	1970-80	1980-90
80	0.12375	0.11812	0.11135	0.09762	0.09996	0.09024	0.07768	0.06229
81	0.13501	0.12910	0.12099	0.10694	0.11007	0.10020	0.08694	0.07038
82	0.14700	0.14039	0.13129	0.11663	0.12112	0.11093	0.09692	0.07901
83	0.16019	0.15278	0.14258	0.12687	0.13336	0.12259	0.10784	0.08852
84	0.17393	0.16535	0.15445	0.13780	0.14594	0.13487	0.11938	0.09890
85	0.18886	0.17946	0.16713	0.14959	0.15958	0.14812	0.13173	0.11015
86	0.20456	0.19387	0.18059	0.16243	0.17354	0.16199	0.14463	0.12222
87	0.22059	0.20956	0.19459	0.17577	0.18811	0.17649	0.15847	0.13525
88	0.23664	0.22515	0.20915	0.18971	0.20293	0.19132	0.17329	0.14940
89	0.25279	0.24142	0.22482	0.20445	0.21844	0.20712	0.18886	0.16445
90	0.26951	0.25872	0.24161	0.22011	0.23391	0.22324	0.20515	0.18024
91	0.28712	0.27721	0.25931	0.23660	0.25097	0.24038	0.22217	0.19656
92	0.30530	0.29587	0.27719	0.25349	0.26797	0.25800	0.23962	0.21358
93	0.32292	0.31455	0.29453	0.27117	0.28622	0.27625	0.25760	0.23126
94	0.34241	0.33315	0.31246	0.28901	0.30416	0.29440	0.27552	0.24899
95	0.35969	0.35207	0.32943	0.30647	0.32349	0.31365	0.29441	0.26718
96	0.37923	0.37021	0.34683	0.32254	0.34459	0.33228	0.31259	0.28475
97	0.39821	0.38841	0.36266	0.33665	0.36560	0.35241	0.33030	0.30203
98	0.42916	0.41536	0.38985	0.35525	0.38799	0.36870	0.34995	0.32008
99	0.46279	0.43908	0.41987	0.38272	0.41359	0.39101	0.37159	0.34178
100	0.46778	0.45966	0.44678	0.40722	0.43047	0.40625	0.39197	0.36303
101	0.46917	0.46530	0.45725	0.42429	0.44247	0.42024	0.40886	0.38178
102	0.46597	0.47745	0.47090	0.43994	0.45559	0.43344	0.42267	0.39911
103	0.48199	0.50734	0.48349	0.44719	0.46412	0.45087	0.44259	0.41533
104	0.50223	0.51795	0.51641	0.45313	0.47324	0.47420	0.46810	0.43608
105	0.52089	0.55455	0.51472	0.45007	0.45571	0.48798	0.49030	0.44605
106	0.43367	0.52227	0.52337	0.46706	0.51422	0.52783	0.50786	0.46008
107	0.49399	0.46671	0.55305	0.50435	0.56456	0.54700	0.54240	0.49362
108	0.64550	0.53162	0.66771	0.61106	0.75443	0.63104	0.59097	0.54393
109	...	0.37778	0.82680	0.52926	...	0.60088	0.50833	0.59583

[1]) Austria, Denmark, England & Wales, Finland, France, Germany (West), Iceland, Italy, Japan, Netherlands, Norway, Sweden, Switzerland.
[2]) For original rates, see Annex Table 2.

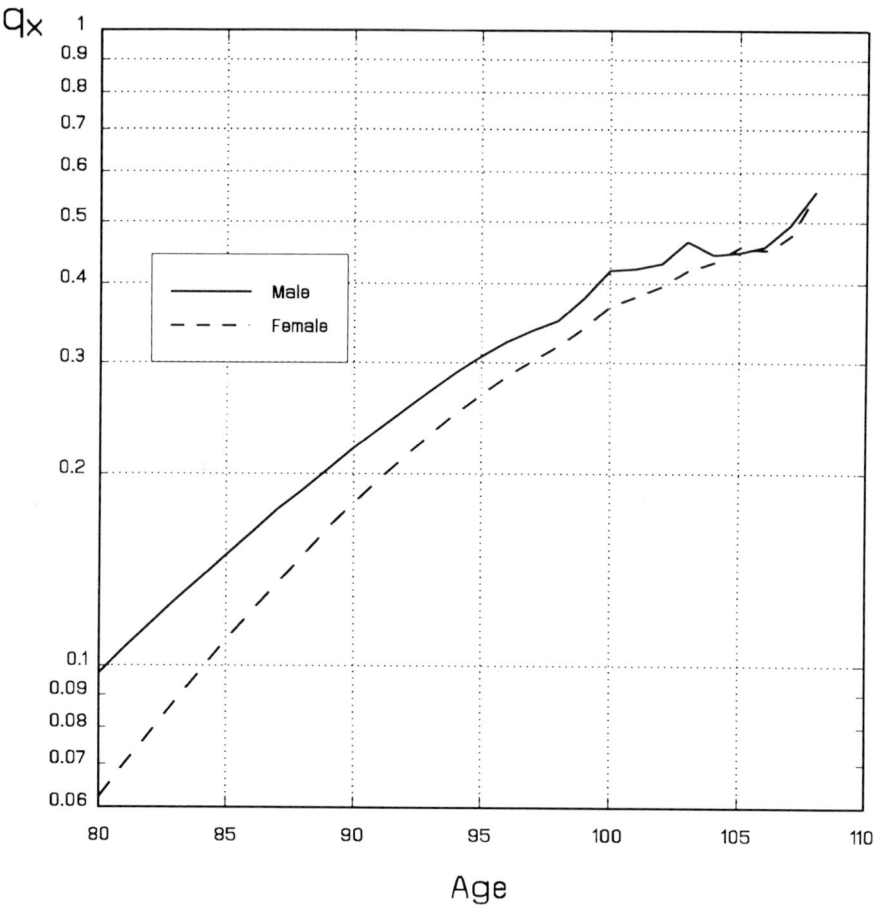

Figure 1. PROBABILITY OF DYING BY AGE AND SEX.
Thirteen countries with good data, 1980-1990.

Figure 1 depicts in logarithmic scale the course of the risk of dying as age advances and shows that it continues to increase as far as it is today measurable, namely close to age 110, without indicating a point where it might peak or stabilize. The increase is, however, less than exponential and displays a curvature well known to demographers and actuaries.

The risk of dying is at all ages higher for men than women. The apparently narrowing gap between the two curves might lead one to expect the two lines eventually to merge or intersect but the absolute difference in the risks does not decline. It actually grows slightly in the early 80s and then remains stationary at least a few years past age 100 after which the picture becomes uncertain due to small numbers. Table 24 in Chapter 11 shows, however, that the female advantage in survival continues till age 110 at least.

Table 3. PROBABILITY OF DYING BY AGE AND SEX, 1980-1990.
Groups of countries with good data[1].

Age	Mortality level							
	Low and medium combined		Low		Medium		High	
	M	F	M	F	M	F	M	F
80	0.0976	0.0623	0.0901	0.0561	0.1055	0.0678	0.1298	0.0942
81	0.1068	0.0701	0.0995	0.0637	0.1146	0.0759	0.1409	0.1043
82	0.1164	0.0787	0.1090	0.0722	0.1244	0.0846	0.1519	0.1157
83	0.1267	0.0882	0.1193	0.0813	0.1348	0.0945	0.1651	0.1277
84	0.1375	0.0987	0.1301	0.0916	0.1458	0.1052	0.1788	0.1426
85	0.1492	0.1099	0.1419	0.1025	0.1576	0.1166	0.1928	0.1555
86	0.1620	0.1219	0.1545	0.1144	0.1708	0.1290	0.2050	0.1706
87	0.1760	0.1349	0.1699	0.1274	0.1832	0.1420	0.2212	0.1863
88	0.1892	0.1489	0.1823	0.1417	0.1974	0.1558	0.2346	0.2029
89	0.2039	0.1644	0.1980	0.1572	0.2108	0.1712	0.2521	0.2178
90	0.2202	0.1800	0.2142	0.1729	0.2274	0.1869	0.2702	0.2355
91	0.2362	0.1963	0.2305	0.1905	0.2429	0.2019	0.2897	0.2552
92	0.2533	0.2133	0.2468	0.2074	0.2609	0.2190	0.3099	0.2747
93	0.2709	0.2311	0.2636	0.2254	0.2794	0.2367	0.3325	0.2976
94	0.2893	0.2493	0.2818	0.2452	0.2979	0.2534	0.3521	0.3128
95	0.3069	0.2665	0.3007	0.2631	0.3139	0.2699	0.3691	0.3396
96	0.3233	0.2857	0.3175	0.2842	0.3299	0.2871	0.3814	0.3479
97	0.3375	0.3020	0.3336	0.3014	0.3417	0.3027	0.4126	0.3681
98	0.3492	0.3184	0.3425	0.3211	0.3566	0.3157	0.4202	0.3897
99	0.3791	0.3398	0.3702	0.3332	0.3889	0.3464	0.4435	0.4198
100	0.4199	0.3671	0.4139	0.3674	0.4261	0.3669	...	...
101	0.4227	0.3821	0.4208	0.3785	0.4246	0.3857	...	...
102	0.4303	0.3961	0.4222	0.3892	0.4388	0.4028	...	...
103	0.4668	0.4191	0.4629	0.4256	0.4710	0.4126	...	...
104	0.4444	0.4308	0.4429	0.4248	0.4461	0.4367	...	...
105	0.4481	0.4583	0.4694	0.4460	0.4262	0.4708	...	...
106	0.4576	0.4491	0.4435	0.4269	0.4711	0.4722	...	...
107	0.4760	0.4729	0.5172	0.4985	0.4706	0.4455	...	...
108		0.5589		0.4483		0.6645		...
109		0.6000		0.5833		0.6279		...

[1] Recorded data without smoothing. Low mortality: Denmark, France, Iceland, Japan, Netherlands, Norway, Sweden, Switzerland.
Medium mortality: Austria, England & Wales, Finland, Germany (West), Italy.
High mortality: Czechoslovakia, Germany (East), Hungary.

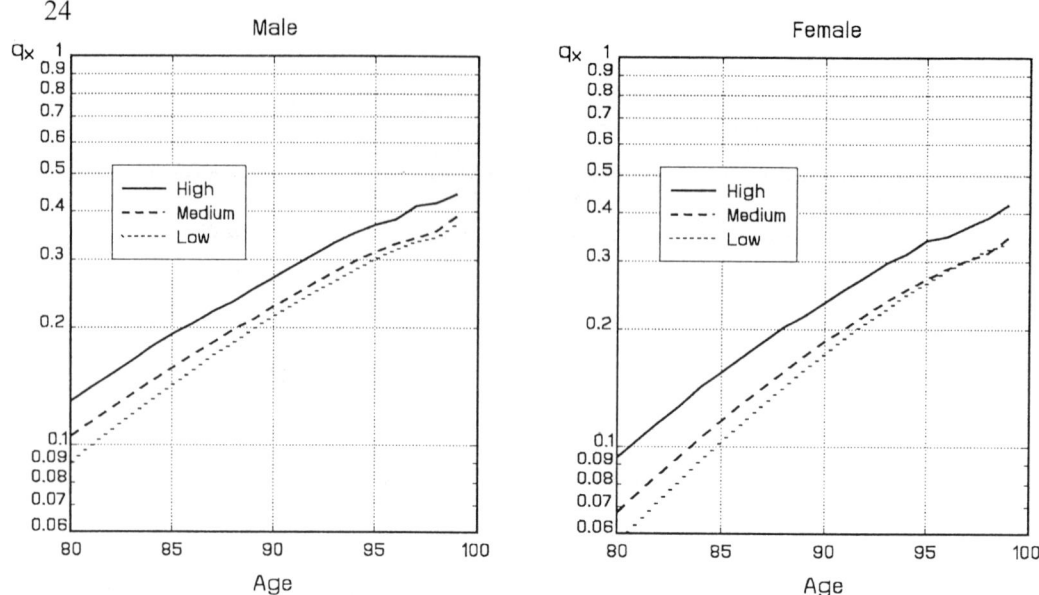

Figure 2. PROBABILITY OF DYING BY AGE AND SEX.
Countries with high, medium and low mortality, 1980-1990.

Table 3 and Figure 2 give the corresponding results for the high-, medium- and low-mortality groups to which the most reliably documented countries were divided. The curves are drawn only to age 99 because the data for the first group do not go beyond it. All curves display the same general form and the logical relative positions but the differences between the low and medium groups which together form the group of thirteen, are small.

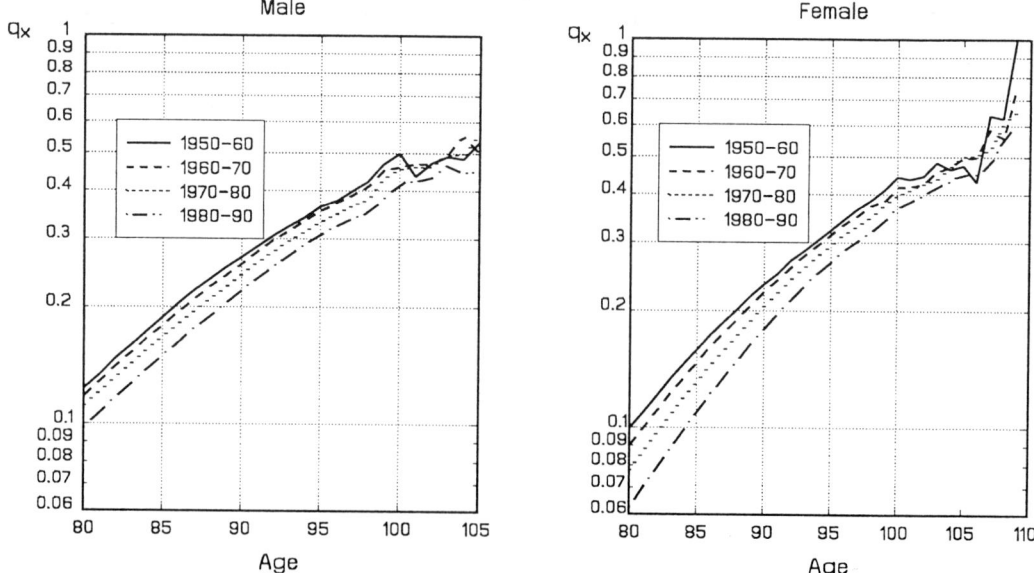

Figure 3. PROBABILITY OF DYING BY AGE AND SEX.
Thirteen countries with good data, by decade.

Finally, the mortality decline can be seen in Figure 3. The curves of successive decades move gradually to lower positions while maintaining the same typical form. The decennial differences show a tendency to increase indicating an accelerating mortality decline, particularly between the 1970s and 1980s. At the same time, the curves for females have become slightly steeper while the male ones have stayed roughly parallel. These phenomena will be elaborated in later chapters.

4. Old age life tables

The old age life tables published in this book were constructed from cohort observations, specified by country, sex, age and year, each with the number exposed-to-risk and the number of deaths, and straddling two calendar years. About 50,000 such double observations were used.

The first life table presented here (Table 4) summarizes the contemporary human longevity in advanced countries. The greatest interest may be centered on the very oldest of whom substantial numbers are now on record. However, they contribute very little to the entire old age experience. Of the 6.27 years of life remaining for an 80-year-old man, only 0.01 year ($T_{100} = 0.0107$) is lived above age 100, and of the 7.83 years of a woman, 0.03 year. Continuing to play with numbers and calculating survivival with greater precision we find that, divided equally between all 80-year-old women, the time to be lived above age one-hundred-and-ten amounts to 26 minutes for each. A closer examination of this and other life tables is the subject of the following chapters.

Slightly more than one hundred decennial life tables for individual countries are given in Annex Table 2 and a few tables for aggregates in Annex Table 3. For reasons of space, the columns L_x and T_x are omitted from these since, if needed, the user can calculate them. Any resulting inconvenience is regretted.

When probabilities of dying cannot be calculated above age 99, as is the case with several countries of the database, the life expectancy at age 100 needs to be estimated. Basing on evidence from countries with complete data, the following approximation was found reasonable:

$$e_{100} = 1.026 + 6.22 \cdot {}_5p_{95}$$

and was applied to "short" life tables for the calculation of:

$$T_{100} = e_{100} \cdot l_{100}$$

Table 4. OLD AGE LIFE TABLE
Thirteen countries with good data, 1980 - 1990
(Male)

x	N_x	D_x	q_x	l_x	d_x	L_x	T_x	e_x
80	6171300	602450	0.0976	1.0000	0.0976	0.9512	6.2670	6.2670
81	5386660	575263	0.1068	0.9024	0.0964	0.8542	5.3158	5.8909
82	4637269	539856	0.1164	0.8060	0.0938	0.7591	4.4616	5.5354
83	3935705	498531	0.1267	0.7122	0.0902	0.6671	3.7025	5.1989
84	3300704	453904	0.1375	0.6220	0.0855	0.5792	3.0354	4.8804
85	2718510	405671	0.1492	0.5364	0.0800	0.4964	2.4562	4.5788
86	2203932	357107	0.1620	0.4564	0.0739	0.4194	1.9598	4.2943
87	1755371	309010	0.1760	0.3824	0.0673	0.3488	1.5404	4.0279
88	1367630	258807	0.1892	0.3151	0.0596	0.2853	1.1917	3.7817
89	1048111	213666	0.2039	0.2555	0.0521	0.2294	0.9064	3.5476
90	790000	173994	0.2202	0.2034	0.0448	0.1810	0.6769	3.3280
91	586574	138558	0.2362	0.1586	0.0375	0.1399	0.4959	3.1268
92	426200	107969	0.2533	0.1211	0.0307	0.1058	0.3560	2.9391
93	302759	82024	0.2709	0.0905	0.0245	0.0782	0.2502	2.7667
94	209593	60627	0.2893	0.0659	0.0191	0.0564	0.1721	2.6090
95	142067	43595	0.3069	0.0469	0.0144	0.0397	0.1156	2.4673
96	93741	30306	0.3233	0.0325	0.0105	0.0272	0.0760	2.3383
97	60141	20295	0.3375	0.0220	0.0074	0.0183	0.0487	2.2165
98	37828	13209	0.3492	0.0146	0.0051	0.0120	0.0305	2.0908
99	23170	8784	0.3791	0.0095	0.0036	0.0077	0.0184	1.9444
100	13066	5486	0.4199	0.0059	0.0025	0.0047	0.0107	1.8263
101	7048	2979	0.4227	0.0034	0.0014	0.0027	0.0061	1.7862
102	3732	1606	0.4303	0.0020	0.0008	0.0015	0.0034	1.7278
103	1958	914	0.4668	0.0011	0.0005	0.0009	0.0019	1.6553
104	963	428	0.4444	0.0006	0.0003	0.0005	0.0010	1.6667
105	482	216	0.4481	0.0003	0.0001	0.0003	0.0005	1.6001
106	236	108	0.4576	0.0002	0.0001	0.0001	0.0003	1.4933
107	109	54	0.4954	0.0001	0.0000	0.0001	0.0001	1.3314
108	50	28	0.5600	0.0001	0.0000	0.0000	0.0001	1.1478
109	18	14	0.7778	0.000	0.0000	0.0000	0.0000	0.9722
110	4	1	0.2500	0.0000	0.0000	0.0000	0.0000	1.6250
111	2	1	0.5000	0.0000	0.0000	0.0000	0.0000	1.0000
112	1	1	1.0000	0.0000	0.0000	0.0000	...	0.5000

x = age
N_x = persons who reached exact age x
D_x = of these, died before age x + 1
q_x = probability of dying at age x
l_x = proportion alive at exact age x
d_x = proportion dying at age x
L_x = years lived at age x
T_x = years lived at age x or later
e_x = life expectancy at exact age x

Table 4. (cont.)
(Female)

x	N_x	D_x	q_x	l_x	d_x	L_x	T_x	e_x
80	11016260	686248	0.0623	1.0000	0.0623	0.9689	7.8267	7.8267
81	10006889	701865	0.0701	0.9377	0.0658	0.9048	6.8578	7.3134
82	8995877	708061	0.0787	0.8719	0.0686	0.8376	5.9530	6.8274
83	7996893	705263	0.0882	0.8033	0.0708	0.7679	5.1154	6.3679
84	7039045	694516	0.0987	0.7325	0.0723	0.6963	4.3475	5.9355
85	6100389	670136	0.1099	0.6602	0.0725	0.6239	3.6512	5.5305
86	5205902	634694	0.1219	0.5877	0.0716	0.5518	3.0273	5.1513
87	4364637	588790	0.1349	0.5160	0.0696	0.4812	2.4754	4.7971
88	3581333	533373	0.1489	0.4464	0.0665	0.4132	1.9942	4.4672
89	2880082	473395	0.1644	0.3799	0.0624	0.3487	1.5810	4.1614
90	2272608	409177	0.1800	0.3175	0.0572	0.2889	1.2323	3.8816
91	1763145	346114	0.1963	0.2603	0.0511	0.2348	0.9434	3.6242
92	1336032	285000	0.2133	0.2092	0.0446	0.1869	0.7087	3.3873
93	987352	228189	0.2311	0.1646	0.0380	0.1456	0.5218	3.1702
94	710422	177138	0.2493	0.1265	0.0316	0.1108	0.3762	2.9728
95	499268	133062	0.2665	0.0950	0.0253	0.0823	0.2654	2.7941
96	340859	97381	0.2857	0.0697	0.0199	0.0597	0.1831	2.6277
97	226248	68334	0.3020	0.0498	0.0150	0.0423	0.1234	2.4787
98	146702	46706	0.3184	0.0347	0.0111	0.0292	0.0811	2.3349
99	92505	31437	0.3398	0.0237	0.0080	0.0197	0.0519	2.1920
100	55761	20472	0.3671	0.0156	0.0057	0.0128	0.0322	2.0630
101	32349	12361	0.3821	0.0099	0.0038	0.0080	0.0195	1.9698
102	18150	7189	0.3961	0.0061	0.0024	0.0049	0.0115	1.8788
103	10035	4206	0.4191	0.0037	0.0015	0.0029	0.0066	1.7830
104	5295	2281	0.4308	0.0021	0.0009	0.0017	0.0037	1.7088
105	2723	1248	0.4583	0.0012	0.0006	0.0009	0.0020	1.6237
106	1325	595	0.4491	0.0007	0.0003	0.0005	0.0010	1.5744
107	645	305	0.4729	0.0004	0.0002	0.0003	0.0005	1.4502
108	297	166	0.5589	0.0002	0.0001	0.0001	0.0003	1.3026
109	115	69	0.6000	0.0001	0.0001	0.0001	0.0001	1.3196
110	35	22	0.6286	0.0000	0.0001	0.0000	0.0001	1.5490
111	11	4	0.3636	0.0000	0.0000	0.0000	0.0000	2.3242
112	5	1	0.2000	0.0000	0.0000	0.0000	0.0000	2.3667
113	3	0	0.0000	0.0000	0.0000	0.0000	0.0000	1.8333
114	3	1	0.3333	0.0000	0.0000	0.0000	0.0000	0.8333

x = age
N_x = persons who reached exact age x
D_x = of these, died before age x + 1
q_x = probability of dying at age x
l_x = proportion alive at exact age x
d_x = proportion dying at age x
L_x = years lived at age x
T_x = years lived at age x or later
e_x = life expectancy at exact age x

Comparison with official life tables

The validity of the life tables produced from the Odense database was checked by comparing them with official life tables of the same countries. Available for comparison purposes was a large file in the United Nations Statistical Division in New York, containing life expectancies at various ages in a very large number of countries around the world since the beginning of the century. Among them, were life expectancies at age 80 according to nearly one thousand life tables from 125 countries. About two hundred e_{80} values for each sex in 26 countries are listed in Annex Table 4 and were used in the comparison.

Although regular demographic statistics are usually not reliable enough for the calculation of death rates or life expectancies after age 90 or 100, they are in most Western countries good for calculating it at age 80 with sufficient precision. This is because only 10 to 15 percent of the lifetime after age 80 is lived after 90, and less than one percent after age 100. The other side of the coin is that the comparison cannot validate any calculations regarding centenarian life.

Comparison of life expectancies at age 80 in official life tables with values derived from Odense data is nevertheless a meaningful operation regarding at least octogenarians and may corroborate the validity of both sources or reveal weaknesses in one or the other.

It should be borne in mind that makers of official life tables are expected to treat their data with caution and have considerable freedom in adjusting the results to what they believe to be a good approximation of reality. In so doing, they frequently use smoothing or extrapolation rather freely or apply a theoretical model of their choice. All in all, there is a good deal of subjective choice involved regarding the values at high ages. The Odense life tables, on the other hand, are constructed adhering strictly to the official data on deaths and leave room for subjective input only in the estimation of current survivors. We have made extensive corrections to official data on survivors at ages approaching or exceeding 100 years but they have relatively little impact at age 80.

In cases where age overstatement was considered serious, population data even for octogenarians were corrected in Odense to conform with survival data but when also the latter suffered from age exaggeration, mortality remained artificially low and life expectancy too high.

A comparison was carried out graphically for 26 countries in the period 1950-1990 and is shown in Figure 4 on seven pages. The official data are expressed with an 0 in the single year or central year of the life table period. The basic data are given in Annex Table 4.

The following interpretation is suggested.

a) Good agreement between the two sources:

    Austria   Germany, West
    Belgium   Japan
    Denmark   Netherlands
    England & Wales   Norway
    Finland   Scotland
    France   Sweden
                             Switzerland

b) Good agreement but insufficient evidence:

    Australia
    Estonia

c) Good agreement but some volatility:

    Iceland, due to small numbers

d) Official life tables more cautious suggesting awareness of age overstatement in deaths:

    Ireland, in all periods
    Italy in 1950s only but strongly
    New Zealand, until the most recent
    Portugal, until about 1980

e) Official life tables too optimistic, inconsistent with data on deaths:

    Czechoslovakia, all periods with few exceptions
    Germany (East), in two tables of the 1960s;
    otherwise good agreement
    Hungary, in about half of the cases
    Poland, in female tables

f) Likelihood of age overstatement in deaths:

    Spain, suggested by more cautious official tables in 1950 and 1960 and by high values in the 1980s.

g) Evidence insufficient

    Luxembourg

30

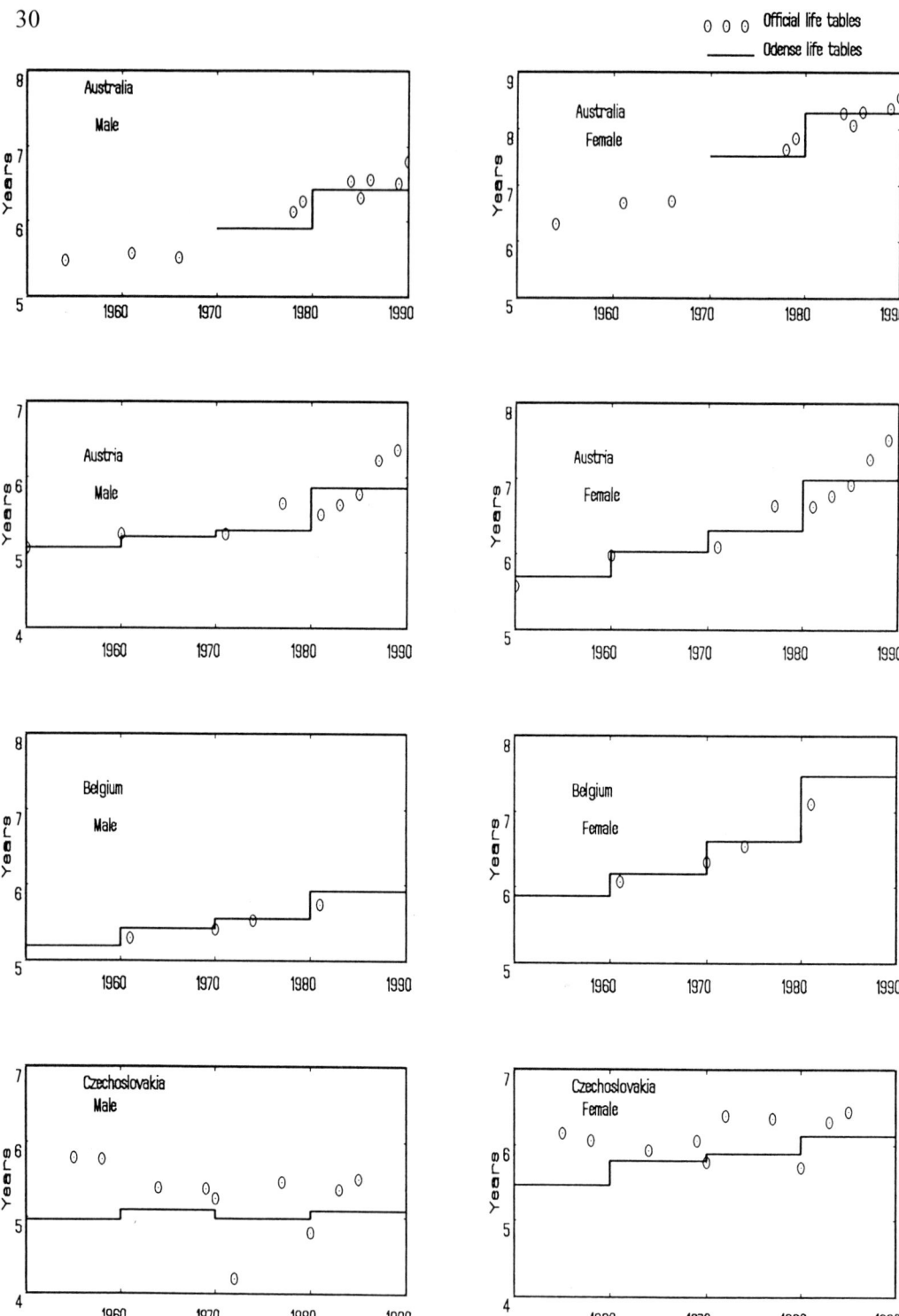

Figure 4. LIFE EXPECTANCY AT AGE 80 ACCORDING TO
OFFICIAL AND ODENSE LIFE TABLES.

31

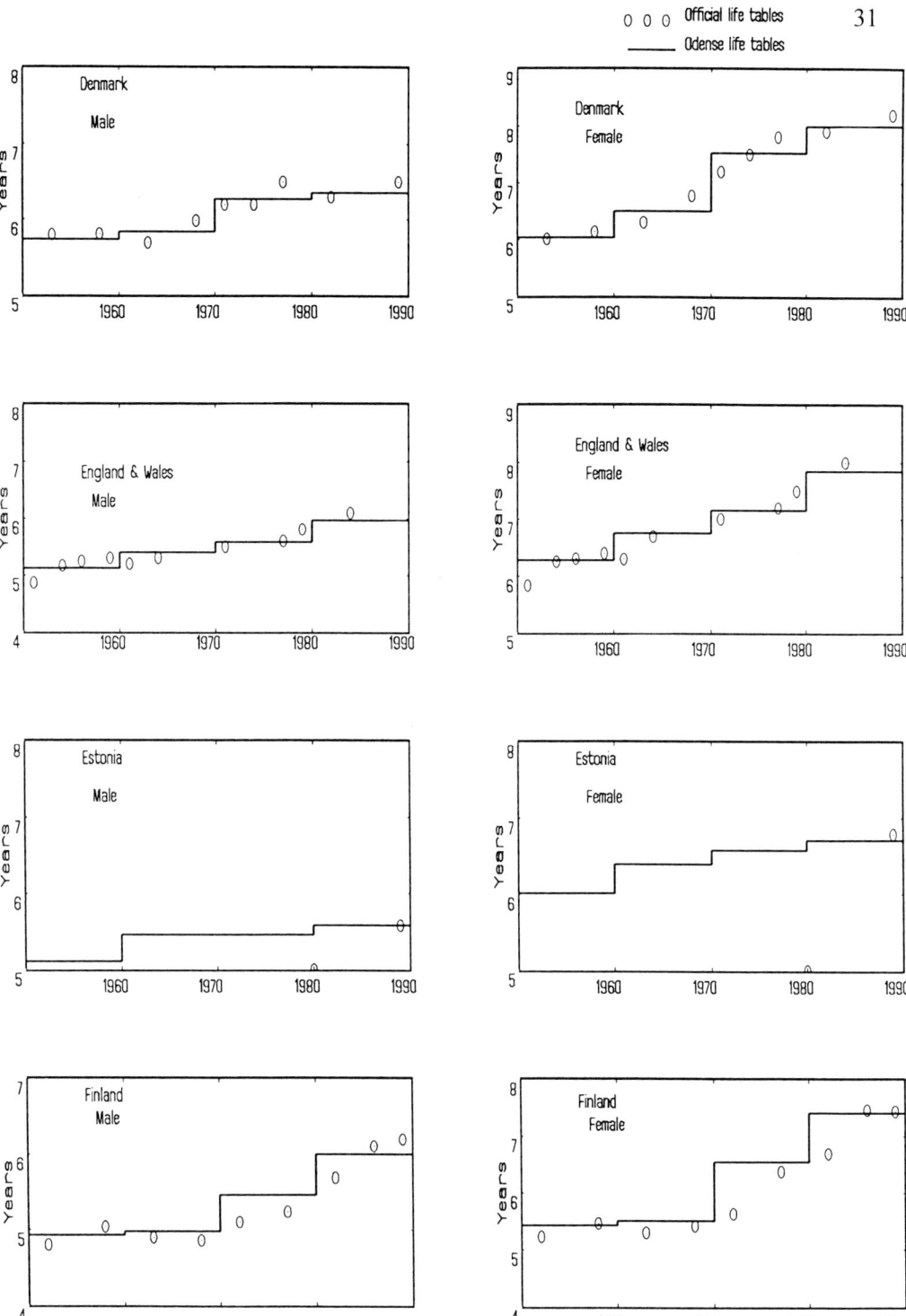

Figure 4 (cont.). LIFE EXPECTANCY AT AGE 80.

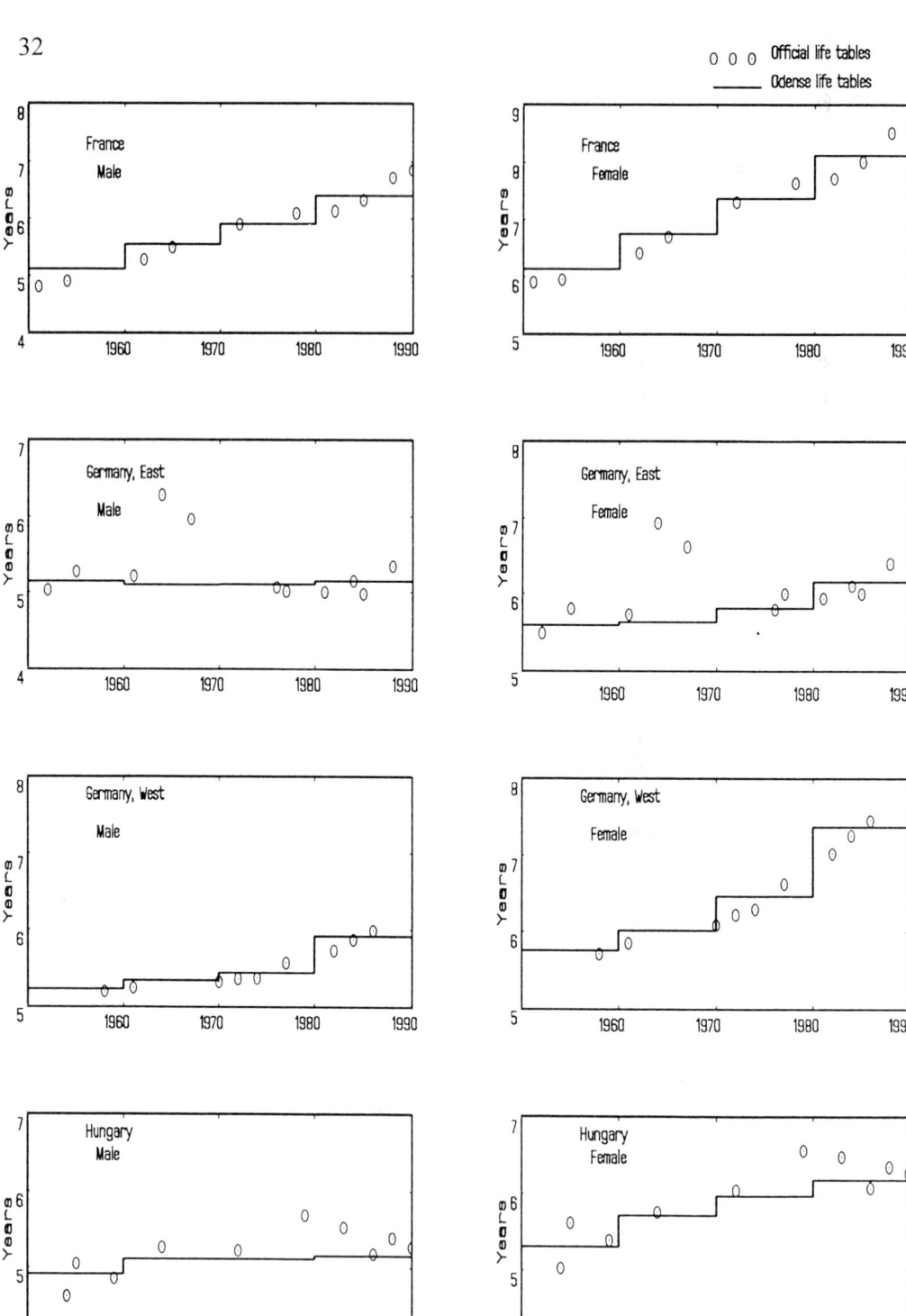

Figure 4(cont.). LIFE EXPECTANCY AT AGE 80.

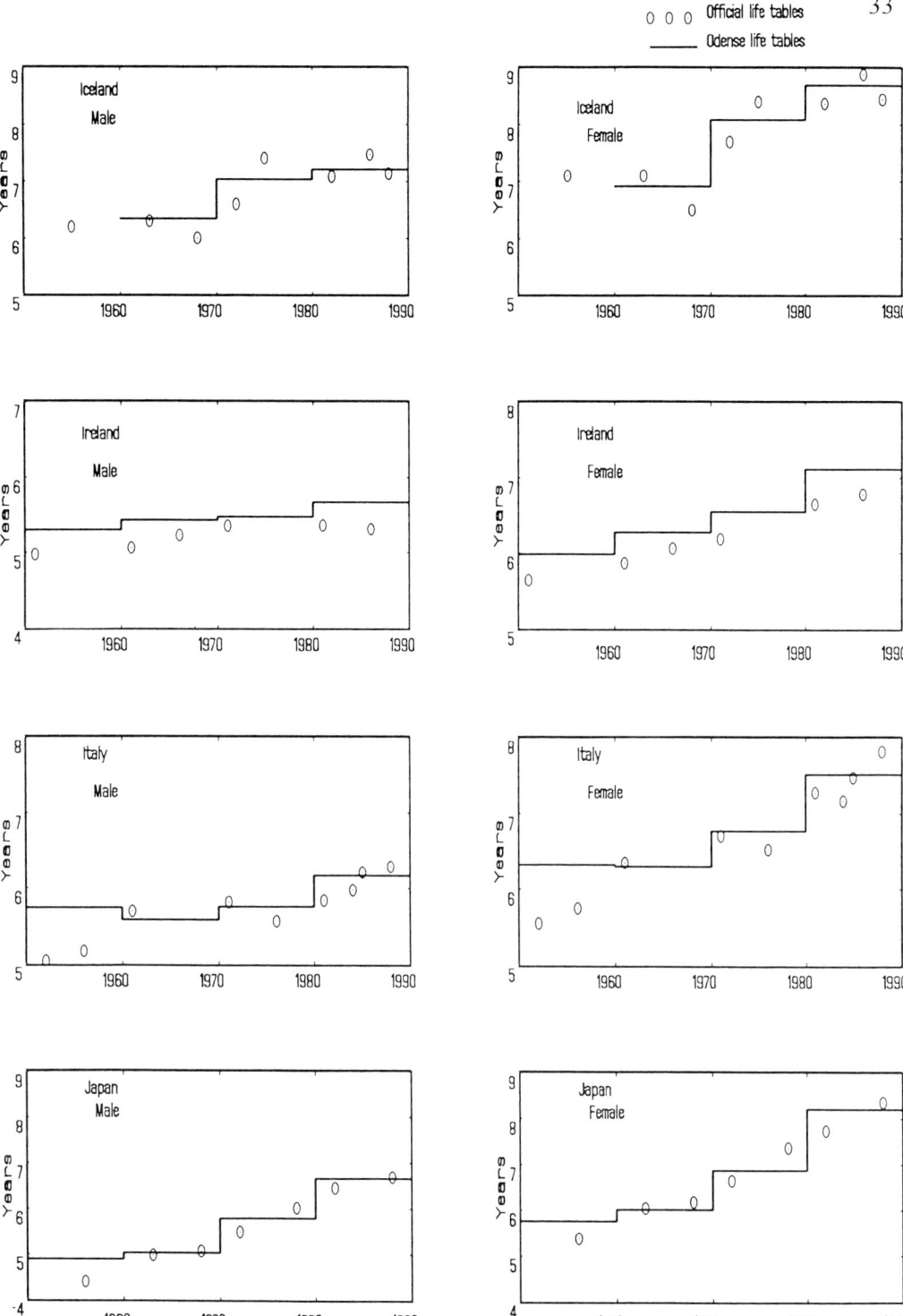

Figure 4(cont.). LIFE EXPECTANCY AT AGE 80.

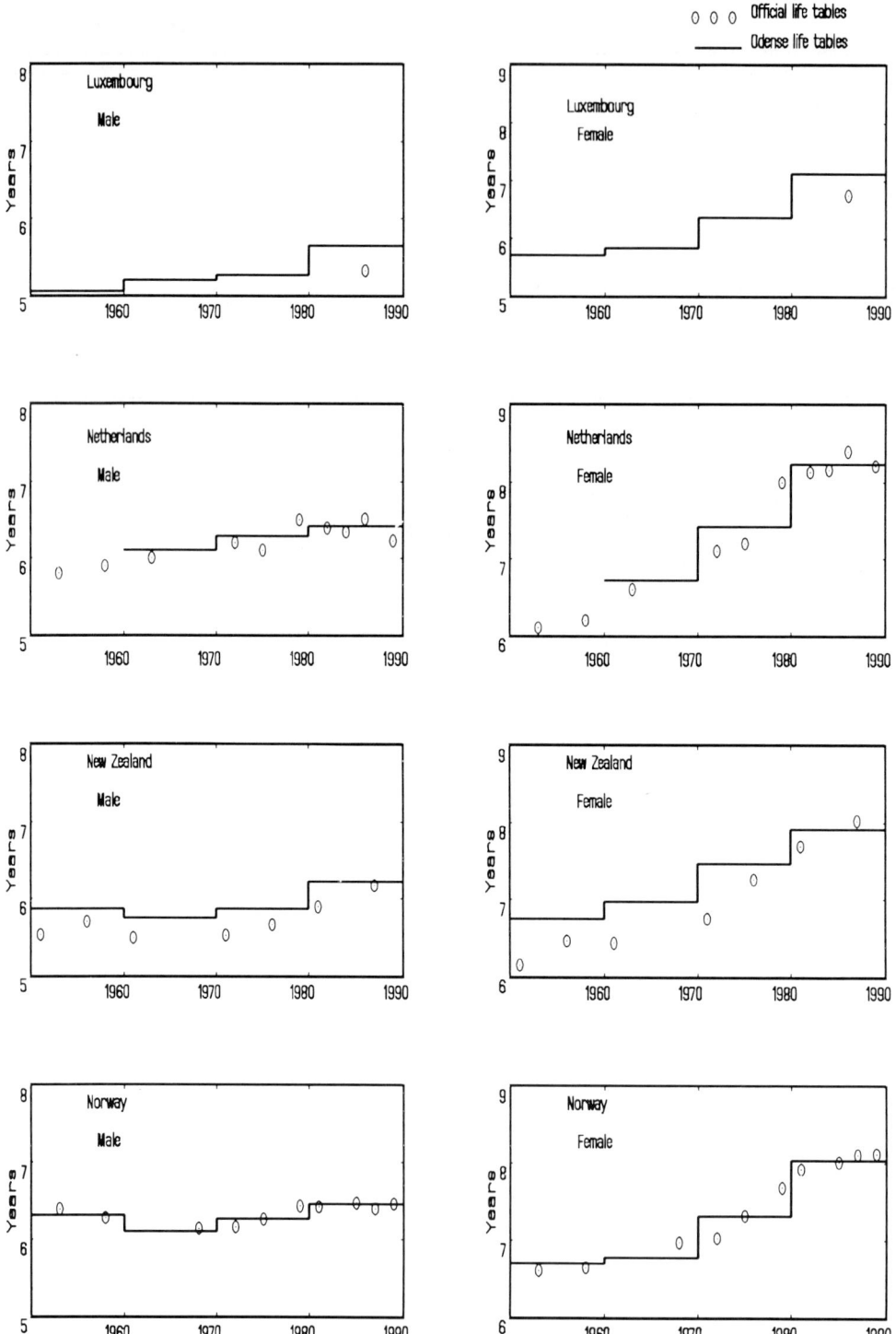

Figure 4 (cont.). LIFE EXPECTANCY AT AGE 80.

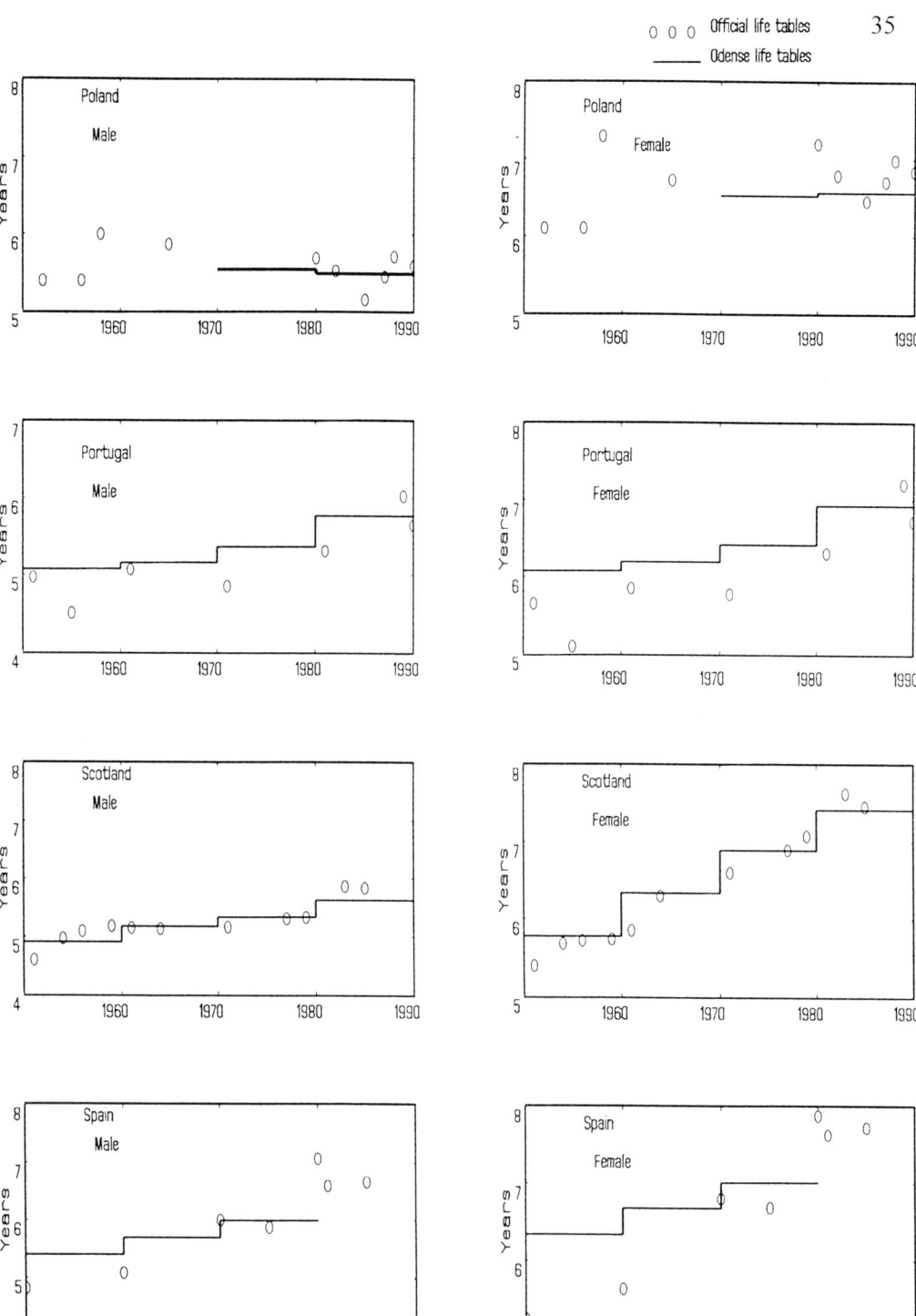

Figure 4(cont.). LIFE EXPECTANCY AT AGE 80.

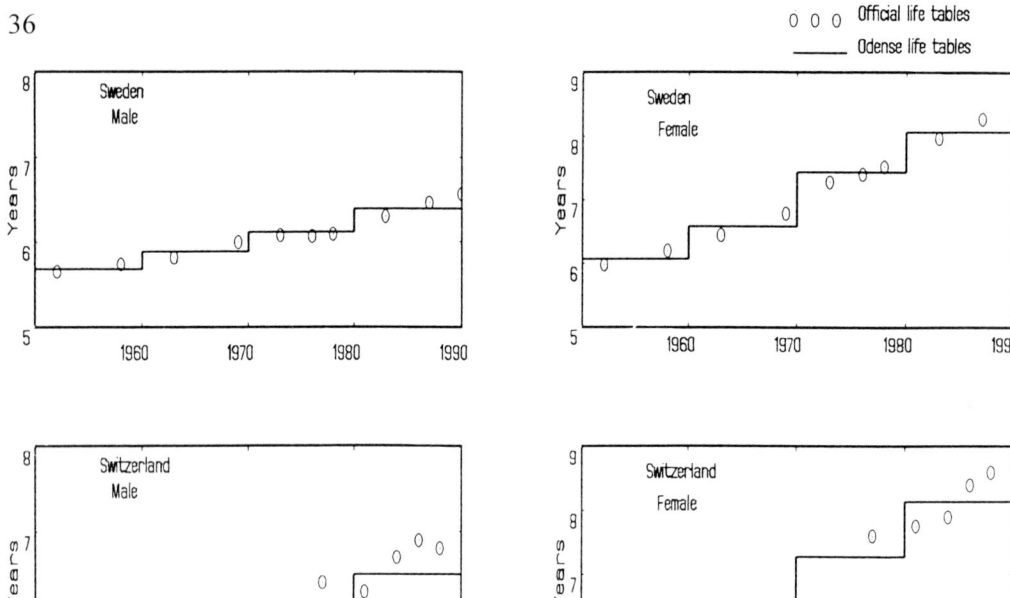

Figure 4(cont.). LIFE EXPECTANCY AT AGE 80.

Of the countries constituting the prime group of thirteen, eleven are in group a) (good agreement), one in c) (good agreement but volatility) and one, Italy, in d) (age overstatement in 1950s). Age overstatement is suggested in the six countries of groups d) and f). Other evidence suggests it as present also in Estonia and Poland.

The findings corroborate generally very well the results of the data quality assessment in Chapter 2.

5. Changing mortality

During the post-war period, the mortality of the oldest-old has declined substantially. It may therefore be helpful to examine at this point the general nature of this decline in order to better appreciate the changing parameters in the later chapters. A general view of the change emerges in Figure 5 which shows the progress made from one decade to the next, by detailed age in the core group of thirteen countries. The decline has accelerated notably over time for both sexes and at all ages below 100 years. Throughout the period, the decline has been faster for women than men.

The age pattern of decline is very clear and consistent for women, the relative benefits for the 80-year-old being always more than twice that for 95-year-old.

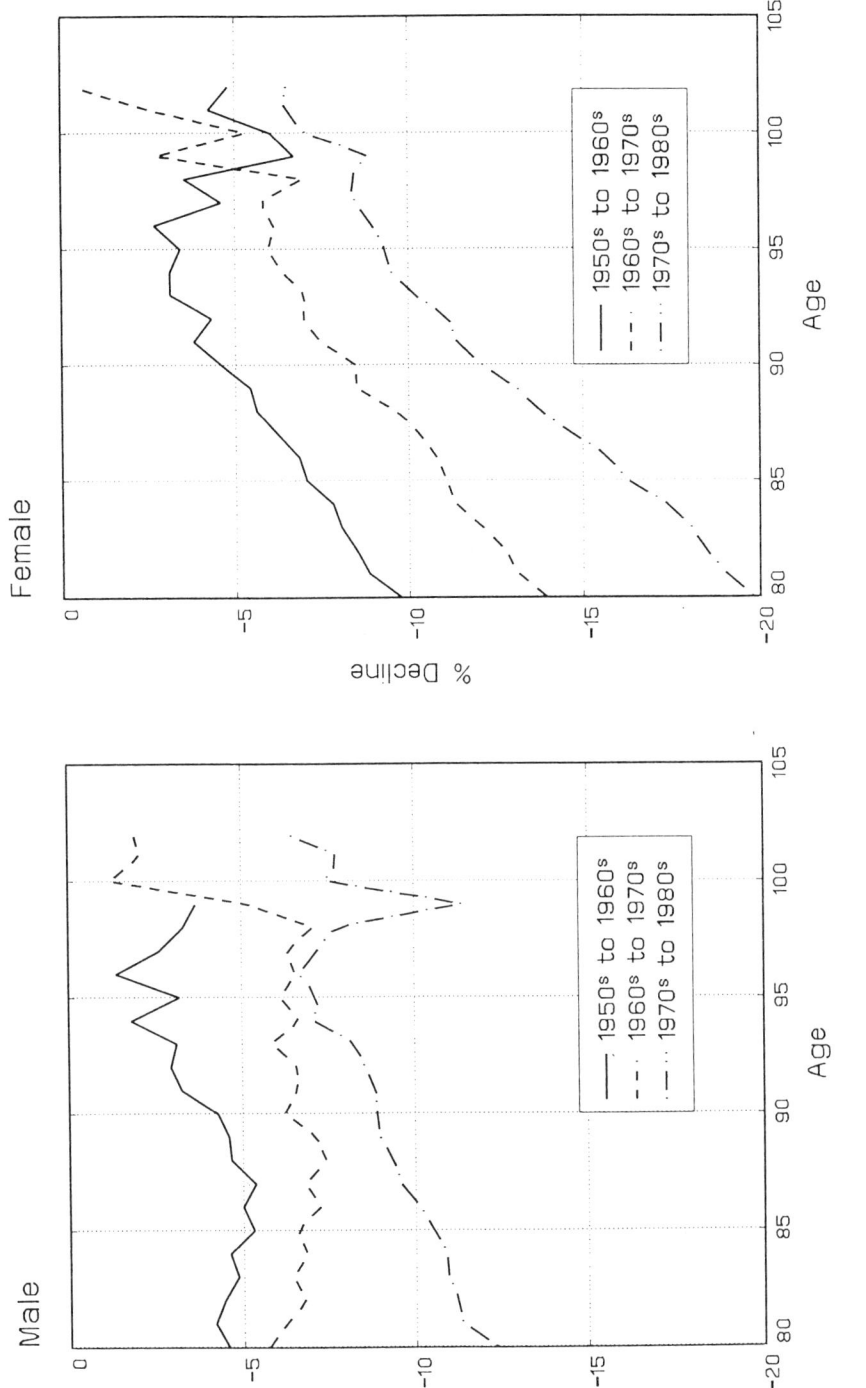

Figure 5. DECLINE OF MORTALITY BY AGE BETWEEN SUCCESSIVE DECADES. Thirteen countries with good data.

Table 5. PERCENT CHANGE IN MORTALITY BETWEEN 1960 - 70 AND 1980 - 90.
Based on mean values of q (x) in Annex Table 5.

Country and aggregate	Male				Female			
	80 - 84	85 - 89	90 - 94	95 - 99	80 - 84	85 - 89	90 - 94	95 - 99
Austria	14.3	12.9	13.0	6.3	21.6	15.0	11.7	6.5
Belgium	9.7	13.0	13.0	6.7	25.9	21.6	18.3	15.4
Czechoslovakia	-1.5	3.3	2.0	3.5	7.8	7.1	3.2	-1.6
Denmark	9.0	13.6	13.2	15.5	29.3	25.0	17.7	15.0
England & Wales	11.7	12.6	11.4	10.6	22.0	18.7	14.0	10.9
Estonia	1.8	4.8	7.1	13.7	5.0	8.2	4.9	3.4
Finland	21.1	21.6	17.4	6.1	35.6	31.7	24.8	21.0
France	18.4	16.0	12.0	3.5	28.2	21.9	15.4	7.9
Germany, East	0.8	1.9	3.5	9.4	12.8	9.2	7.6	13.0
Germany, West	12.0	13.0	11.7	13.7	27.2	22.4	17.8	15.8
Hungary	-0.9	4.8	5.2	11.7	10.3	10.0	6.4	11.1
Iceland	16.2	16.8	6.7	16.4	31.1	29.2	23.7	24.2
Ireland	5.1	6.4	-0.3	-2.0	17.8	15.0	5.9	13.6
Italy	11.2	13.6	14.2	22.5	24.6	20.8	16.9	20.3
Japan	32.3	26.9	21.7	15.6	40.7	33.2	24.9	19.8
Latvia	-6.1	-2.3	5.1	3.5	1.0	1.6	0.6	-0.1
Luxembourg	10.0	9.2	2.0	5.4	27.4	21.7	17.4	24.7
Netherlands	4.3	8.7	12.0	11.6	29.1	24.2	18.4	14.9
New Zealand	10.3	11.9	5.4	6.8	17.1	18.8	13.4	16.0
Norway	6.3	8.2	10.5	5.9	26.0	20.0	14.7	14.7
Portugal	13.9	11.7	10.4	3.2	15.6	14.0	8.2	6.5
Scotland	9.1	11.2	13.4	8.2	21.2	18.8	14.4	17.4
Spain	18.2	17.3	15.7	18.0	21.3	15.2	8.3	6.1
Sweden	10.2	10.1	10.3	9.6	30.2	23.9	16.4	10.7
Switzerland	20.1	17.2	13.3	13.7	34.6	28.6	20.3	12.6
Low mortality (8 countries)	21.8	18.3	14.8	9.1	33.3	26.2	18.7	12.0
Medium mortality (5 countries)	11.8	13.0	12.6	16.3	24.4	19.9	15.5	15.0
High mortality (3 countries)	-0.3	3.1	3.6	8.4	10.9	8.9	6.2	8.7
Thirteen countries (low & medium)	17.0	16.0	14.2	14.0	28.6	23.0	17.2	13.5

Around age 100 a definite decline is still observed but it is more modest and an acceleration is not obvious. The pattern for men is more ambiguous. Up to 1970s, the decline was hardly at all age-selective but between the last decades it took on the form observed for women.

The decline by country and aggregate is given in Table 5 by age groups and illustrated in Figures 6a and b. The curves in Figure 6a, showing a 20-year change in individual countries, produce for males a rather ambivalent picture which includes some contrasting patters. In the first frame, England & Wales, West Germany and Italy display an almost level decline of 10 - 15 percent while the reductions in France and Japan are strongly concentrated among the youngest. In the second frame, Sweden shows an even 10 percent decline while in Norway and Denmark the reduction increases, in Finland and Iceland decreases with age. In the third group, the East European countries show actual mortality increase at younger ages and slight decline after that but Scotland and New Zealand a fairly constant 10 percent decrease.

In the last frame, a contrast is evident between gains that increase in the Netherlands, stay level in Belgium and Austria and decrease in Portugal and particularly in Switzerland. In a general way, where the decline is concentrated on oldest ages, it is altogether slight, vz. Eastern Europe, the Netherlands and Norway. In countries with largest overall gains, these are most impressive among the 80-year-old as witnessed by Japan, Switzerland, France and Finland.

These diverging age patterns are connected with what happens to the younger elderly men. In Monograph I in this series, a connection was made with death rates at ages 60 - 79 published in the United Nations Demographic Yearbook, (various editions), and it showed that in countries with large declines for octogenarian men (Japan, France, Finland), as large or still larger declines were recorded for the younger elderly. On the other hand, in the Netherlands, Norway, Denmark and Eastern Europe where the decline was smaller for octogenarians, there was some actual increase in the mortality of the younger elderly men (Kannisto, 1994, p.46).

The changes regarding females are confirmed in Figure 6b as adhering closely to one single pattern of large declines at age 80 which then become gradually smaller. This common pattern operates on widely different levels. Relatively small gains are recorded for Eastern and Southern Europe and Austria. The countries with the largest gains are the same four as with males though in a different order: Switzerland, Finland, France and Japan. In Norway and the Netherlands, the slight gains for men, particularly the younger, contrast with large gains for women, and again particularly the younger ones. The mean values of q_x by age group and country are given in Annex Table 5.

40

a. Males

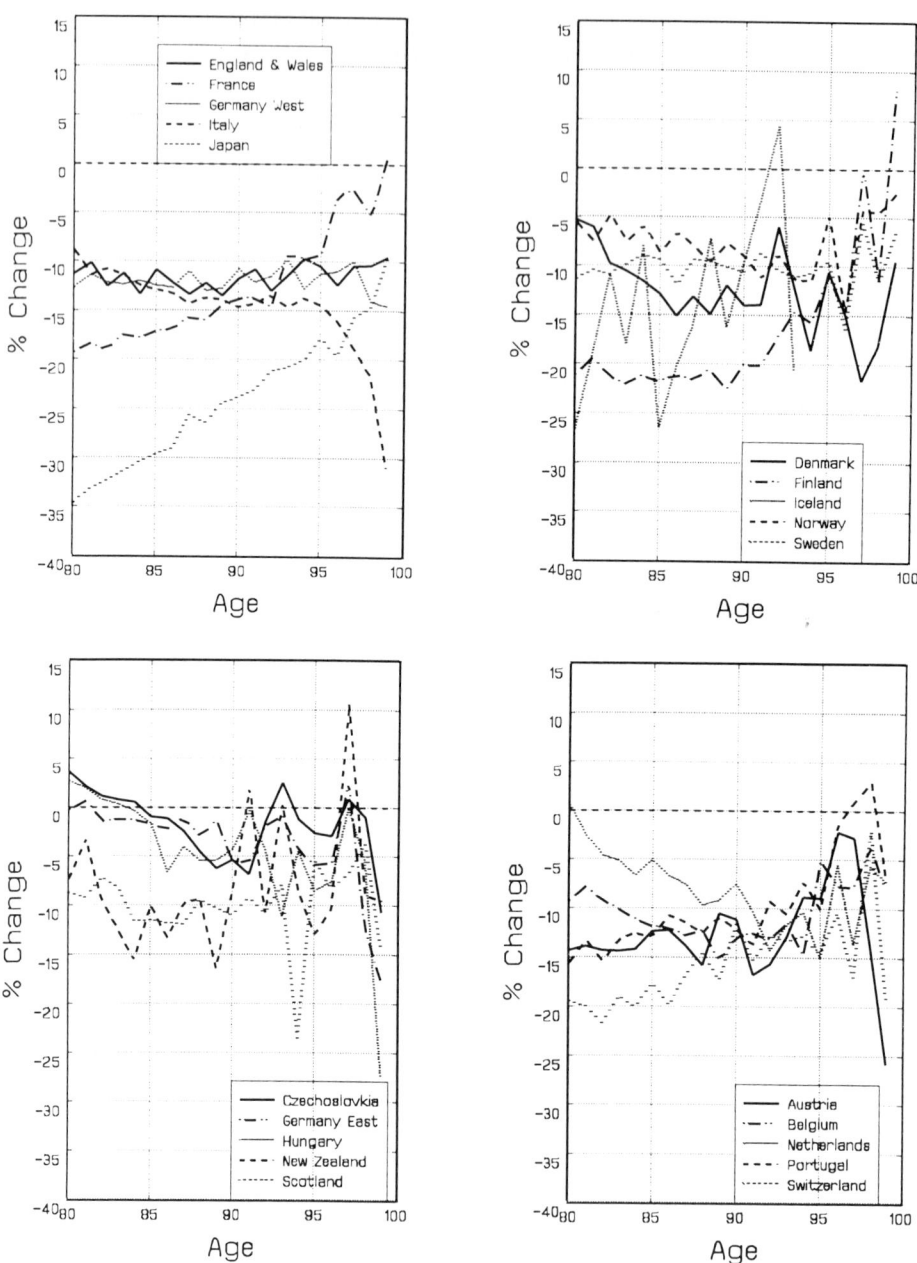

Figure 6.   PERCENT CHANGE IN MORTALITY FROM 1960-70 TO 1980-90.

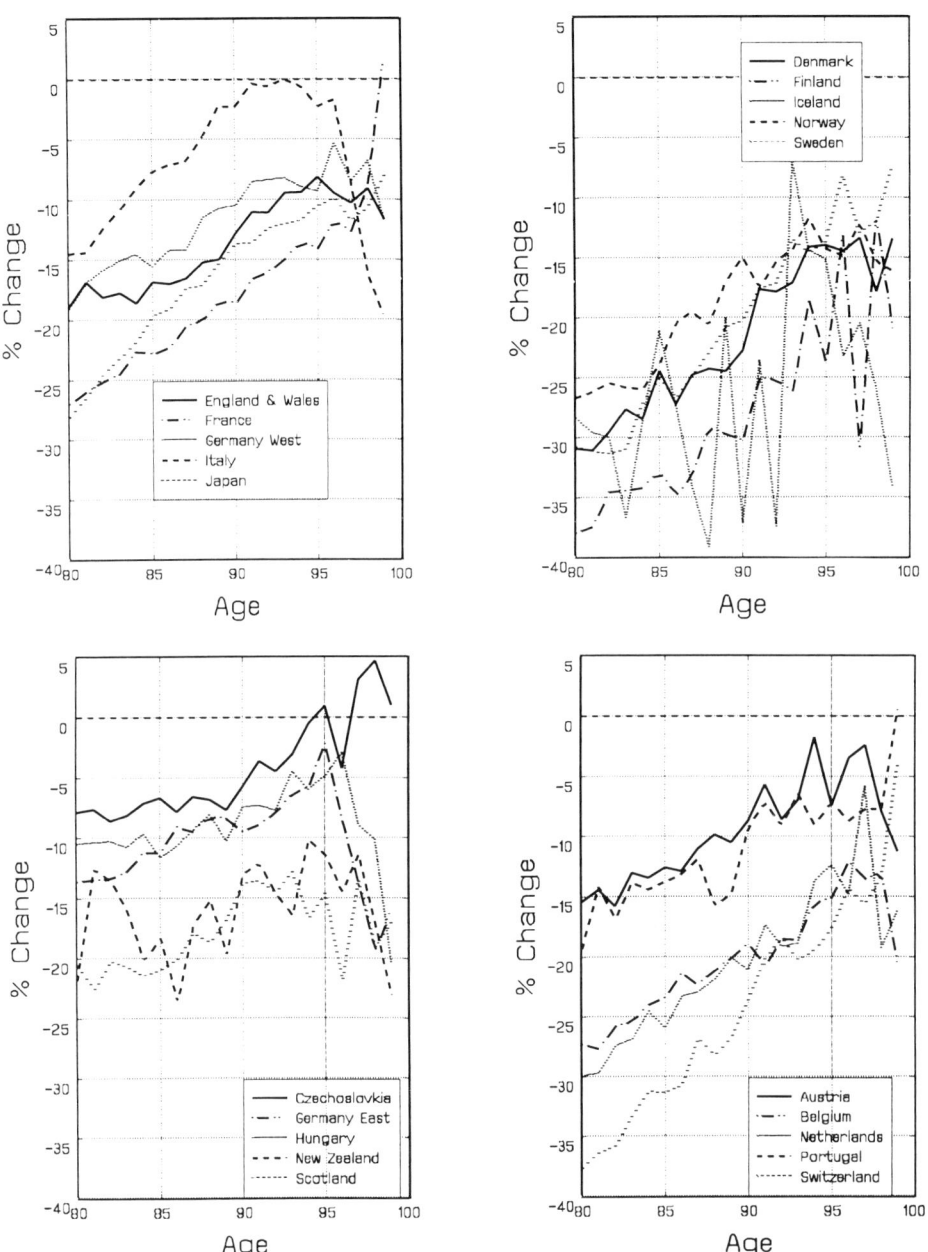

Figure 6. PERCENT DECLINE OF MORTALITY FROM 1960-70 TO 1980-90.

If the present stage of epidemiological transition is a manifestation of delayed senescence or at least delayed terminal frailty, then it can be expected to have more effect on the relatively younger elderly and less at older ages where vitality ebbs. The characteristic age pattern of the new stage of mortality transition is therefore one of larger gains among the younger, observed among women in all countries of the database and among men where overall progress has been good. In some countries, a contrasting tendency of obviously different etiology has caused the death rates of middle-aged and elderly men to stagnate or rise, sending ripple effects to older ages and so interfering with the general decline.

6. Life expectancy at age 80

One single indicator, life expectancy at age 80, summarizes old age mortality very well and certainly much better than the life expectancy at birth describes the mortality as a whole. The reason is that the same causes of death dominate the scene throughout the old age span, and all persons at these ages are subject to the same underlying force: senescence. The death rate rises in old age monotonically and even the differences in the pattern of change, observed in Chapter 5, fail to diminish the value of this indicator as an overall expression of death and survival at old ages. It was demonstrated in the first monograph in this series that all notable changes in mortality in the post-war era not only were observed in all old age groups but even took place simultaneously (Kannisto, 1994, pp. 55-59).

Table 6 gives the life expectancy at 80 in 26 countries for which it can be considered at least approximately correct. However, the figures for Ireland, Italy, New Zealand and Portugal are probably too high in the 1950s and possibly in the 1960s, and those for Estonia, Latvia and Poland probably somewhat too high in all periods. The Australian figures should be considered tentative.

Table 6. LIFE EXPECTANCY AT AGE 80 BY COUNTRY, AGGREGATE AND SEX, EACH DECADE.

Country and aggregate	Both sexes				Males				Females			
	1950-60	1960-70	1970-80	1980-90	1950-60	1960-70	1970-80	1980-90	1950-60	1960-70	1970-80	1980-90
Australia	5.48	...	6.96	7.64	5.07	...	5.91	6.43	5.70	...	7.52	8.29
Austria	5.64	5.75	5.96	6.59	5.19	5.21	5.29	5.86	5.88	6.03	6.31	6.99
Belgium	5.64	5.91	6.24	6.93	5.19	5.42	5.55	5.92	5.88	6.18	6.61	7.48
Czechoslovakia	5.30	5.56	5.57	5.77	4.97	5.10	4.99	5.09	5.48	5.80	5.89	6.13
Denmark	5.94	6.27	7.08	7.43	5.74	5.84	6.27	6.36	6.04	6.50	7.52	8.00
England & Wales	5.87	6.27	6.60	7.19	5.12	5.40	5.58	5.97	6.28	6.75	7.15	7.85
Estonia	5.69	6.07	6.19	6.31	5.11	5.46	5.46	5.58	6.01	6.40	6.58	6.71
Finland	5.25	5.32	6.16	6.92	4.93	4.98	5.46	6.00	5.43	5.51	6.54	7.42
France	5.78	6.33	6.85	7.52	5.12	5.55	5.91	6.40	6.14	6.75	7.36	8.13
Germany, East	5.44	5.44	5.57	5.81	5.15	5.10	5.11	5.15	5.59	5.63	5.81	6.16
Germany, West	5.57	5.78	6.12	6.87	5.23	5.34	5.44	5.92	5.76	6.02	6.48	7.38
Hungary	5.18	5.51	5.68	5.83	4.92	5.12	5.12	5.16	5.31	5.72	5.98	6.19
Iceland	...	6.72	7.72	8.18	...	6.34	7.04	7.21	...	6.92	8.08	8.70
Ireland	5.75	5.98	6.17	6.61	5.30	5.43	5.47	5.67	5.99	6.28	6.55	7.12
Italy	6.13	6.05	6.43	7.05	5.75	5.59	5.76	6.17	6.33	6.30	6.78	7.52
Japan	5.46	5.68	6.50	7.67	4.90	5.04	5.79	6.66	5.76	6.02	6.87	8.21
Latvia	6.25	6.47	6.47	6.44	5.63	5.93	5.83	5.74	6.59	6.76	6.81	6.81
Luxembourg	5.48	5.61	5.98	6.61	5.05	5.20	5.26	5.65	5.71	5.83	6.37	7.13
Netherlands	...	6.51	7.02	7.60	...	6.11	6.29	6.42	...	6.72	7.42	8.24
New Zealand	6.44	6.54	6.91	7.32	5.87	5.75	5.87	6.22	6.75	6.97	7.47	7.92
Norway	6.57	6.54	6.95	7.49	6.32	6.11	6.27	6.46	6.70	6.78	7.32	8.04
Poland	...	...	6.18	6.19	...	...	5.54	5.49	...	...	6.53	6.57
Portugal	5.73	5.84	6.05	6.53	5.08	5.16	5.37	5.77	6.08	6.20	6.42	6.93
Scotland	5.47	5.94	6.34	6.80	4.91	5.18	5.33	5.63	5.78	6.34	6.89	7.42
Sweden	5.93	6.34	6.97	7.48	5.68	5.89	6.12	6.39	6.07	6.58	7.44	8.07
Switzerland	5.70	6.08	6.84	7.57	5.28	5.58	6.05	6.50	5.92	6.36	7.27	8.14
AGGREGATES												
Low (8)	5.72	6.12	6.76	7.59	5.18	5.49	5.95	6.52	6.01	6.47	7.20	8.16
Medium (5)	5.79	6.02	6.35	7.00	5.30	5.42	5.57	6.00	6.06	6.33	6.77	7.54
High (3)	5.33	5.48	5.59	5.80	5.03	5.10	5.07	5.13	5.48	5.69	5.87	6.16
Thirteen	5.76	6.06	6.53	7.28	5.25	5.45	5.75	6.27	6.04	6.39	6.96	7.83

The 19 countries with most reliable data are ranked in Table 7 according to life expectancy for both sexes combined, in periods 30 years apart. This interval has been sufficient to extensively alter the relative positions. Iceland has remained the undisputed leader but the three countries of Scandinavia proper, while progressing, have lost ground to others and now occupy the sixth to eight positions. They have been replaced in the leading group by rapidly advancing Japan, Switzerland and France. Finland has risen rapidly from a low level while several countries of Central and Southern Europe have made more moderate progress and lost some rank, and the countries of the former East bloc have remained far behind. The ranking in 1980-90 was used for dividing the countries into low-, medium- and high-mortality groups but Belgium, Luxembourg and Scotland were excluded from the middle group due to unavailability of data above age 100 for a part or all of the study period.

Table 7. **RANKING OF COUNTRIES ACCORDING TO LIFE EXPECTANCY AT 80 FOR BOTH SEXES, 1950-60 AND 1980-90.**
19 countries with good quality data.

Rank	1950-1960[1]		1980-1990[2]	
1	Iceland	6.72	Iceland	8.18
2	Norway	6.57	Japan	7.67
3	Netherlands	6.51	Netherlands	7.60
4	Italy	(6.13)[3]	Switzerland	7.57
5	Denmark	5.94	France	7.52
6	Sweden	5.93	Norway	7.49
7	England & Wales	5.87	Sweden	7.48
8	France	5.78	Denmark	7.43
9	Switzerland	5.70	England & Wales	7.19
10	Belgium	5.64	Italy	7.05
11	Germany, West	5.57	Belgium	6.93
12	Austria	5.48	Finland	6.92
13	Luxembourg	5.48	Germany, West	6.87
14	Scotland	5.47	Scotland	6.80
15	Japan	5.46	Luxembourg	6.61
16	Germany, East	5.44	Austria	6.59
17	Czechoslovakia	5.30	Hungary	5.83
18	Finland	5.25	Germany, East	5.81
19	Hungary	5.18	Czechoslovakia	5.77

[1] Germany, East 1954-60; Germany, West 1956-60; Iceland 1961-70; Italy 1952-60; Luxembourg 1953-60; Netherlands 1960-70.
[2] Italy and Luxembourg 1980-89.
[3] Probably too high.

Figure 7 gives the life expectancies by sex in the 19 countries in the order of the length for both sexes combined. It facilitates spotting cases where the male expectancy is particularly low in relation to the female, namely the Netherlands, England and Wales, and Scotland, as well as the opposite situation in Austria.

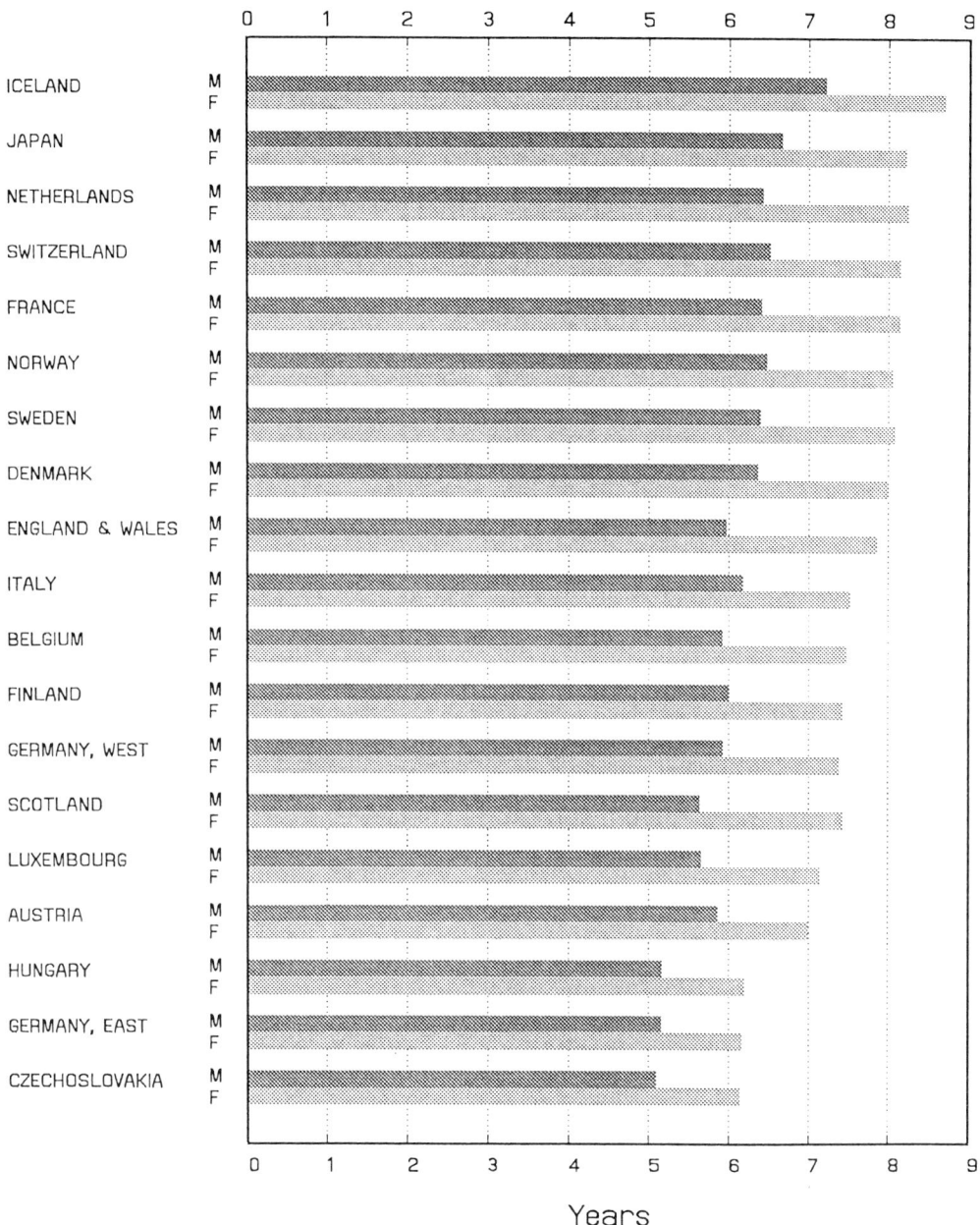

Figure 7. **LIFE EXPECTANCY AT AGE 80 IN 1980-90 BY SEX.**
Nineteen countries with good data.

The increase in old age life expectancy is sketched in Figure 8 for the three aggregates. The growth has tended to accelerate over time and the advantage of women over men has increased in all groups. The low and medium groups, in their present composition, began to separate only in the 1960s because high initial mortality in Japan adversely affected the rate of the low group in 1950-60. The increase in individual countries is given in Table 8 which places Japan far ahead of the others. As the advantage among women has been considerable in virtually every country, the overall life expectancy has increased most in those countries - Japan, Switzerland, France and Finland - in which also males have gained substantially. In spite of good gains for women, Norway and the Netherlands rank low in overall progress due to very small gains for men, and the case is even worse for the former East bloc. The figures for Italy are distorted by too high values in 1950-60.

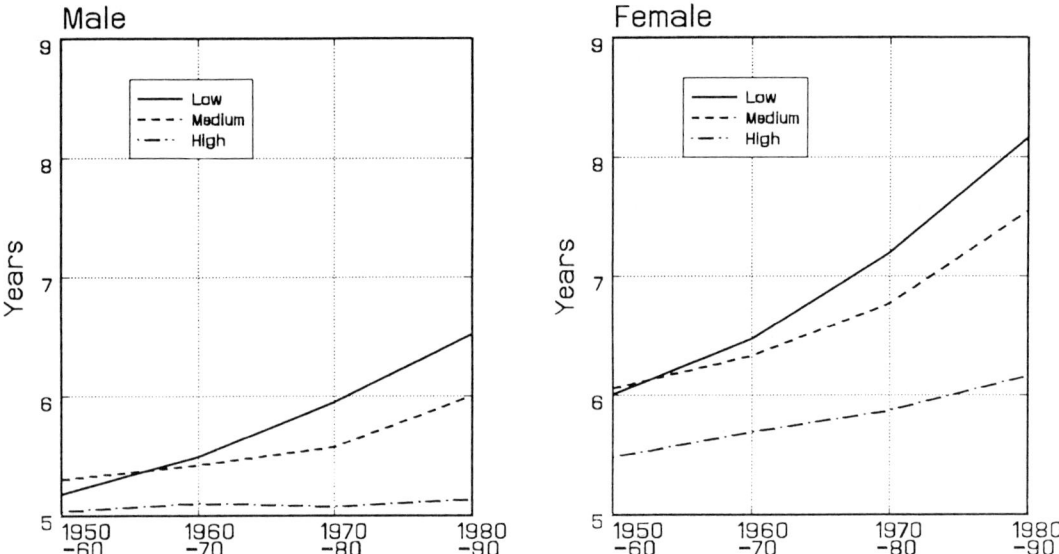

Figure 8. LIFE EXPECTANCY AT AGE 80 BY SEX AND DECADE.
Low, medium and high mortality countries.

Table 8. **INCREASE IN LIFE EXPECTANCY AT AGE 80 FROM 1950-60 TO 1980-90, YEARS.**
19 countries with good data.

Country[1]	Both sexes	Male	Female
Japan	2.21	1.76	2.45
Switzerland	1.87	1.23	2.22
France	1.74	1.28	1.99
Finland	1.67	1.07	1.99
Sweden	1.55	0.71	2.01
Denmark	1.49	0.62	1.96
Iceland	1.46	0.87	1.78
Scotland	1.32	0.85	1.58
Germany, West	1.30	0.69	1.62
England & Wales	1.29	0.72	1.59
Belgium	1.29	0.72	1.59
Luxembourg	1.13	0.60	1.42
Austria	1.11	0.79	1.29
Netherlands	1.09	0.31	1.52
Norway	0.92	0.14	1.34
Italy	0.92	0.42	1.19
Hungary	0.65	0.23	0.88
Czechoslovakia	0.47	0.12	0.65
Germany, East	0.37	0.00	0.57

[1] Same exceptions to periods apply as in Table 7.

The increase in life expectancy has not been at all dependent on its initial level as is proven in Figure 9. The correlation coefficient is for men an insignificant -0.27 and for women +0.23. There has therefore been no tendency towards convergence between countries. If there is a natural limit to human survival, it is not visible at present levels.

Resorting to historical data, a tendency towards growing life expectancy in old age can be observed in Nordic countries since late last century at least (Figure 10) but the increase was slow and interrupted by setbacks. Around 1970, the development suddenly accelerated in all three countries shown in the figure, particularly among women. At the same time, a notable transformation took place. Until then, the three countries were set apart so that Norwegians of both sexes had higher life expectancy than Swedes of either sex who, in turn, had higher expectancy than Finns of either sex. In the new situation, women of all three countries have higher life expectancy than men in any of them.

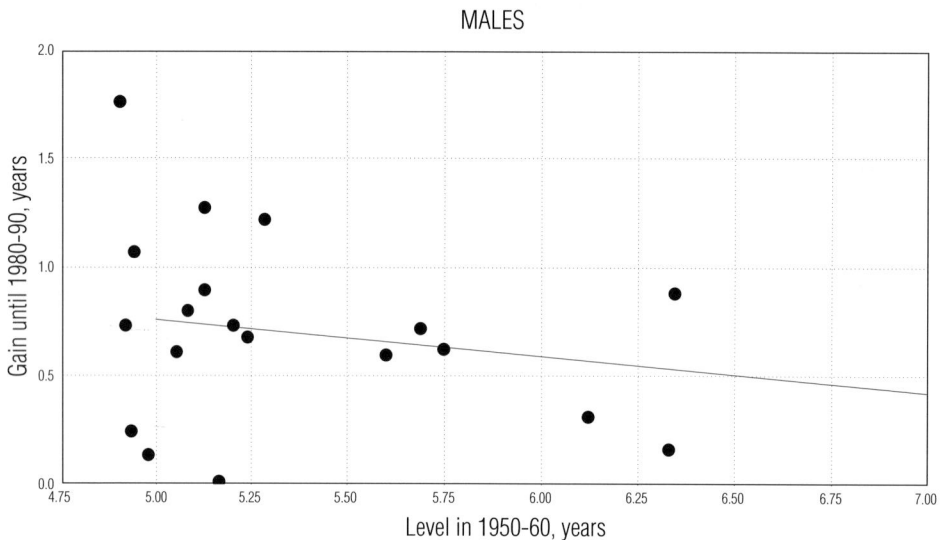

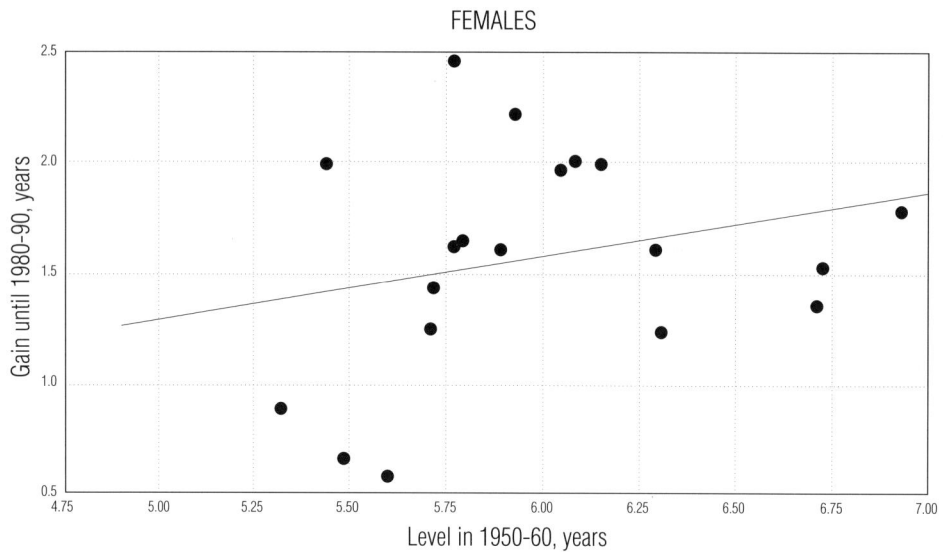

Figure 9. CORRELATION BETWEEN LIFE EXPECTANCY AT AGE 80 IN 1950-60 AND ITS GAIN UNTIL 1980-90.
Nineteen countries with good data.

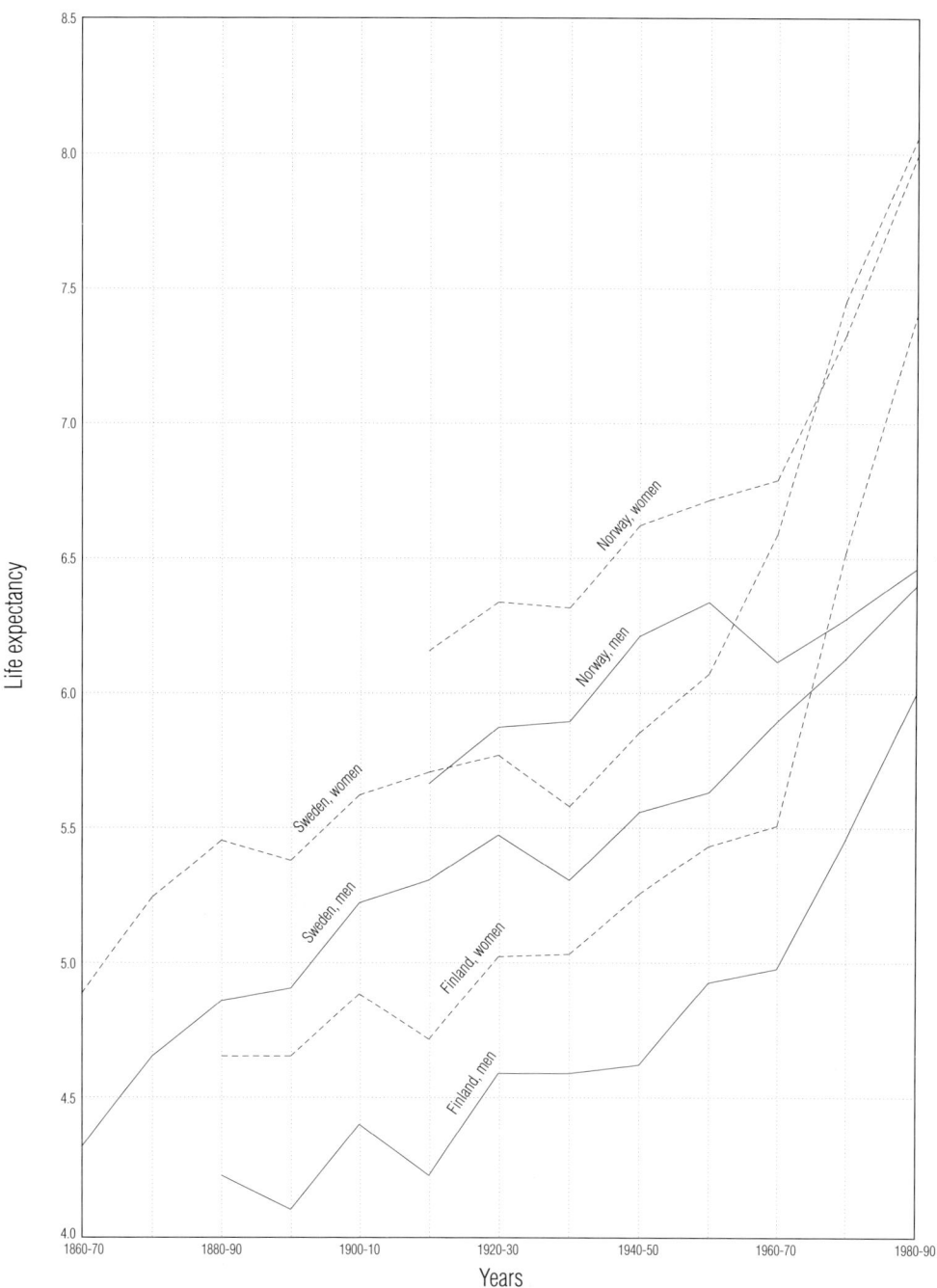

Figure 10. LONG TERM DEVELOPMENT OF LIFE EXPECTANCY AT 80 IN SWEDEN, FINLAND AND NORWAY.

7. Other longevity parameters

The most commonly used parameters of the length of life in a total population are the mean, median and mode. They have their equivalents in an oldest-old population also although their significance varies. The mean was the subject of Chapter 6. The median, mode and some other measures will be discussed here.

Table 9. MEDIAN, QUARTILES AND INTER-QUARTILE RANGE OF AGE AT DEATH AFTER 80 IN LIFE TABLE POPULATION.
Thirteen countries with good data.

Period	Males				Females			
	Q1	M	Q3	IQR	Q1	M	Q3	IQR
1950-60	82.08	84.46	87.63	5.55	82.53	85.26	88.74	6.21
1960-70	82.17	84.65	87.92	5.75	82.76	85.65	89.24	6.48
1970-80	82.31	84.92	88.37	6.06	83.14	86.26	90.02	6.88
1980-90	82.60	85.45	89.11	6.51	83.75	87.23	91.20	7.45

Among those who reach 80, the median length of life, shown in Table 9, has followed closely the mean while remaining slightly shorter. This stems from the skewed distribution of deaths, open to the right which also determines the relative positions of the quartiles. As a consequence of mortality decline, all three measures have been moving upward, the third quartile most of all so that the inter-quartile range has progressively widened.

More interesting is perhaps the mode. The distribution of deaths in a complete population is usually bi-modal with one mode immediately after birth and another in late life which is considered to describe the *typical* length of life. A third mode may appear among young adults where it is due to specific causes of death such as accidents, tuberculosis or maternity. Before the secular mortality transition, the infant mortality peak was the highest but in modern low-mortality populations, the late-life mode tends to be higher.

Only one of the length-of-life parameters of the total population, the late-life mode, can be observed in oldest-old life tables, and then only if it exceeds the starting age. That this is possible, is because true multiple modes - not caused by chance or age heaping - have not been observed in late life.

In life table terms, the mode is the age corresponding to the highest frequency of d_x. A more exact value can be pinpointed as:

$$M = x + \frac{d_x - d_{x-1}}{(d_x - d_{x-1}) + (d_x - d_{x+1})}$$

In the following, modes of 80 years are ignored as non-significant and therefore all values shown (81 or higher) are modal values for the whole population, not only for the oldest-old.

Table 10 shows the emergence of modes equalling or exceeding 81 years. In the 1950s, such cases were a rarity, reliably observed only in Norway and Denmark, surpassed by Iceland when data became available in the next decade. Among women, this situation is now commonplace. It deserves to be stressed that in almost all advanced countries a woman's typical length of life is now more than 80 years, and in nine countries more than 85 years reaching 86.7 in Switzerland. Among men, the 81-year limit is surpassed only in five countries of the low-mortality group.

The transformation of the survival curve which has led to the emergence of the 80-plus mode, is shown in Figure 11. For females the cycle has been completed and the curve is advancing to the right. Among males, the mode is about to emerge. The latest d(80) for the group of thirteen is now between the values registered for females in 1950-60 and 1960-70.

Figure 12 shows some of the international variety in regard to the late-life mode. The shape of the curves is very closely connected with life expectancy at 80. The delay of Czechoslovakia is evident in the female curve not yet peaking at 80 and in the precipitous fall of the male curve.

In every population on record, the mode of the length of life is several years higher than the mean which is pulled down by premature deaths.

Table 10. MODAL LENGTH OF LIFE.

Country and aggregate	Male				Female			
	1950-60	1960-70	1970-80	1980-90	1950-60	1960-70	1970-80	1980-90
Australia	-	-	-	-	-	-	-	86.3
Austria	-	-	-	-	-	-	81.8	83.7
Belgium	-	-	-	-	-	81.3	83.1	84.5
Czechoslovakia	-	-	-	-	-	-	-	-
Denmark	-	-	-	-	81.5	81.1	84.5	85.4
England & Wales	-	-	-	-	-	82.7	83.4	84.6
Estonia	-	-	-	-	-	-	82.5	81.5
Finland	-	-	-	-	-	-	82.9	83.7
France	-	-	-	81.2	-	82.9	84.3	86.1
Germany East	-	-	-	-	-	-	-	81.6
Germany West	-	-	-	-	-	-	82.4	84.5
Hungary	-	-	-	-	-	-	-	81.2
Iceland	-	-	81.7	81.7	-	83.5	84.7	86.3
Ireland	-	-	-	-	-	-	-	-
Italy	-	-	-	-	81.3	81.8	83.3	84.9
Japan	-	-	-	81.7	-	-	83.5	86.2
Latvia	-	-	-	-	-	-	-	-
Luxembourg	-	-	-	-	-	-	-	-
Netherlands	-	-	-	-	-	81.8	83.9	86.4
New Zealand	-	-	-	-	-	-	-	84.5
Norway	81.5	-	-	-	81.8	83.4	84.6	86.3
Poland	-	-	-	-	-	-	81.1	82.4
Portugal	-	-	-	-	-	-	82.5	83.6
Scotland	-	-	-	-	-	81.2	-	82.8
Singapore	-	-	-	-	-	-	-	81.7
Spain	-	-	-	-	-	-	82.8	84.7
Sweden	-	-	-	81.3	-	82.6	85.3	85.6
Switzerland	-	-	-	81.1	-	82.3	84.4	86.7
Good quality (13)	-	-	-	-	-	81.8	83.4	85.2
Low mortality (8)	-	-	-	81.2	-	81.9	84.1	86.1
Medium mortality (5)	-	-	-	-	-	82.0	82.8	84.5
High mortality (3)	-	-	-	-	-	-	-	81.3

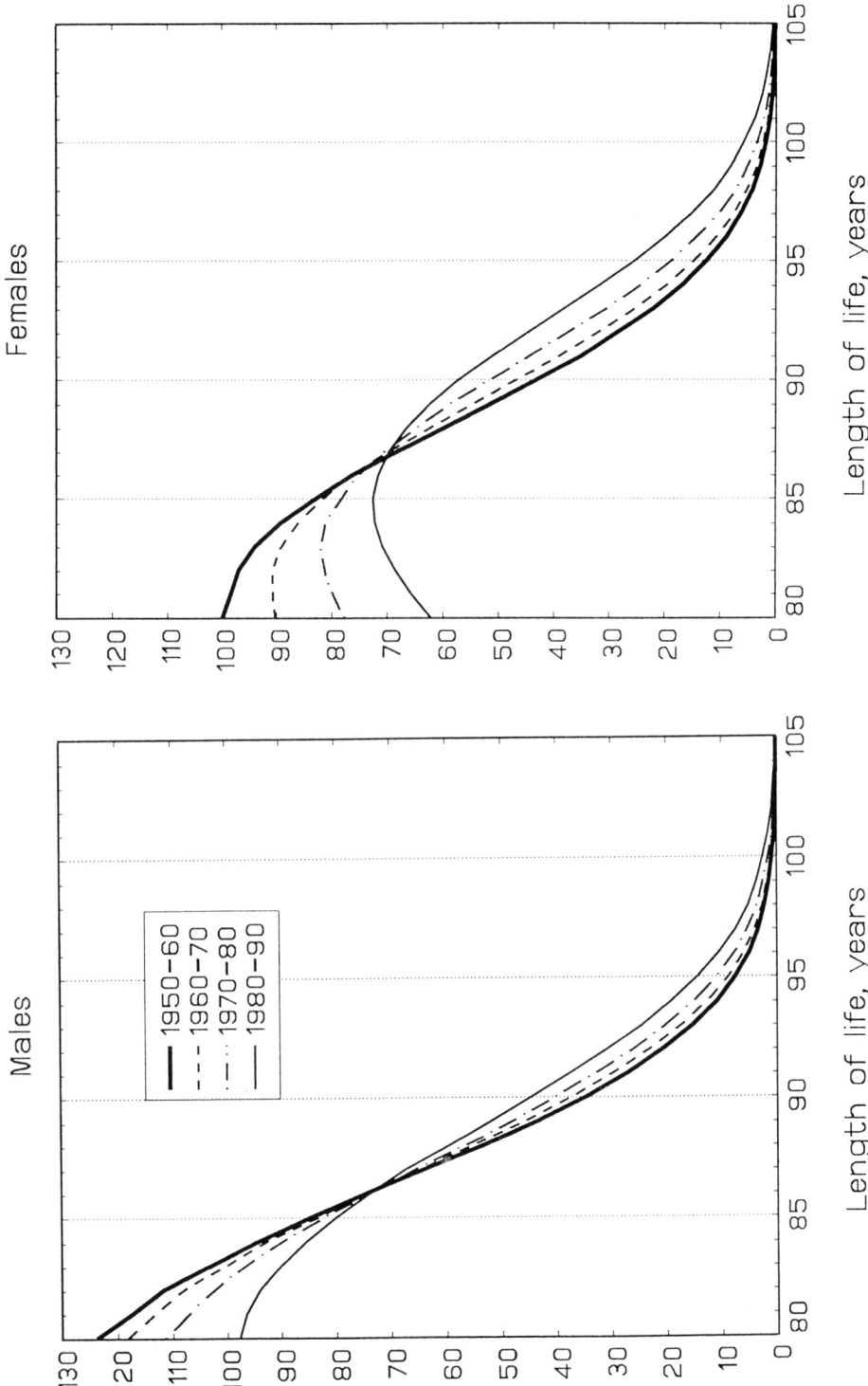

Figure 11. LENGTH OF LIFE OF 1000 PERSONS WHO REACHED AGE 80. Thirteen countries with good data.

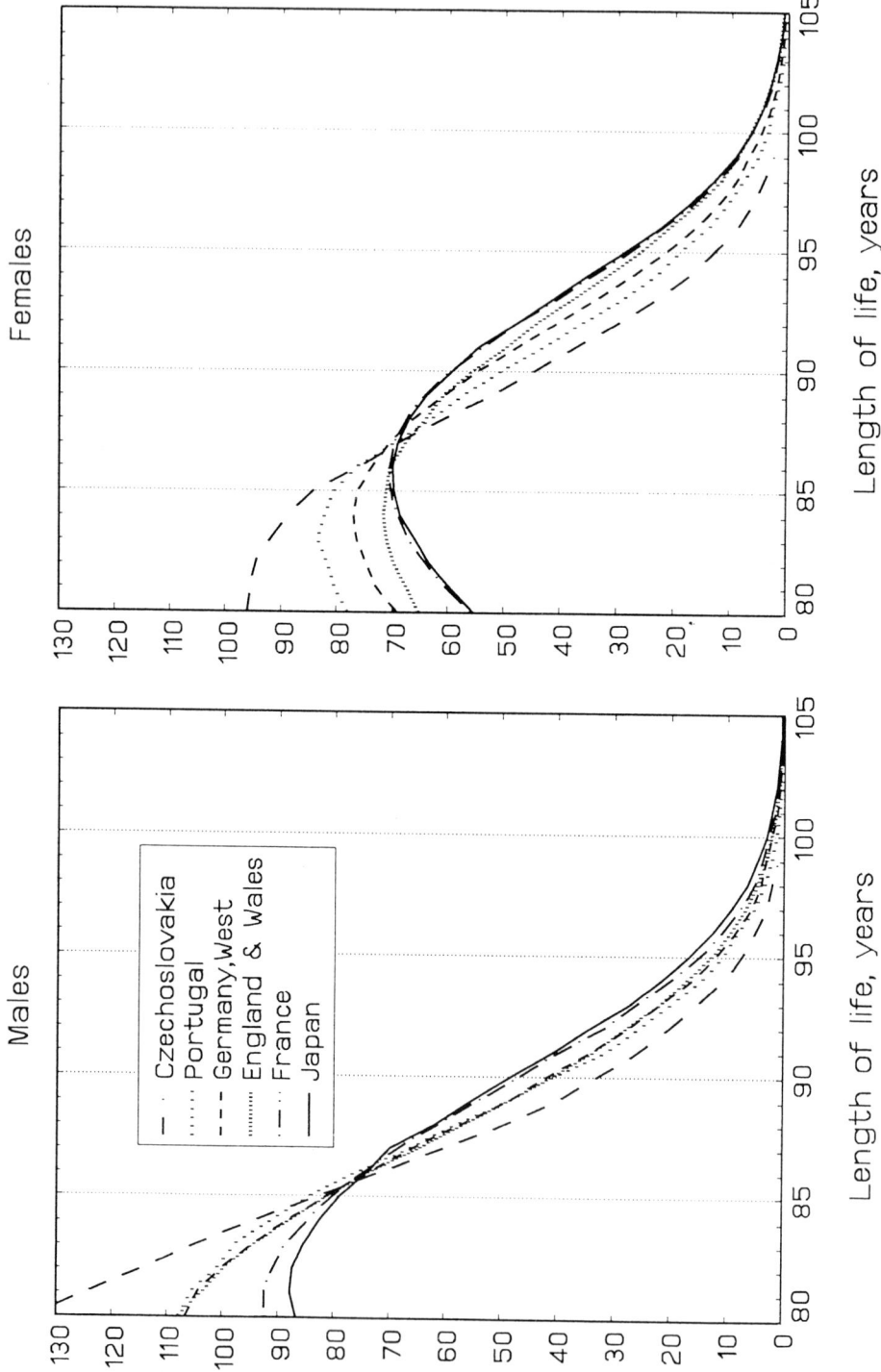

Figure 12. LENGTH OF LIFE OF 1000 PERSONS WHO REACHED AGE 80. Selected countries, 1980-90.

Table 11. AGE WHEN LIFE EXPECTANCY EQUALS A GIVEN NUMBER OF YEARS.
Low, medium and high mortality countries.

Period	Male			Female		
	Low	Medium	High	Low	Medium	High
Life expectancy 5 years						
1950 - 60	80.55	80.90	80.10	82.74	82.92	81.36
1960 - 70	81.47	81.27	80.31	83.79	83.50	81.85
1970 - 80	82.76	81.78	80.04	85.23	84.46	82.29
1980 - 90	84.13	83.01	80.43	86.84	86.00	82.98
Life expectancy 2 years						
1950 -60	96.56	95.14	94.59	97.41	97.20	94.94
1960 - 70	97.29	95.46	94.20	98.67	97.28	95.60
1970 - 80	97.71	96.74	95.64	99.43	98.79	96.97
1980 - 90	98.86	98.35	95.29	100.94	100.47	96.95

Low mortality countries: Denmark, France, Iceland, Japan, Netherlands, Norway, Sweden, Switzerland.
Medium mortality countries: Austria, England & Wales, Finland, Germany (West), Italy.
High mortality countries: Czechoslovakia, Germany (East), Hungary.

A life table parameter introduced by VAUPEL and LUNDSTRÖM (1993) is the age at which the remaining life expectancy equals a certain number of years. In our material, this can be determined e.g. in relation to 5 or 2 years. These points in life are given in Table 11 for three aggregates and illustrated in Figure 13 regarding the 5-year point ($e = 5$). The shifting of this point which arguably may be interpreted as evidence of delayed aging, has been nothing less than remarkable in the vanguard populations - up to four years. This brings us to the topic of the next chapter, the age shift in mortality.

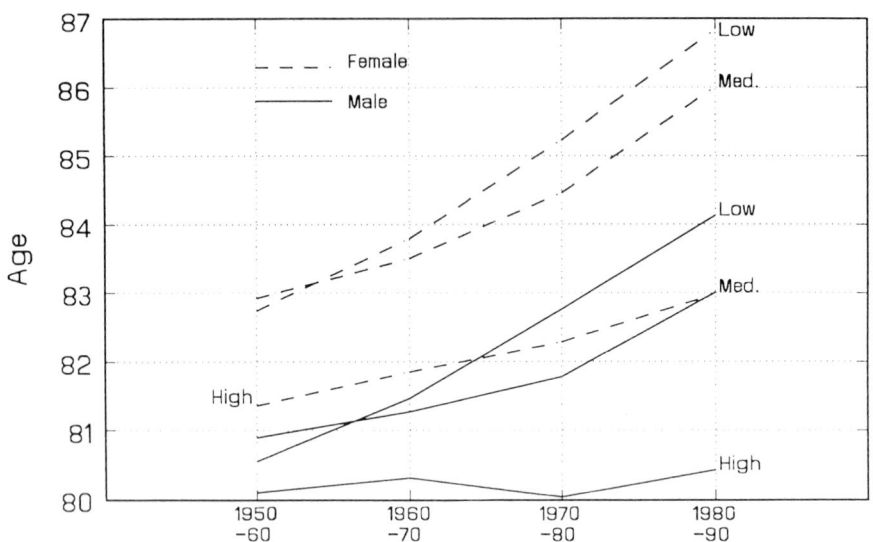

Figure 13. AGE WHEN LIFE EXPECTANCY EQUALS 5 YEARS.
Low, medium and high mortality countries.

8. Age shift in mortality

Figure 3 in Chapter 3 demonstrated how mortality curves of successive periods moved generally to the right while essentially maintaining their characteristic form. In other words, *mortality shifted to higher age*. The magnitude of this shift is measurable in years of age. The shift may be considered indicative of a similar shift in the physical health or robustness of a population. It may mean a commensurate delay in the aging process.

At young ages, the age shift has few if any practical applications but starts to have meaning in middle age when mortality begins to rise monotonically. It is perhaps most meaningful in old age.

The age shift could be measured in relation to given mortality levels expressed in m_x or q_x or μ_x or other parameters but is more easily visualized when expressed in relation to age itself. In the following, we therefore start with mortality by age in a given period and observe at which ages the same mortality levels are reached in a later period. We shall call the difference *the age shift in mortality*. When mortality declines, the shift is positive; when it rises, it is negative.

To illustrate the procedure, we find in the life table for Austrian females in 1950-60 the value $q(85) = 0.1721$. Assuming that mortality rises from age x to x + 1 linearly, we can pinpoint the exact age at which q equals 0.1721 in later life tables and obtain the following:

Period	$q_x = 0.1721$	Age shift	Cumulative shift
1950-60	85.00		
		0.96	0.96
1960-70	85.96		
		0.48	1.44
1970-80	86.44		
		1.25	2.65
1980-90	87.69		

In the same way, two contemporary populations can be compared by observing at which age the death rates found in a population of higher mortality are reached by a population of lower mortality. The difference may be called *age delay in mortality*. Likewise, we may measure the *age delay of female mortality* in relation to male.

It is advantageous to calculate the age shift or age delay from smoothed - or originally smooth - age series in order to avoid meaningless irregularities. The smoothing can be considered fully justified at ages where mortality is generally linked to aging.

As an introduction, the age shift is illustrated in Figure 14 for the aggregate of thirteen countries. The curves for males rise with advancing age. In the first period, it progressed between 0.7 years at age 80 and about twice as much at 95-97. In the combined 20-year period, the age shift was more than twice as large but the rise by age relatively and even absolutely more modest, namely from 2.2 to 2.7 years.

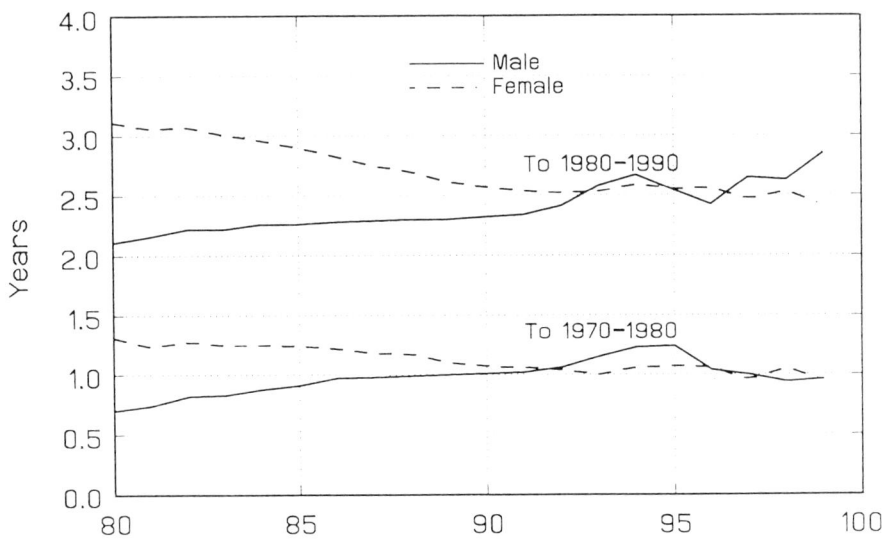

Figure 14. AGE SHIFT IN MORTALITY, FROM 1960-70 TO SPECIFIED PERIODS. Thirteen countries.

The age shift for women had the opposite, descending profile with age. Among octogenarians it was much greater for women than men but declined thereafter. Around age 95 the shift was approximately equal for both sexes, namely 2.7 years in twenty years' time. The generally ascending curve for men means that for them the ascent of mortality by age became less steep while the opposite form for women indicates a steepening of the mortality curve by age.

Figure 15 demonstrates a great variety in the shifting of age between countries. For men, both the level and the form contrast widely. In some countries, the shift is very steady over the entire age range, declining only slightly while in some others it is very low or negative near age 80 and then climbs gradually. To these belong on one hand the Netherlands, Norway and Denmark (not shown), on the other, the former East bloc, exemplified here by Hungary. Though the level of mortality was very different in these two groups, common to both was that they recorded little progress among the relatively younger men.

The curves for women vary widely between the limits of one and five years but display a common tendency to a slow descent by age. The rise recorded at oldest ages is not very significant in Finland because of small numbers, nor in Japan because of uncertain age information on the very oldest in the 1960s.

The actual data for 22 countries and 4 aggregates are given in Annex Table 6 and summarized by 5-year age groups in Table 12. Only the age range 80-94 (as of 1960-70) can be effectively observed because for the older the comparable 1980-90 rates are found at ages where data are not available or in some cases more erratic. The largest shift, surpassing 4 years, is registered for Finnish women and for Japanese men and women, shifts of over 3 years for Icelandic and Swiss women and Finnish men. In Eastern Europe, the shift was generally less than one year.

That the age shift in mortality is an indicator independent from change in life expectancy is shown by the large difference in their magnitude and a less than strict correlation be-tween the two. The two indicators are juxtaposed in Figure 16 for the 22 countries in Table 17 plus Ireland which was omitted from it because heavy age heaping made the details questionable.

The age shift proves to be throughout much larger than the gain in life expectancy. This can be well understood from the fact that if in a life table we move a certain number of years up or down, the corresponding life expectancy changes much less.

The second observation is the looseness of the correlation. When the countries are ranked by increase in life expectancy, the profile of the age shift is jagged. The former is a more robust measure while the latter is more sensitive to the age pattern of mortality and also to small numbers. Above all, however, they measure mortality from different points of view.

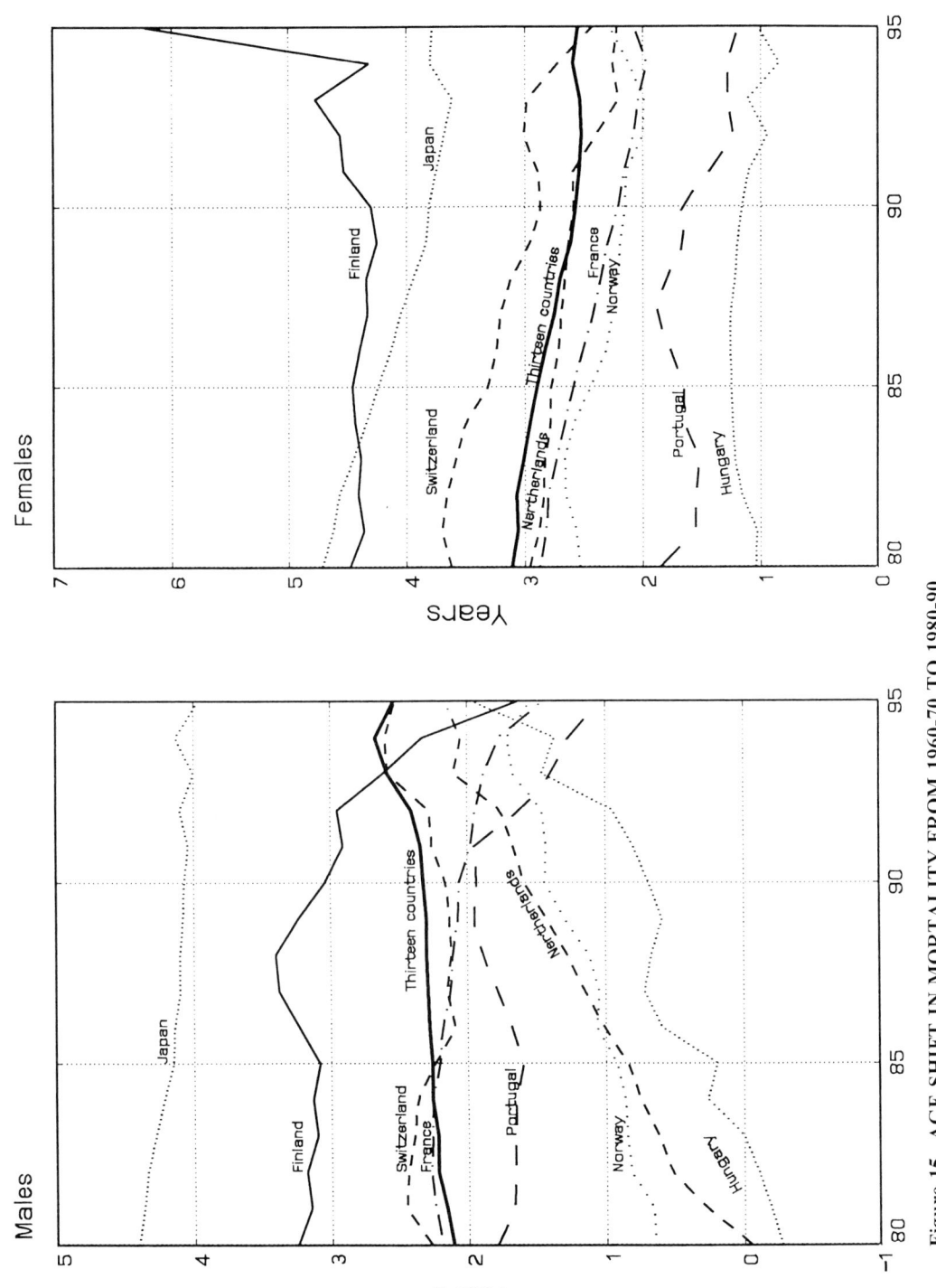

Figure 15. AGE SHIFT IN MORTALITY FROM 1960-70 TO 1980-90.

Table 12. MEAN AGE SHIFT IN AGE GROUPS FROM 1960 - 70 TO 1980 - 90

Country	Male				Country	Female				F - M[1]
	80-84	85-89	90-94	Mean 80-94		80-84	85-89	90-94	Mean 80-94	
Japan	4.32	4.11	4.07	4.17	Finland	4.42	4.36	4.50	4.43	1.36
Finland	3.16	3.27	2.77	3.07	Japan	4.54	4.04	3.73	4.10	-0.07
Switzerland	2.38	2.15	2.38	2.30	Iceland	3.00	3.94	4.28	3.74	2.07
France	2.24	2.14	1.93	2.10	Switzerland	3.61	3.17	2.89	3.22	1.02
Austria	1.81	1.98	1.93	1.91	Luxembourg	3.08	2.45	3.09	2.87	1.88
Italy	1.40	1.87	2.42	1.90	Denmark	3.20	2.86	2.48	2.85	1.20
Germany, West	1.60	1.80	2.22	1.87	Germany, West	2.84	2.70	2.92	2.82	0.95
England & Wales	1.58	1.82	2.00	1.80	Belgium	2.76	2.74	2.85	2.78	1.00
Belgium	1.28	1.91	2.14	1.78	Sweden	3.03	2.76	2.24	2.68	1.29
Portugal	1.69	1.78	1.63	1.70	Netherlands	2.86	2.69	2.41	2.65	1.52
Iceland	2.15	1.75	1.11	1.67	Italy	2.53	2.45	2.50	2.49	0.59
Denmark	1.24	1.82	1.97	1.65	France	2.78	2.44	2.09	2.44	0.34
Scotland	1.28	1.71	1.97	1.65	Scotland	2.48	2.31	2.51	2.43	0.72
Sweden	1.19	1.28	1.69	1.39	Norway	2.59	2.28	2.08	2.32	1.19
New Zealand	1.29	1.62	1.13	1.35	England & Wales	2.41	2.28	2.05	2.25	0.45
Netherlands	0.42	1.14	1.83	1.13	New Zealand	1.96	2.18	1.96	2.03	0.68
Norway	0.77	1.09	1.54	1.13	Austria	2.16	1.82	1.60	1.86	0.05
Luxembourg	1.62	1.37	-0.01	0.99	Ireland	2.30	2.03	0.90	1.74	1.21
Estonia	0.12	0.49	2.15	0.92	Portugal	1.62	1.75	1.39	1.59	-0.11
Ireland	0.89	0.71	-0.08	0.53	Germany, East	1.28	1.17	1.13	1.19	0.83
Hungary	-0.07	0.55	1.05	0.51	Hungary	1.14	1.24	1.03	1.14	0.63
Germany, East	0.10	0.33	0.06	0.34	Estonia	0.58	1.02	0.81	0.80	-0.12
Czechoslovakia	-0.22	0.48	0.36	0.24	Czechoslovakia	0.82	0.85	0.49	0.72	0.48
Unweighted mean	1.40	1.62	1.69	1.57	Unweighted mean	2.49	2.41	2.26	2.40	0.83

[1] Difference between female and male means.

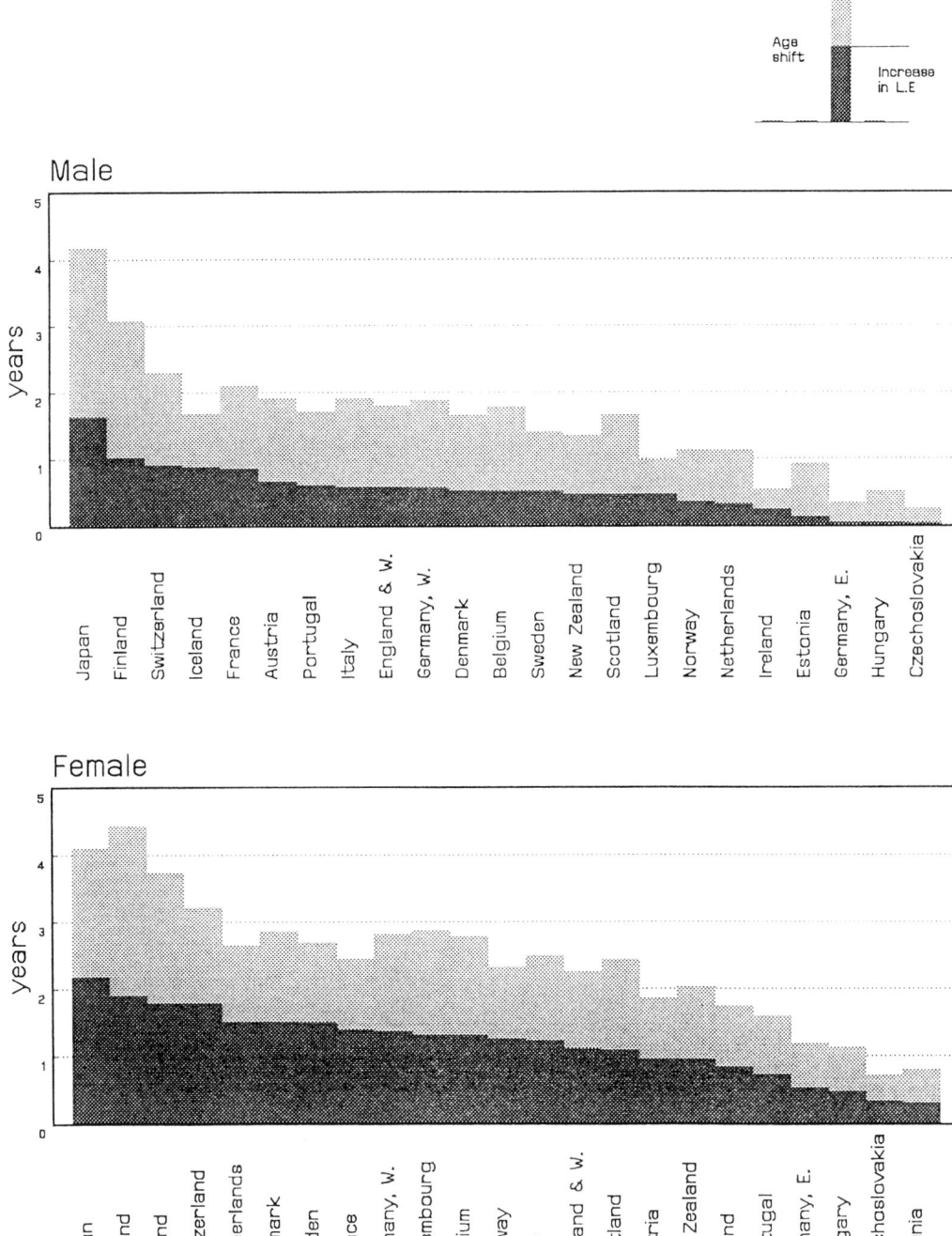

Figure 16. COMPARISON OF AGE SHIFT WITH INCREASE IN LIFE EXPECTANCY AT 80 FROM 1960-70 TO 1980-90.

9. Slope of mortality

The trajectory of mortality in old age, plotted in logarithmic scale, is a convex curve. Its level varies between populations and over time a great deal but its form very little. The remarkable regularity of this form has led generations of actuaries and demographers to search for a formula which would express it neatly and be universally valid. Leaving this question aside, we shall simply give indications of the steepness of the arch as observed in the countries of the database. We shall call it slope as we can do about a hill without implying that it is linear.

This increase by advancing age can be measured by the parameter k defined by HORIUCHI and COALE (1990) as the relative derivative of $\mu(x)$:

$$k(x) = \frac{d\mu(x)/dx}{\mu(x)}$$

The force of mortality is obtained by the approximate formula:

$$\mu(x+0.5) = -\ln p(x)$$

where $p = 1 - q$. For greater stability we averaged the p (x) values which were already smoothed by 5-year moving averages, over 5-year age periods by:

$$p(x/x+4) = \sqrt[5]{p(x)p(x+1)\ldots p(x+4)}$$

A value for the force of mortality was this way calculated for the approximate ages 83, 88, 93, 98 and 103, and from them, the values of k for the intervals as shown in Table 13 for the aggregate of thirteen countries. The same are illustrated in Figure 17.

Table 13. **LIFE TABLE AGING RATE k IN SPECIFIED AGE INTERVALS, BY DECADE.**
Thirteen countries with good data.

Sex and period	Age interval				
	83 - 88	88 - 93	93 - 98	98 - 103	83 - 98
Male					
1950 - 1960	.0889	.0757	.0718	.0432	.0788
1960 - 1970	.0876	.0798	.0714	.0595	.0796
1970 - 1980	.0855	.0806	.0706	.0651	.0789
1980 - 1990	.0884	.0829	.0693	.0651	.0802
Increase 1960 - 70 to 1980 - 90	.0008	.0031	-.0011	.0056	.0006
Female					
1950 - 1960	.0948	.0808	.0757	.0567	.0838
1960 - 1970	.0996	.0860	.0725	.0574	.0864
1970 - 1980	.1048	.0919	.0769	.0642	.0912
1980 - 1990	.1135	.0999	.0805	.0692	.0980
Increase 1960 - 70 to 1980 - 90	.0139	.0139	.0080	.0118	.0116

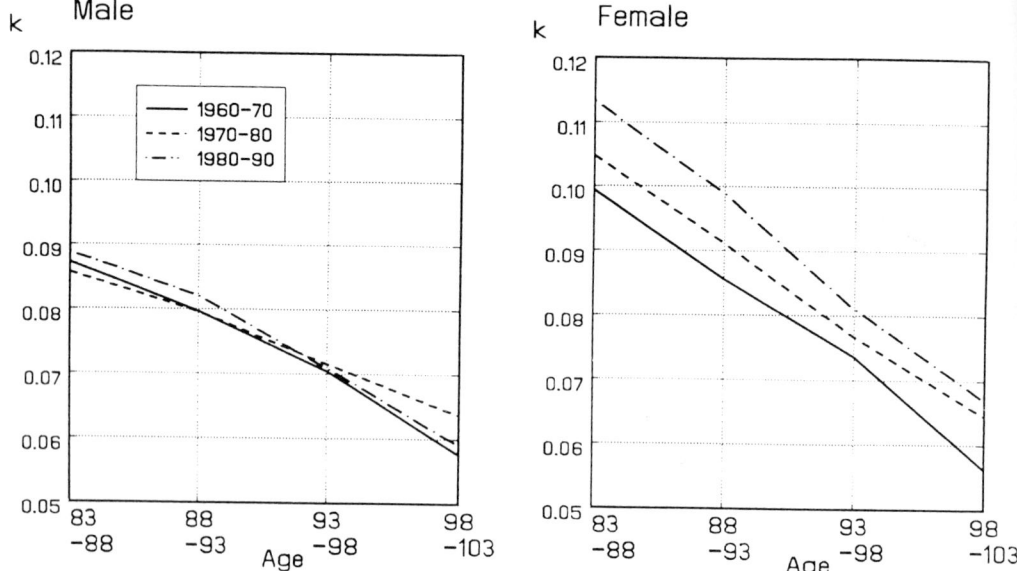

Figure 17. SLOPE OF MORTALITY (k) IN 5 YEAR AGE INTERVALS.
Thirteen countries with good data.

Certain characteristics of the mortality curve (expressed in q_x, m_x, or μ_x) and of the k curve which is defined as the slope of ln (μ_x), correspond in the following way:

	Mortality curve	k curve
1)	ascends with age	positive values
2)	decelerates in log. scale	declines
3)	regular convex form	linear decline
4)	steeper over time or vice versa	higher over time or vice versa

Though the first two characteristics are obvious in both presentations, the features are generally better perceived and become measurable in the k curve. Correspondence 3) is meaningful only from k to mortality curve. Altogether, k is a good analytical tool which facilitates seeing and measuring facets that are imbedded but not very apparent in the mortality curve.

For the thirteen countries, the k values of the last three decades (the somewhat irregular 1950-60 data are excluded) in Figure 17 show the principal features of the slope of mortality in the post-war era. The slope of the female curve is steeper (k is larger) than that of the male over most of the age range but approximates it in the proximity of 100 years. Its steepness has further increased noticeably from one decade to the next while the male curve shows only the slightest tendency in this direction. All lines are fairly linear which can be interpreted as a certain basic regularity in the well-known curvature that characterizes the ascent of mortality.

The 15-year age interval 83-98 summarizes the situation and the development best because, in spite of double smoothing, the interval 98-103 is not entirely free from irregularity. This summary measure is given in the last column in Table 13. We will note for males a near-complete immobility of k but for females a steady and accelerating increase from decade to decade, namely .0026, .0048 and .0068. This aggravation of the slope of female mortality is of course a consequence of greater reduction in death rates of the relatively younger old.

For individual countries, the k function was calculated for the 83-98 year interval by the same method which makes

$$k = \frac{1}{15} (\ln \mu_{98} - \ln \mu_{83})$$

In the ensuing international comparison, presented in Table 14, it is noteworthy that the slope is found in a relatively narrow range: for men mostly between .07 and .09, for women between .08 and slightly over .10. In all cases, with one insignificant exception, k has been larger for women than men, a feature which is closely associated with the lower mortality level of women.

The countries with steepest slopes for men are Iceland, Switzerland, France and Sweden while those where the slope has increased most are Japan, France and Finland, all three of them countries with a large mortality decline for men. Lack of a uniform tendency by men is shown by the fact that in eleven countries, k has increased, in nine others decreased. In the criss-crossing movements among the 20 countries, the unweighted mean of k as well as the standard deviation remained virtually unchanged.

Table 14. LIFE TABLE AGING RATE k BETWEEN AGES 83 AND 98.

Country	Male		Female		Change	
	1960 - 70	1980 - 90	1960 - 70	1980 - 90	Male	Female
Austria	.0768	.0762	.0862	.0953	-.0006	.0091
Belgium	.0751	.0765	.0869	.0929	.0014	.0060
Czechoslovakia	.0808	.0758	.0818	.0885	-.0050	.0067
Denmark	.0902	.0826	.0893	.1011	-.0076	.0118
England & Wales	.0756	.0747	.0852	.0930	-.0009	.0078
Estonia	.0798	0682	.0802	.0822	-.0116	.0020
Finland	.0721	.0807	.0785	.0911	.0086	.0126
France	.0750	.0856	.0888	.1036	.0106	.0148
Germany, East	.0888	.0795	.0920	.0892	-.0093	-.0028
Germany, West	.0777	.0766	.0850	.0928	-.0011	.0078
Hungary	.0833	.0695	.0895	.0857	-.0138	-.0038
Iceland	.0847	.0891	.0875	.0949	.0044	.0074
Japan	.0684	.0829	.0845	.1032	.0145	.0187
Netherlands	.0840	.0775	.0896	.1000	-.0065	.0104
New Zealand	.0767	.0819	.0913	.0924	.0052	.0011
Norway	.0837	.0813	.0921	.0995	-.0024	.0074
Portugal	.0738	.0807	.0789	.0876	.0069	.0087
Scotland	.0775	.0750	.0798	.0816	-.0025	.0018
Sweden	.0854	.0855	.0871	.1023	.0001	.0152
Switzerland	.0818	.0858	.0894	.1010	.0040	.0116
Mean	.0796	.0792	.0860	.0938	-.0004	.0078
Standard deviation	.0057	.0059	.0048	.0071	.0002	.0023

Among women, the slope became steeper with only two exceptions in Eastern Europe. The magnitude of the change varied widely between countries and both the mean and the standard deviation increased significantly, the former from .0860 to .0938 and the latter from .0048 to .0071. The steepest slopes for women are found in France, Japan, Sweden, Denmark and Switzerland which all boast low death rates. The increase in k in the past 20 years has been largest in Japan, Sweden, France, Finland and Denmark.

It can thus be observed that countries with lowest mortality tend to exhibit relatively steep slopes in it. This is confirmed by respective correlation coefficients which are for males +0.75 and for females +0.73, both of them significant at more than 99 percent level. The regression lines of k by e(80) in Figure 18 are almost parallel for both sexes but that for women lies on a higher level. Even with equal life expectancy the female slope of mortality tends to be slightly steeper. For the most part, however, the steeper slopes for women are associated with their higher life expectancy.

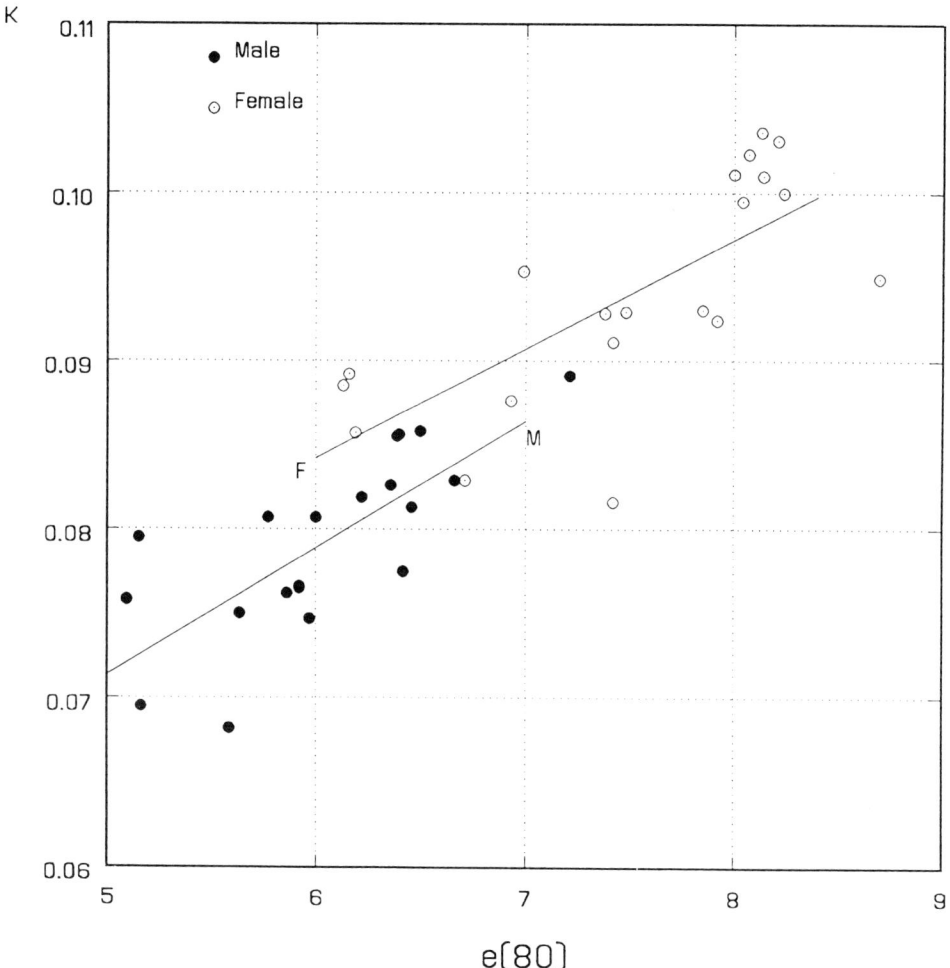

Figure 18. CORRELATION BETWEEN LIFE EXPECTANCY AT AGE 80 AND SLOPE OF MORTALITY (k) BETWEEN AGES 83 AND 98.
Twenty countries in 1980-90.

A closer look at the changes of the last 20 years in Figure 19 reveals different patterns of development between men and women. Though both show a high positive correlation between increase in life expectancy and increase in steepness (for males, r = +0.87, for females +0.74), the regression lines intersect. The slope has changed in the female populations more uniformly while the male populations are very sharply divided, and low overall progress has been accompanied by an actual reduction in the slope. Such reduction has not been caused by unusually large gains at highest ages but by stagnation or slow progress among the relatively younger.

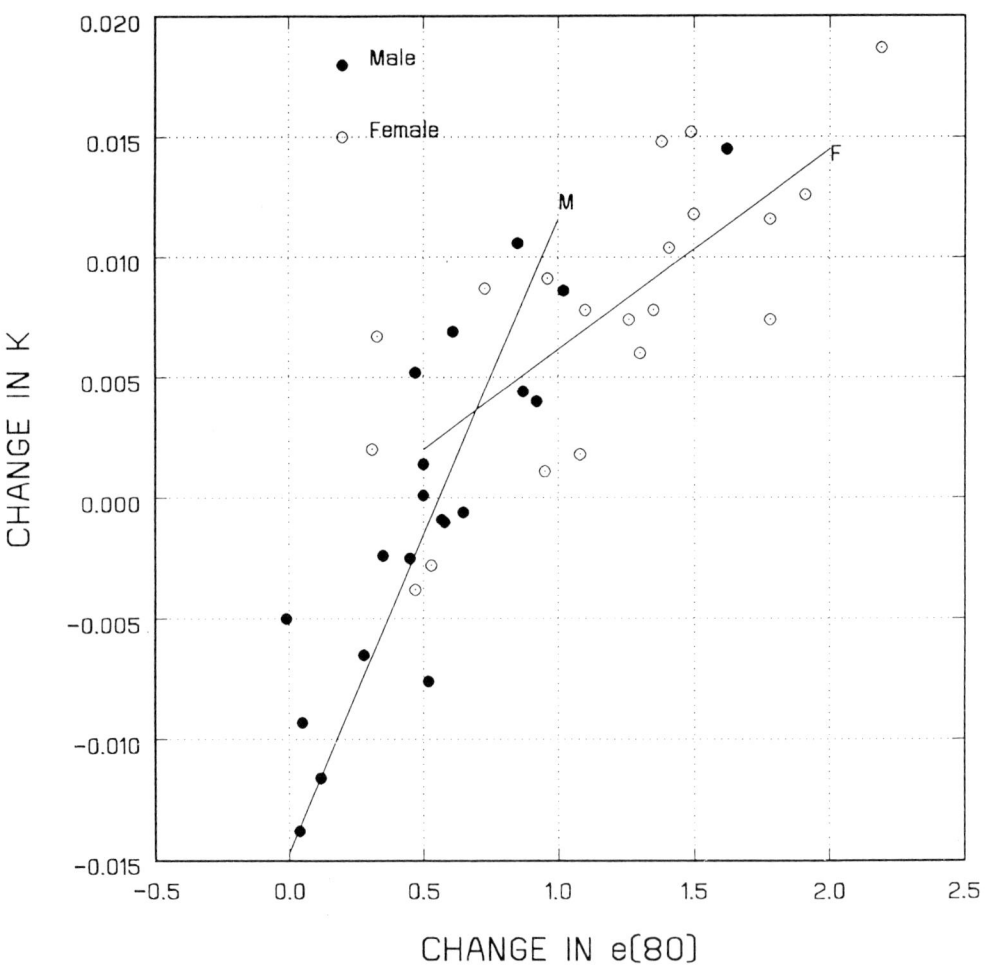

Figure 19. CORRELATION BETWEEN CHANGE IN LIFE EXPECTANCY AT AGE 80 AND IN SLOPE OF MORTALITY (k) FROM 1960-70 TO 1980-90.
Twenty countries.

10. The road from 80 to 100

A person's or a cohort's advance from age eighty towards one hundred is of a certain interest because it separates the individuals of true longevity from the merely old in a process which is seen by many as a selection of the fittest or the more robust, by some as an accumulation of wear and tear, and by others as a more complicated and less deterministic interaction of many forces and influences.

The road from 80 to 100 may be visualized as a long march or an uphill struggle which separates the few successful from the many unsuccessful, the graduates from the candidates. Though few of the persons involved would consciously set such a goal for themselves, most of the people in this situation carry on with their daily living with the will or the instinct to survive which is intrinsic in every species.

Whatever our view, or lack of it, of this process, the simple prosaic figure indicating the probability of an 80-year-old to live to the age 100 is an important indicator of the force of survival in a population. The data will show that the odds in this process, though still overwhelmingly against survival, have lately undergone deep transformations and are in today's low-mortality populations undoubtedly much more favourable than ever before in the history of mankind.

We have seen in Chapter 5 how the decline in the probability of dying was generally greatest near age 80 and gradually declined with age. Viewed from the opposite angle, that of survival, the change has a totally opposite form: it is smallest near age 80 and grows rapidly as age advances because the ever smaller chances of survival are affected relatively more by even small improvements. For the thirteen countries, the data are given in Table 15 and shown graphically in Figure 20.

The relative decline in mortality was very much larger for octogenarian women than for men of the same age but their increase in survival, shown in Figure 20, was only narrowly greater than that for men. In mortality decline, the rates of the two sexes merged just before age 100 but in survival increase, the lines cross at age 92 after which the male gains stay higher. As far as it is possible to determine, the survival gains made in the last twenty years seem to reach their maximum values around age 100 - about nine percent for men and seven percent for women.

Table 15. PROBABILITY OF SURVIVAL BY AGE AND SEX AND INCREASE FROM 1960-70 TO 1980-90. Thirteen countries with good data; 5-year moving averages.

Age x	Male				Female			
	p (x)		Growth factor		p (x)		Growth factor	
	1960-70	1980-90	x	80 to x	1960-70	1980-90	x	80 to x
80	0.8819	0.9024	1.0232	1.0232	0.9098	0.9377	1.0307	1.0307
81	0.8709	0.8931	1.0254	1.0493	0.8998	0.9296	1.0331	1.0648
82	0.8590	0.8830	1.0279	1.0786	0.8885	0.9204	1.0360	1.1030
83	0.8470	0.8727	1.0304	1.1112	0.8770	0.9109	1.0386	1.1454
84	0.8338	0.8616	1.0334	1.1483	0.8645	0.9005	1.0417	1.1934
85	0.8202	0.8497	1.0360	1.1896	0.8514	0.8893	1.0445	1.2465
86	0.8055	0.8372	1.0394	1.2365	0.8377	0.8771	1.0471	1.3051
87	0.7904	0.8239	1.0425	1.2889	0.8233	0.8640	1.0495	1.3696
88	0.7745	0.8097	1.0455	1.3474	0.8080	0.8500	1.0519	1.4408
89	0.7579	0.7949	1.0488	1.4132	0.7926	0.8351	1.0536	1.5180
90	0.7404	0.7794	1.0528	1.4876	0.7762	0.8194	1.0556	1.6025
91	0.7227	0.7631	1.0558	1.5108	0.7591	0.8030	1.0577	1.6952
92	0.7043	0.7460	1.0593	1.6638	0.7416	0.7860	1.0598	1.7967
93	0.6853	0.7287	1.0633	1.7691	0.7239	0.7687	1.0619	1.9079
94	0.6667	0.7113	1.0668	1.8874	0.7049	0.7508	1.0651	2.0321
95	0.6485	0.6944	1.0709	2.0211	0.6865	0.7331	1.0678	2.1701
96	0.6298	0.6788	1.0778	2.1783	0.6672	0.7156	1.0725	2.3275
97	0.6062	0.6608	1.0901	2.3746	0.6494	0.6975	1.0741	2.4999
98	0.5849	0.6382	1.0912	2.5909	0.6285	0.6774	1.0777	2.6944
99	0.5652	0.6183	1.0939	2.8342	0.6117	0.6581	1.0759	2.8989
100	0.5492	0.5998	1.0921	3.0952	0.5966	0.6493	1.0715	3.1062
101	0.5315	0.5762	1.0842	3.3558	0.5799	0.6191	1.0676	3.3161
102	0.5101	0.5632	1.1042	3.7055	0.5624	0.6009	1.0686	3.5436
103	0.5019	0.5575	1.1109	4.1165	0.5467	0.5827	1.0658	3.7768
104	0.4745	0.5505	1.1601	4.7755	0.5309	0.5693	1.0724	4.0502

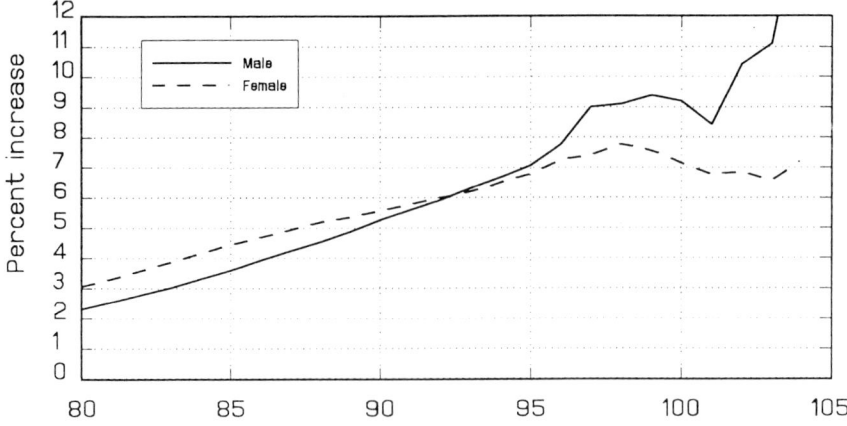

Figure 20. INCREASE FROM 1960-70 TO 1980-90 IN AGE-SPECIFIC PROBABILITY OF SURVIVAL. Thirteen countries with good data.

Over longer age spans, however, the gains in survival at single ages are compounded and may reach impressive proportions. At high ages, where the chances of further survival are dwindling, even a moderate decline in death rates causes vigorous relative expansion of these chances as becomes manifest from a perusal of Table 16.

Table 16. **5-YEAR PROBABILITIES OF SURVIVAL BY AGE AND SEX AND INCREASE BETWEEN SPECIFIED PERIODS.**
Thirteen countries with good data.

Sex and age	$5 p_x$			Growth factor of $p(x)$		
	1960 - 70	1970 - 80	1980 - 90	1960 - 70 to 1970 - 80	1970 - 80 to 1980 - 90	1960 - 70 to 1980 - 90
Male						
80 - 85	0.4659	0.4911	0.5351	1.0541	1.0896	1.1485
85 - 90	0.3065	0.3357	0.3772	1.0953	1.1236	1.2307
90 - 95	0.1722	0.1969	0.2300	1.1434	1.1681	1.3357
95 - 100	0.0818	0.0978	0.1229	1.1956	1.2566	1.5024
100 - 105	0.0354	0.0408	0.0598	1.1525	1.4657	1.6893
80 - 100	0.00201	0.00317	0.00571	1.5771	1.8013	2.8408
Female						
80 - 85	0.5515	0.5965	0.6581	1.0816	1.1033	1.1933
85 - 90	0.3760	0.4178	0.4784	1.1112	1.1450	1.2723
90 - 95	0.2230	0.2522	0.2985	1.1309	1.1836	1.3386
95 - 100	0.1144	0.1325	0.1631	1.1582	1.2309	1.4257
100 - 105	0.0565	0.0613	0.0789	1.0850	1.2871	1.3965
80 - 100	0.00529	0.00833	0.01532	1.5747	1.8391	2.8960

While the one-year probabilities of survival had increased between two and nine percent, the five-year probabilities increased by between 15 and 50 percent, the highest increases always with the oldest. Exceptions to this rule appear among centenarians, and these may be due either to small numbers or to actually different development. All we really know is that death rates at 100-104 have indeed declined but the precise extent remains uncertain for the time being.

The chances to survive the entire 80-100-year age span continue to be slim - 0.5 percent for men and 1.5 percent for women even in 1980-90 but they have increased in the last 20 years by no less than 180 percent for each sex.

A comparison of the three decades, given in the table, shows that the progress in survival has accelerated over this period in every age group of each sex. The logarithmic scale presentation in Figure 21 illustrates the relatively ever wider differences between successive age groups and the likewise relatively faster changes in them over time as well as the special case of longterm survival at the bottom. By coincidence, the men have reached in each case approximately the same survival level as the women had twenty years earlier. To make a finer point, this catching up with women has been slightly more successful for the very oldest.

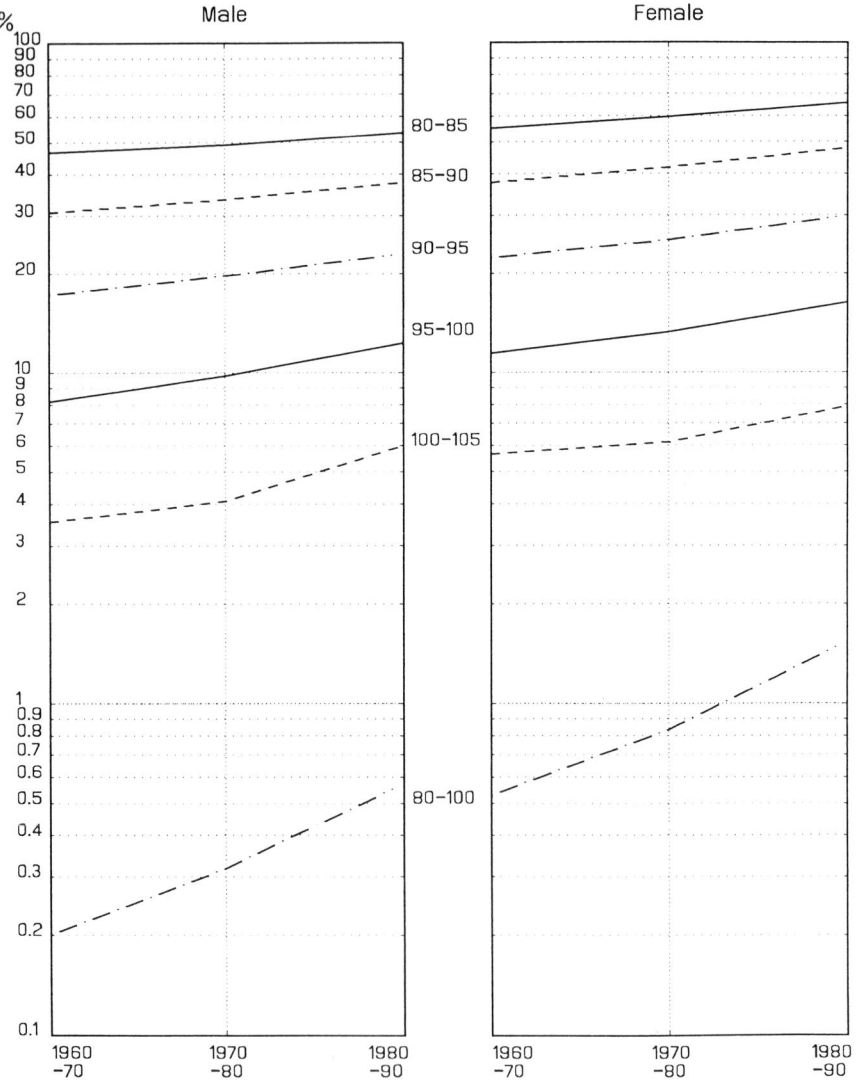

Figure 21. PERCENT SURVIVING THROUGH SPECIFIED AGE INTERVALS.
Thirteen countries with good data.

Table 17. PERSONS REACHING AGE 100 OUT OF 1000 80-YEAR-OLD.

Data quality and country	Males				Females			
	1950 -60	1960 -70	1970 -80	1980 -90	1950 -60	1960 -70	1970 -80	1980 -90
A. Good quality								
Austria	1	1	2	4	2	3	4	7
Belgium	2	2	2	5	3	4	5	13
Czechoslovakia	1	1	2	1	2	3	3	3
Denmark	3	2	5	6	3	5	13	17
England & Wales	1	2	3	5	5	8	11	18
Finland	1	1	2	4	2	2	7	13
France	1	3	4	6	4	8	11	17
Germany, East	1	1	1	1	2	1	3	3
Germany West	1	2	2	4	2	4	5	12
Hungary	1	1	1	2	1	2	3	4
Iceland	...	6	8	13	...	9	26	36
Italy	2	1	3	5	4	3	6	12
Japan	1	2	3	8	3	3	7	18
Luxembourg	0	1	3	2	2	2	5	11
Netherlands	...	4	5	8	...	7	12	20
Norway	4	4	5	7	6	7	11	17
Scotland	1	1	2	3	3	6	9	16
Sweden	2	3	4	6	3	6	12	17
Switzerland	2	2	4	6	3	5	10	16
B. Acceptable								
Australia	...	...	5	6	...	...	14	21
New Zealand	4	3	4	6	6	8	14	20
Portugal	1	2	2	3	5	5	5	9
C. Conditionally acceptable								
Estonia	2	2	4	4	4	6	9	8
Ireland	2	1	1	1	5	4	5	10
Latvia	5	6	7	6	11	10	10	10
Poland	...	...	5	5	...	...	9	8
Spain	3	3	5	10	7	9	10	15
D. Weak quality								
Canada	5	7	9	12	10	15	24	36
Chile	...	...	...	11	...	...	...	19

An international comparison reveals again substantial differences both in the level and the improvement of the indicator. Table 17 gives the numbers that would survive to age 100 out of 1000 persons of age 80 according to successive decennial life tables. The ratio is given also for countries with not fully reliable data, classified accordingly.

Until 1970, not even one percent of the 80-year-old in any well-documented population would make it to a full hundred. After 1970, the proportions have increased rapidly, and by the 1980s, the one percent level was surpassed by women in almost all countries while some reached two and Iceland 3.6 percent. The men began in the 1950s mostly at one-promille level and have since made large gains while still remaining far behind women. Very small chances to reach age 100 continue to be recorded in those countries of the former East bloc which produce fully reliable data.

For greater certainty, we have also tabulated the 80-to-100 evidence for actual cohorts which have already been fully observed over this age span. Joined into groups of ten cohorts each, the data are given in Annex Table 7 and summarized in Table 18. Being necessarily less up-to-date than the latest period data, they show somewhat lower ratios but the overall picture regarding international and gender differentials and the recent trends is the same.

Table 18. **SURVIVORS FROM AGE 80 TO 100 IN ACTUAL COHORTS, PER 1000.**

Country	Male cohorts		Female cohorts	
	1870 - 1879	1880 - 1889	1870 - 1879	1880 - 1889
Austria	1.63	2.15	3.27	4.55
Belgium	1.83	3.04	3.63	6.91
Czechoslovakia	1.75	1.36	3.10	2.83
Denmark	3.43	5.38	7.07	11.53
England & Wales	2.30	3.49	8.28	12.05
Finland	1.32	2.40	2.82	7.32
France	2.74	4.01	7.15	11.20
Germany, East	1.32	1.31	2.21	2.57
Germany, West	1.67	2.84	3.31	6.17
Hungary	1.00	1.63	2.63	3.31
Iceland	...	8.38	...	27.21
Italy	2.31	3.44	4.44	7.15
Japan	1.80	3.75	4.10	8.15
Netherlands	...	7.05	...	12.88
Norway	4.93	6.03	8.35	12.13
Scotland	1.75	2.45	5.89	11.55
Sweden	3.69	4.40	7.08	12.27
Switzerland	2.34	4.34	4.86	9.58

11. The centenarians

To live one hundred years has no particular significance to the organism as it is simply a fortuitous product of the speed of the earth on its orbit around the sun, and the way man began to use his fingers to count things. Yet, already in remote times, he became intrigued with the possibility of living ten times ten cycles of the sun, undoubtedly because it was perceived as being at or close to the maximum possible. The length of the solar year was for both agricultural and religious purposes painstakingly measured with great accuracy by civilizations which did not learn it from each other. Even today, to live to the age of 100 years carries with it a distinction and is the source of such prestige and pride that where strict records have not been kept, most claims to such age are false.

The recent increase in the number of centenarians has given rise to a debate on whether true centenarians are a new phenomenon or whether some of the historical claims to such age can be credited. VAUPEL and JEUNE (1994) argued that centenarians must have been very rare in most countries before the modern era, and demonstrated that the growth in their number is mostly due to improved chances of surviving from age 80 to 100. This finding is supported by our data in Chapter 17 and since the substantial improvement of these chances is a very recent development, the probability of reaching age 100 must have been very much smaller in the recent past. Basing on the view that the tail end of the survival distribution has been moving to the right, JEUNE (1994a) made the rather provocative assertion that no person lived to age 100 before 1800, nor to 110 before 1950. In sharp contrast to this is the calculation of WILMOTH that the first centenarians appeared when the world population reached 100 million and life expectancy at age 50 was 14 years; according to him, the two conditions were met around 2500 BC (Wilmoth, 1995). Most of the sources he cites, however, would indicate 12 years as a more likely value for $e(50)$ during the early agricultural era of mankind but if, as most historical demographers are inclined to believe, there were prolonged periods of higher and lower mortality, 14 years may have been characteristic of some better period.

How rare then is a centenarian today? The answer is: still quite rare but less and less so. In low-mortality countries, there is today one centenarian per about 20,000 people while thirty years ago, there was only one per 200,000. In the rest of the world, despite claims here and there to the contrary, a true centenarian is much more difficult to find. This author estimated that there were in 1985 about 30,000 centenarians in the world (Kannisto, 1990).

Table 19. PROPORTION OF CENTENARIANS IN TOTAL POPULATION, 1960 AND 1990.

Country	1.1.1960		1.1.1990	
	Number	Per million	Number	Per million
Austria	25	3.5	232	29.8
Belgium	...	...	474	48.1
Denmark	19	4.1	323	62.8
England & Wales	531	11.6	3890	76.3
Estonia	...	...	42	26.7
Finland	11	2.5	141	28.3
France	371	8.1	3853	67.9
Germany, West	119	2.2	2528	40.0
Iceland	3	17.0	17	66.7
Ireland	...	...	87	24.8
Italy	265	5.4	2047	35.5
Japan	155	1.7	3126	25.3
Netherlands	62	5.4	818	54.7
New Zealand	18	7.6	198	59.2
Norway	73	20.4	300	70.7
Portugal	...	...	268	27.2
Singapore	...	...	41	15.2
Sweden	72	9.6	583	68.1
Switzerland	29	5.4	338	50.4
14 countries	1753	5.3	18 394	45.1
19 countries	...	...	19 306	44.3

The number and proportion of centenarians in the countries of the Odense database are given in Table 19. Female centenarians are much more numerous than male (Table 20) outnumbering them at age 100 by 4:1 and at still higher ages even more.

Table 20. SEX RATIO OF CENTENARIANS.
Thirteen countries with good data.

Period and age	Number reaching age		Females per male
	Male	Female	
1980-1989			
100	13 066	55 761	4.1
101	7 048	32 349	4.6
102	3 732	18 150	4.9
103	1 958	10 035	5.1
104	963	5 295	5.5
105	482	2 723	5.6
106	236	1 325	5.6
107	109	645	5.9
108	50	297	5.9
109	18	115	6.4
110+	7	57	8.1
Total	27 669	126 752	4.6
1970-1979	15 136	59 504	3.9
1960-1969	7 061	28 218	4.0
1950-1959	3 184	12 086	3.8

A centenarian life table is presented as Table 21 for an aggregate of fourteen countries by adding to the usual thirteen Belgium for which the requisite data are not available for earlier decades. The life table is relatively accurate for men up to age 107, for women to 109 - ages where the numbers of observations are not less than 100. Beyond these ages, all rates become so unsteady as to give nothing more than rough indications at best. It can be expected that the above-mentioned limits (107 and 109) will be pushed ahead by one or two years in each decade as long as the mortality decline continues at present speed.

Table 21. CENTENARIAN LIFE TABLE, 1980-1990.
Fourteen countries with good data [1].

x	N_x	D_x	q_x	l_x	d_x	L_x	T_x	e_x
Male								
100	13433	5658	0.4213	1.0000	0.4213	0.7894	1.8227	1.82
101	7293	3097	0.4247	0.5787	0.2458	0.4558	1.0333	1.79
102	3856	1657	0.4297	0.3329	0.1430	0.2614	0.5775	1.73
103	2032	942	0.4636	0.1899	0.0880	0.1459	0.3161	1.66
104	1007	445	0.4419	0.1019	0.0450	0.0794	0.1702	1.67
105	495	223	0.4505	0.0569	0.0256	0.0441	0.0908	1.60
106	243	110	0.4527	0.0313	0.0142	0.0242	0.0467	1.49
107	109	53	0.4862	0.0171	0.0083	0.0129	0.0225	1.32
108	53	29	0.5472	0.0088	0.0048	0.0064	0.0096	
109	19	15	0.7895	0.0040	0.0032	0.0024	0.0032	
110	5	2	0.4000	0.0008	0.0003	0.0006	0.0008	
111	2	1	0.5000	0.0005	0.0003	0.0002	0.0002	

x	N_x	D_x	q_x	l_x	d_x	L_x	T_x	e_x
Female								
100	56926	20927	0.3676	1.0000	0.3676	0.8162	2.0571	2.06
101	33003	12646	0.3832	0.6324	0.2423	0.5112	1.2409	1.96
102	18547	7363	0.3970	0.3901	0.1549	0.3127	0.7297	1.87
103	10249	4308	0.4203	0.2352	0.0989	0.1857	0.4170	1.77
104	5382	2332	0.4333	0.1363	0.0590	0.1068	0.2313	1.70
105	2759	1267	0.4592	0.0773	0.0355	0.0595	0.1245	1.61
106	1342	610	0.4545	0.0418	0.0190	0.0323	0.0650	1.56
107	644	307	0.4767	0.0228	0.0109	0.0173	0.0327	1.43
108	297	167	0.5623	0.0119	0.0067	0.0085	0.0154	1.29
109	116	70	0.6034	0.0052	0.0031	0.0036	0.0069	1.33
110	40	21	0.5250	0.0021	0.0011	0.0015	0.0033	
111	14	5	0.3571	0.0010	0.0004	0.0008	0.0018	
112	6	2	0.3333	0.0006	0.0002	0.0005	0.0010	
113	4	1	0.2500	0.0004	0.0001	0.0003	0.0005	
114	3	1	0.3333	0.0003	0.0001	0.0002	0.0002	

[1] Austria, Belgium, Denmark, England and Wales, Finland, France, Germany (West), Iceland, Italy, Japan, Netherlands, Norway, Sweden, Switzerland.

N_x = reached age x in 1980-89
D_x = of these, died before age x+1
q_x = probability of dying at age x
l_x = proportion alive at exact age x
d_x = proportion dying at age x
L_x = years lived in age x
T_x = years lived in age x or later
e_x = life expectancy at exact age x

Table 22 presents a Nordic centenarian life table in which the five countries are separated from the main group of 14 on the grounds that the accuracy of age information is in them more rigorous because the age of every deceased is routinely verified against a permanent population register where the date of birth is based on a birth certificate. The drawback is that in this group, the numbers are much smaller, about one-tenth of the larger group.

Table 22. NORDIC CENTENARIAN LIFE TABLE, 1980-1990.
Denmark, Finland, Iceland, Norway, Sweden.

x	N_x	D_x	q_x	l_x	d_x	L_x	T_x	e_x
Male								
100	1340	542	0.4045	1.0000	0.4045	0.7978	1.8249	1.82
101	752	315	0.4189	0.5955	0.2495	0.4707	1.0271	1.72
102	413	190	0.4600	0.3460	0.1592	0.2664	0.5564	1.61
103	201	98	0.4876	0.1868	0.0911	0.1412	0.2900	1.55
104	97	52	0.5361	0.0957	0.0513	0.0700	0.1488	1.55
105	37	16	0.4324	0.0444	0.0192	0.0349	0.0788	
106	19	7	0.3684	0.0252	0.0093	0.0205	0.0440	
107	11	5	0.4545	0.0159	0.0072	0.0123	0.0235	
108	5	3	0.6000	0.0087	0.0052	0.0061	0.0112	
109	2	1	0.5000	0.0035	0.0018	0.0026	0.0051	
110	1	-	-	0.0017	-	0.0017	0.0025	
111	1	1	1.0000	0.0017	0.0017	0.0008	0.0008	

x	N_x	D_x	q_x	l_x	d_x	L_x	T_x	e_x
Female								
100	4420	1615	0.3654	1.0000	0.3654	0.8173	2.0508	2.05
101	2622	1001	0.3818	0.6346	0.2423	0.5134	1.2335	1.94
102	1523	597	0.3920	0.3923	0.1538	0.3154	0.7201	1.84
103	848	355	0.4186	0.2385	0.0988	0.1891	0.4047	1.70
104	465	207	0.4452	0.1397	0.0622	0.1086	0.2156	1.54
105	243	125	0.5144	0.0775	0.0399	0.0575	0.1070	1.38
106	105	56	0.5333	0.0376	0.0201	0.0275	0.0495	1.32
107	44	25	0.5682	0.0175	0.0099	0.0125	0.0220	1.26
108	18	11	0.6111	0.0076	0.0046	0.0053	0.0095	1.25
109	8	5	0.6250	0.0030	0.0019	0.0020	0.0042	1.40
110	1	-	-	0.0011	-	0.0011	0.0022	
111	1	-	-	0.0011	-	0.0011	0.0011	

For explanation of symbols, see Table 21.

When the q_x values of both life tables are shown together in Figure 22, the female rates agree very well up to age 104 and the difference after that is not very important. The shape of the male curve for the larger group may, however, raise doubts about its accuracy because of its low initial slope which contrasts with the curve for Nordic males and for both female groups. The existence of some weakness in the basic data can therefore not be excluded.

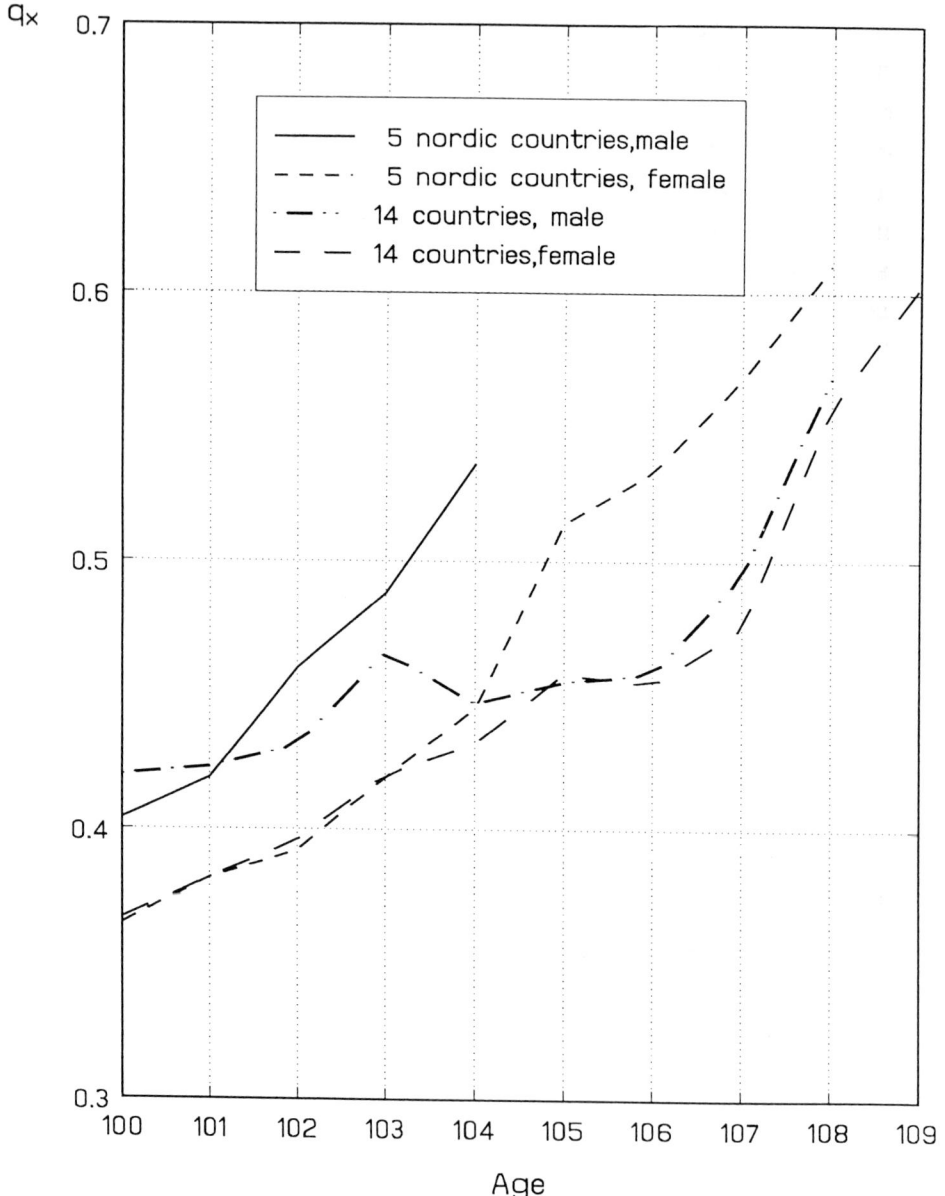

Figure 22. PROBABILITY OF DYING AT AGES 100 AND OVER, 1980-90.

Survival after age 100 is expressed adequately by life expectancy at 100 because significantly different mortality patterns at these ages have so far not been recorded. Even this summary measure is often volatile because of small numbers or due to short term fluctuations. In Table 23, the indicator is given for countries where it is considered meaningful. For the aggregate of thirteen best-documented countries we note in the post-war period a steady increase, slow for men, moderate for women and an acceleration in the last decade. The differences between countries are small and not very consistent from one period to the next. One could perhaps very tentatively single out Japan and Norway as countries with possibly above-average survival of centenarians in case future years confirm the tendency.

Regarding pre-war development, our data indicate since 1930 slow improvement for both sexes in Norway and Sweden as well as among English women. For English men the data show a fall in life expectancy which, however, may be an artefact caused by improving accuracy.

The data which VINCENT (1951) and DEPOID (1973) assembled from France, the Netherlands, Sweden and Switzerland also indicated improvement in life expectancy at age 100:

		Male	Female
Vincent,	pre-1948	1.30	1.42
Depoid,	pre-war	1.26	1.47
	post-war	1.37	1.66

Our own data based on fully extinct cohorts in thirteen countries confirm this trend but, lagging behind period data, do not yet show the recent acceleration:

		Male	Female
Cohorts	1850-59	1.60	1.76
	1860-69	1.64	1.84
	1870-79	1.67	1.92

Table 23. **LIFE EXPECTANCY AT AGE 100.**
Rates based on at least 100 person-years.

Country	1930-40	1940-50	1950-60	1960-70	1970-80	1980-90
Male						
Austria				1.64	1.68	1.76
Belgium					1.52	1.73
Denmark			1.25	1.44	1.65	1.77
England & Wales	1.80	1.85	1.66	1.57	1.68	1.92
Finland						1.67
France			1.38	1.56	1.57	1.68
Germany, West			1.27	1.51	1.52	1.71
Italy					1.62	1.79
Japan			1.94	1.79	1.84	2.02
Netherlands				1.58	1.84	1.99
Norway	1.74	1.79	1.97	1.69	1.89	2.00
Portugal					1.67	1.82
Sweden	1.36	1.40	1.51	1.72	1.68	1.76
Switzerland				1.80	1.73	1.82
Female						
Austria			1.67	1.67	1.71	1.85
Belgium					1.67	2.03
Denmark			1.31	1.77	1.99	1.92
England & Wales	1.71	1.78	1.81	1.93	2.00	2.12
Finland			1.76	1.80	2.01	2.22
France			1.54	1.79	1.93	2.05
Germany, West			1.39	1.60	1.59	2.02
Iceland						2.00
Italy					1.85	1.92
Japan			1.85	1.83	1.93	2.16
Netherlands				1.79	2.05	2.10
Norway	1.52	1.67	1.97	1.78	1.93	2.20
Portugal					2.04	1.95
Sweden	1.46	1.66	1.71	1.84	1.98	2.01
Switzerland			1.58	1.69	1.60	2.00

Figure 23 presents the survival curve after age 100 according to two life tables, 20 years apart. The difference in each pair of curves seems narrow but corresponds at highest ages to a ratio of nearly 1:2. In complete life tables, the two survival curves would reach age 100 at different levels but their form after that point would be equal to the one shown in the graph. In this actual case, the proportion of live-born surviving to age 100 might have grown by a factor of 4 and close to age 110 the growth factor might therefore be 7 or 8. The proportional increase in the number of survivors to extreme ages is therefore quite remarkable but the increase in the highest age reached would probably be modest.

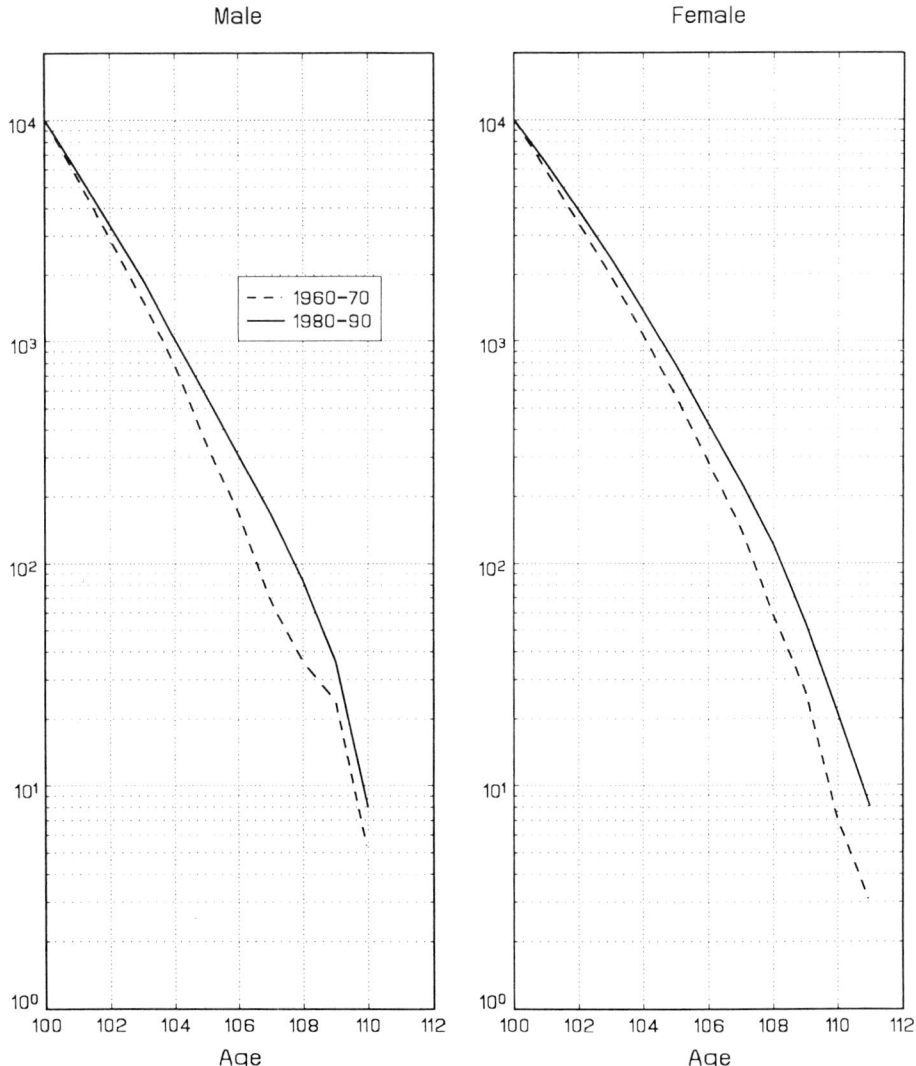

Figure 23. SURVIVAL CURVE OF CENTENARIANS.
Thirteen countries with good data.

If, as is sometimes assumed, mortality reaches a plateau at some advanced age such as 110 years, the survival curve in log. scale would from that point on not bend down any more but fall in straight line. A look at Figure 23 shows that the effect of the plateau on human survival would not be important in practice.

There are by now sufficient observations to trace the probability of a centenarian to survive ten more years and to become what James VAUPEL has termed a super-centenarian. Combining the data for thirteen countries we obtain the probabilities given Table 24.

Though unsteady, particularly on the male side, they bear witness to improvement of the chances. The female survival ratios, based on much larger numbers, show that the relative improvement has been considerably greater in the 105-110 interval. The chances of surviving this interval are now for women one-third of the chances of making it from 100 to 105, and two out of every 1000 female centenarians live to be 110.

Table 24. **THE ROAD FROM 100 TO 110 YEARS.**
Thirteen countries with good data.

Sex and period	Probability of surviving the age interval		
	100 to 105	105 to 110	100 to 110
Male			
1950-60	0.039269	-	-
1960-70	0.034054	0.014170	0.000482
1970-80	0.040671	0.006337	0.000258
1980-90	0.056520	0.014768	0.000835
Female			
1950-60	0.048129	-	-
1960-70	0.056046	0.011611	0.000650
1970-80	0.061910	0.020056	0.001242
1980-90	0.078088	0.027754	0.002167

12. Gender and mortality

Almost all modern data available anywhere on the subject show the human female to have a longer life span than the male, and the exceptions to this rule arise from unusually harsh living conditions for women. This female superiority in survival is very strongly manifest in old age where, therefore, as age advances, women outnumber men in an ever-increasing ratio.

This is also the case in the countries of the database. On the other hand, critical evaluation of the data have shown that where age overstatement occurs, it was always more serious for men. This male preponderance for age overstatement may obscure the true situation in poorly documented populations. Table 25 gives four gender indicators of mortality derived from probabilities of dying in the group of thirteen countries in 1980-90. The data are for single years of age but beginning with age 98, they were averaged over 3-year age periods. As the averages for 104-106 are often out of line with the rest, they should be considered tentative. The corresponding data for earlier decades are given in Annex Table 9.

Table 25. GENDER INDICATORS OF MORTALITY.
Thirteen countries 1980 - 1990.

X	$q_x 10^4$				$p_x 10^4$			Female age delay
	M	F	M/F	M - F	M	F	F/M	
80	976	623	1.567	353	9024	9377	1.039	3.82
81	1069	704	1.520	366	8931	9296	1.041	3.66
82	1170	796	1.470	374	8830	9204	1.042	3.52
83	1273	891	1.429	382	8727	9109	1.044	3.34
84	1384	995	1.391	389	8616	9005	1.045	3.17
85	1503	1107	1.358	396	8497	8893	1.047	3.02
86	1628	1229	1.325	400	8372	8771	1.048	2.86
87	1761	1360	1.295	401	8239	8640	1.049	2.71
88	1903	1500	1.268	402	8097	8500	1.050	2.59
89	2051	1649	1.244	402	7949	8351	1.051	2.48
90	2206	1806	1.221	400	7794	8194	1.051	2.38
91	2369	1970	1.202	399	7631	8030	1.052	2.30
92	2540	2140	1.187	400	7460	7860	1.054	2.27
93	2713	2313	1.173	400	7287	7687	1.055	2.25
94	2887	2492	1.159	395	7113	7508	1.056	2.23
95	3056	2669	1.145	386	6944	7331	1.056	2.15
96	3212	2844	1.129	368	6788	7156	1.054	2.03
97	3392	3025	1.121	367	6608	6975	1.056	1.86
98	3618	3226	1.121	392	6382	6774	1.061	2.05
99	3817	3419	1.116	398	6183	6581	1.064	2.04
100	4002	3607	1.110	395	5998	6393	1.066	2.06
101	4238	3809	1.113	429	5762	6191	1.074	2.48
102	4368	3991	1.095	378	5632	6009	1.067	2.40
103	4425	4173	1.060	252	5575	5827	1.045	1.77
104	4495	4307	1.044	188	5505	5693	1.034	
105	4625	4460	1.037	165	5375	5540	1.031	
106	4811	4740	1.015	71	5189	5260	1.014	
98-100	3812	3417	1.116	395	6188	6583	1.064	
101-103	4344	3991	1.089	353	5656	6009	1.062	
104-106	4644	4502	1.032	141	5356	5498	1.026	

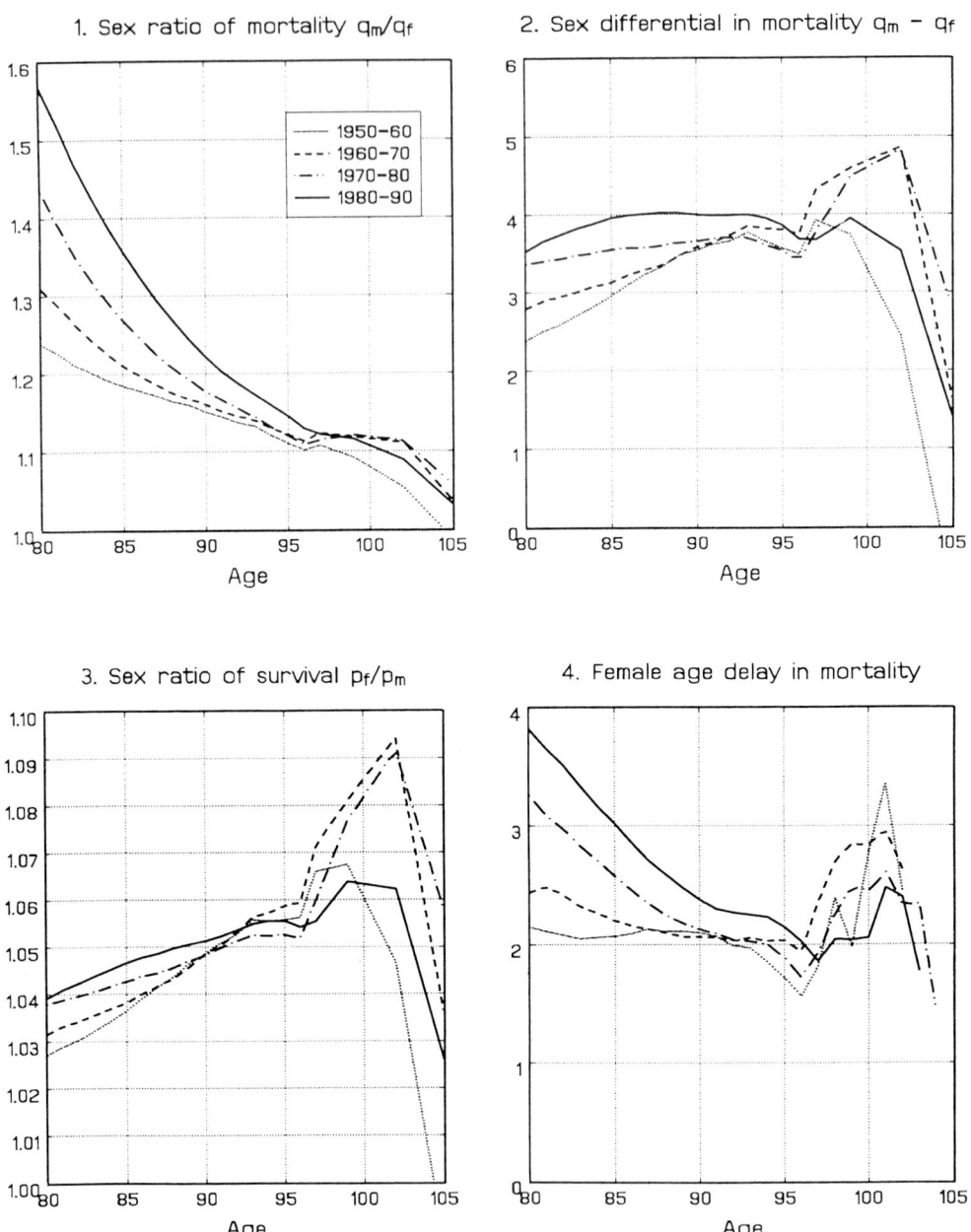

Figure 24. GENDER INDICATORS OF MORTALITY.
   Thirteen countries with good data.

The four indicators give the following account of the situation:

1. Sex ratio of mortality, also called *excess male mortality*, is obtained by dividing a male mortality indicator (q or m or other) by the corresponding female indicator. It is the most commonly used measure of relative mortality of the sexes. Frame 1 in Figure 24 shows how the ratio tends to decline with age and how in the postwar era, this fall has become more abrupt as the male excess has more than doubled at age 80. The form of the curves suggests convergence of the male and female mortality at high ages. Such a conclusion, however, does not stand the test of the following indicators.

2. Sex differential in mortality is the absolute difference of the male and female mortality parameters. Frame 2 shows that this indicator is fairly constant over the age range and that its increase over time has been quite small. What deserves emphasis is that there is no sign of convergence of male and female mortality as was suggested by the sex ratio, except perhaps among the older centenarians.

3. Sex ratio of survival equals the female parameter divided by the male and is therefore a figure normally larger than one. This ratio increases slowly with age, its level slightly higher in each successive decade. More stable by age and over time than the sex ratio of mortality, this may be a better indicator of the gender factor at high ages.

4. Female age delay in mortality tells at how much older age the female parameter equals the male parameter of a specified age. This indicator is therefore akin to the age shift discussed in Chapter 8. In 1950-60, the age delay was very steady at 2 years at all ages until it became volatile with decreasing numbers of observations at high ages. Since then, it has increased at age 80 to exactly 4 years due to the rapidly declining mortality of women at these ages. From this high level, the indicator now declines and reaches around age 90 the former 2-year level. It is a property of this indicator that it does not measure the mortality of the two sexes against a neutral mathematical standard but against each other. If a population has its own characteristic age pattern of mortality, then this indicator can be considered the most suitable one to measure the gender factor.

The observations above leave open the question of whether the female advantage in survival lasts to the highest ages. Three of the four indicators seem to register a sudden drop towards unity by age 105, a drop so abrupt as to raise doubt about its reliability. At these ages, where the number of observations is not large, greater stability is found in survival rates of longer term. Table 24 in Chapter 11 gives for 1980-90 in the age span 100-105 a sex ratio of survival 1.38, and for 105-110, a ratio of 1.88. Another strand of hard evidence is the number of supercentenarians in the thirteen countries: before 1980, there were 2 men and 15 women, after that date, 4 men and 35 women. These facts suggest that the female advantage lasts till the highest ages.

The four gender indicators presented above describe the situation and its development from different angles, and each of them has a justification. The nearly exclusive use of the first indicator by demographers is understandable regarding young and middle age where death rates are low, deaths largely preventable and their causes relatively well definable. This situation begins to change subtly with the onset of old age. First, there is a question of simple mathematics. At death rates of 1 or less per 1000, the sex ratio of deaths may amount to several integers but when the death rate reaches 400 per 1000, this is no longer possible. To observe that the sex ratio of mortality declines with age, is stating the obvious.

As age advances, a person's fate depends less and less on the action of forces of death outside him and increasingly on the waning force of life in himself. BOURGEOIS-PICHAT (1953) saw here endogenous causes of death gradually prevailing over the exogenous. At the same time, death rate rises to levels where its complement, the survival rate, becomes a useful demographic tool. At high ages, therefore, the forces of life and death may be more appropriately measured by the rate of survival which stands for the force of life. The greater stability of the sex ratio of survival in Figure 24 supports this view. The characteristics of these and other mortality parameters will be further discussed in Chapter 16.

For an international comparison of the gender factor in old age mortality we present in Table 26 two summary indicators which together perhaps give a fair overall appraisal of it, namely the difference in life expectancy of the sexes at 80, and the age difference by which the female death rate trails the male death rate, termed *female age delay*. This latter is given in the table as the mean delay from male mortality at ages 80-94. Altogether, 25 countries are listed because these gender indicators were found plausible for several countries where data quality generally is somewhat uncertain.

The difference in life expectancy varies from one to just short of two years. At the top are countries of medium or low mortality but not those of lowest (Iceland and Japan). Clearly, when males are far behind, the average for the two sexes is affected. The smallest gender differences in life expectancy are found in the former East bloc and also in Southern Europe.

Table 26. **FEMALE ADVANTAGE IN LIFE EXPECTANCY AT 80 AND FEMALE AGE DELAY.**

Country	e (80) F-M	Female age delay			
		Mean 80-94	80-84	85-89	90-94
England & Wales	1.89	3.74	4.5	3.7	3.1
Netherlands	1.82	3.08	4.1	3.0	2.1
Scotland	1.79	4.20	4.5	3.7	4.4
France	1.73	3.02	3.6	2.9	2.5
New Zealand	1.70	3.46	3.9	3.3	3.0
Sweden	1.69	2.99	3.5	2.9	2.4
Denmark	1.64	2.86	3.8	2.6	2.1
Switzerland	1.63	2.80	3.4	2.7	2.2
Australia	1.61	3.25	3.8	3.5	2.5
Norway	1.58	2.73	3.5	2.6	2.0
Belgium	1.56	2.97	3.6	2.8	2.4
Japan	1.55	2.59	3.2	2.6	1.8
Iceland	1.49	2.95	2.8	2.8	3.2
Germany, West	1.45	2.82	3.4	2.6	2.4
Finland	1.41	2.76	3.4	2.5	2.3
Italy	1.34	2.41	3.1	2.2	1.8
Portugal	1.17	2.68	2.6	2.6	2.6
Austria	1.13	1.96	2.7	1.8	1.3
Estonia	1.13	2.33	3.0	2.6	1.4
Poland	1.08	2.01	2.8	2.0	1.2
Latvia	1.07	2.06	2.9	2.0	1.2
Spain	1.05	2.13	2.5	2.0	1.9
Czechoslovakia	1.04	2.21	2.9	2.0	1.6
Hungary	1.03	2.31	2.8	2.1	1.8
Germany, East	1.01	2.21	2.6	2.1	1.9

The age delay indicator, measuring the gender difference in terms of the mortality pattern peculiar to each country, gives a somewhat different picture. The two indicators are juxtaposed in Figure 25 and reveal remarkably enough that the four Anglo-Saxon countries have the largest sex differences when measured in their own terms. The smallest differentials are found in countries with not very reliable data (Latvia, Poland and Spain) but also generally in Eastern and Southern Europe.

At ages 80-84, the female age delay is usually between 2.5 and 4 years and thereafter tends to decline to around 2 years by 90-94, a tendency which has a moderating effect on the overall female advantage. When this does not happen, as in Scotland, the gender difference in mortality is strengthened.

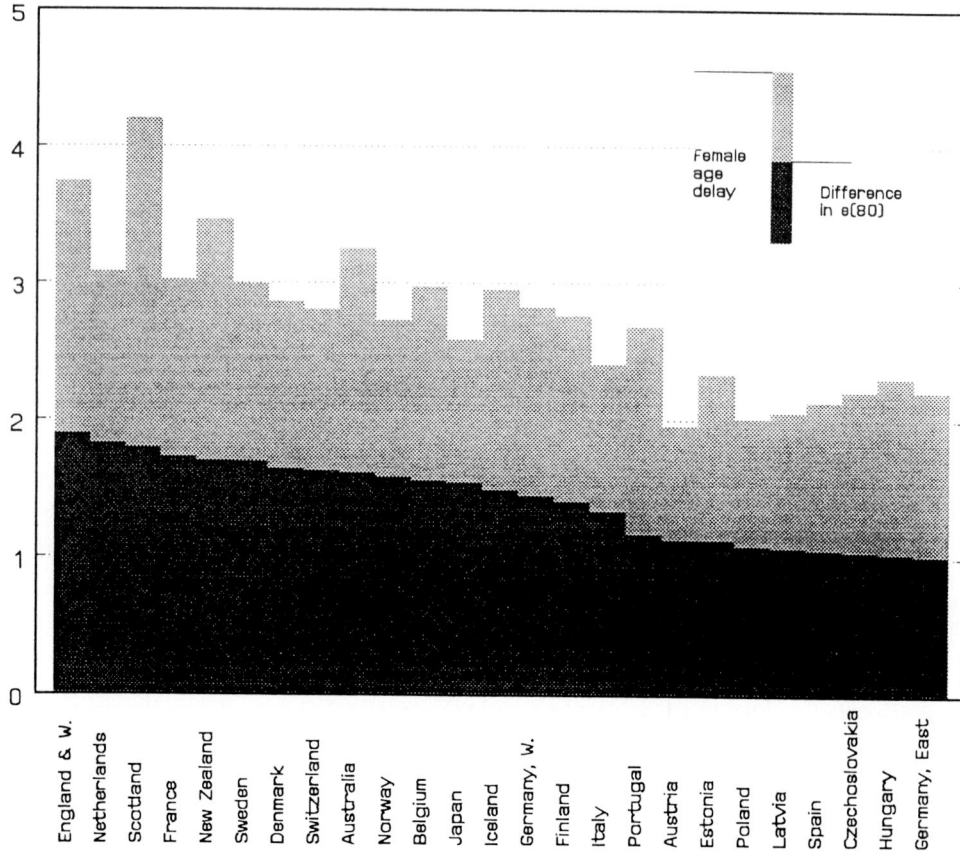

Figure 25. FEMALE ADVANTAGE IN LIFE EXPECTANCY AND FEMALE AGE DELAY IN MORTALITY 1980-90.

The wealth of evidence in this and other studies definitely supports the view that in societies which do not seriously discriminate against either sex, the females tend to live longer than the males. As this must be a genetic factor, result of evolution, it is almost certainly present in all human populations today.

The recent, relatively greater progress by females is, however, subject to period factors and may not continue in the future. Due to a gradual effect of increased smoking by women while smoking by men has decreased, the sex ratio in lung cancer mortality at ages 65 - 74 declined in many countries of Northern and Western Europe between 1979 and 1987 (Waldron 1993).

13. Stationary population

The stationary oldest-old population is shaped by a constant number of persons annually reaching age 80 and then being subject to constant mortality. The following calculations are based on an annual contingent of 10,000 persons of whom 3500 are male and 6500 female - the average proportions observed in the group of thirteen countries in 1950-1990. Two mortality regimes are applied, those of 1960-70 and 1980-90 in the group of thirteen.

The stationary populations resulting from these premises are given in Table 27. The lower mortality schedule of 1980-90 adds of course very little at ages immediately after 80 but swells the ranks from 85 to 95 or so and allows a vanguard to advance in some strength past age 100. In the proportional distribution, which is illustrated by the age pyramid in Figure 26, a significant transformation is noticeable. The pyramid has lost some of its very broad base, compensated by incipient filling of the middle steps in the nineties. Women are now relatively more numerous than before beginning with age 85, the men beginning with 86. Built on an initial sex ratio 35:65, the two sides of the pyramid are not independent and a small relative loss of the male side has occurred in the 20-year period.

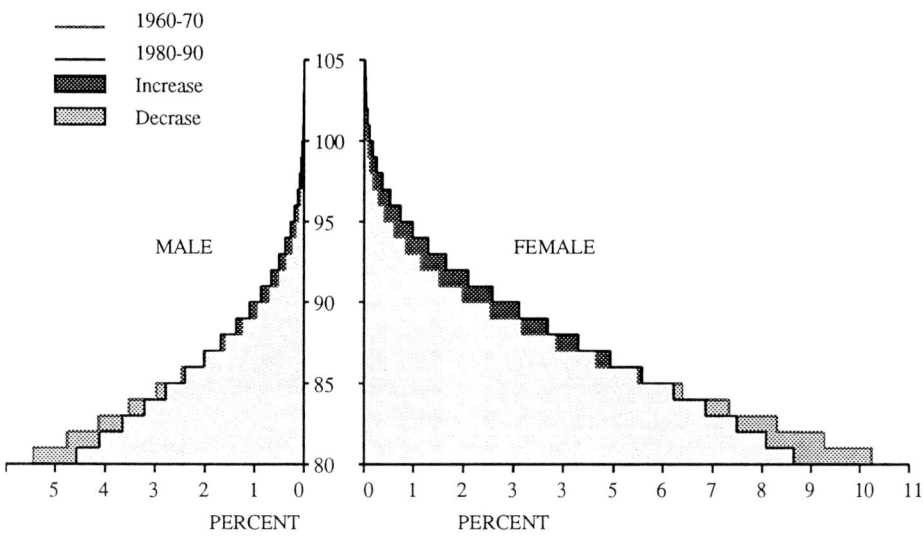

Figure 26. PORPORTIONAL AGE PYRAMID OF THE OLDEST-OLD.
Thirteen countries with good data.

Table 27. **STATIONARY OLDEST-OLD POPULATION.**
Based on 10 000 persons (3500 male and 6500 female) annually reaching age 80 and being subject to life tables of thirteen countries in 1960-70 and 1980-90.

Age	Number				Percent			
	1960-70		1980-90		1960-70		1980-90	
	M	F	M	F	M	F	M	F
80	3321	6207	3329	6298	5.48	10.24	4.57	8.65
81	2880	5619	2989	5881	4.75	9.27	4.11	8.08
82	2501	5029	2657	5444	4.13	8.29	3.65	7.48
83	2136	4445	2335	4991	3.52	7.33	3.21	6.86
84	1798	3875	2027	4526	2.97	6.39	2.78	6.22
85	1490	3331	1737	4055	2.46	5.49	2.39	5.57
86	1192	2816	1468	3587	1.97	4.64	2.02	4.93
87	970	2342	1221	3128	1.60	3.86	1.68	4.30
88	760	1914	999	2686	1.25	3.16	1.37	3.69
89	583	1535	803	2267	0.96	2.53	1.10	3.11
90	439	1206	633	1878	0.72	1.99	0.86	2.58
91	322	928	490	1526	0.53	1.53	0.67	2.10
92	230	698	370	1215	0.38	1.15	0.51	1.67
93	160	513	274	946	0.26	0.85	0.38	1.30
94	108	367	197	720	0.18	0.61	0.27	0.99
95	72	257	139	535	0.12	0.42	0.19	0.73
96	46	174	95	388	0.08	0.29	0.13	0.53
97	29	114	64	275	0.05	0.19	0.09	0.38
98	17	73	42	190	0.03	0.12	0.06	0.26
99	10	45	27	128	0.02	0.07	0.04	0.18
100	6	28	16	83	0.01	0.05	0.02	0.11
101	3	16	9	52	0.00	0.03	0.01	0.07
102	1	9	5	32	0.00	0.01	0.01	0.04
103	1	5	3	19	0.00	0.01	0.00	0.03
104	-	3	2	11	-	0.00	0.00	0.02
105	-	1	1	6	-	0.00	0.00	0.01
106	-	1	-	3	-	0.00	-	0.00
107	-	1	-	2	-	0.00	-	0.00
108	-	-	-	1	-	-	-	0.00
109	-	-	-	1	-	-	-	0.00
80-84	12636	25175	13337	27140	20.84	41.52	18.32	37.28
85-89	4995	11938	6228	15723	8.24	19.69	8.55	21.60
90-94	1259	3712	1964	6285	2.08	6.12	2.70	8.63
95-99	174	663	367	1516	0.29	1.09	0.50	2.08
100-	11	64	36	210	0.02	0.11	0.05	0.29
Total	19075	41552	21932	50874	31.46	68.54	30.12	69.88

The centenarian situation is in these presentations overshadowed by the mass of the younger groups and requires separate accounting which is done in Table 28 and Figure 27.

The stationary centenarian population, based on the observed sex ratio 20:80, has undergone a similar development but, when the number reaching age 100 is held constant, the effect is muted. We note in Table 28 an overall increase in size and a penetration into the supercentenarian age.

Table 28. **STATIONARY CENTENARIAN POPULATION**
Based on 10.000 persons (2000 males and 8000 female) annually reaching age 100 and being subject to life tables of thirteen countries in 1960-70 and 1980-90.

Age	Number				Percent			
	1960-70		1980-90		1960-70		1980-90	
	M	F	M	F	M	F	M	F
100	1549	6386	1600	6557	8.57	35.33	7.86	32.19
101	841	3770	945	4140	4.65	20.86	4.64	20.33
102	441	2162	540	2534	2.44	11.96	2.65	12.44
103	224	1204	303	1506	1.24	6.66	1.49	7.39
104	110	652	168	870	0.61	3.61	0.82	4.27
105	52	338	92	490	0.29	1.87	0.45	2.41
106	26	166	49	267	0.14	0.92	0.24	1.31
107	13	76	24	137	0.07	0.42	0.12	0.67
108	6	32	11	66	0.03	0.18	0.05	0.32
109	2	14	5	31	0.01	0.08	0.02	0.15
110	1	6	2	15	0.00	0.03	0.01	0.07
111	-	2	1	8	-	0.01	0.00	0.04
112	-	1	-	4	-	0.00	-	0.02
113	-	-	-	2	-	-	-	0.01
114	-	-	-	1	-	-	-	0.00
Total	3265	14809	3740	16628	18.06	81.94	18.36	81.64

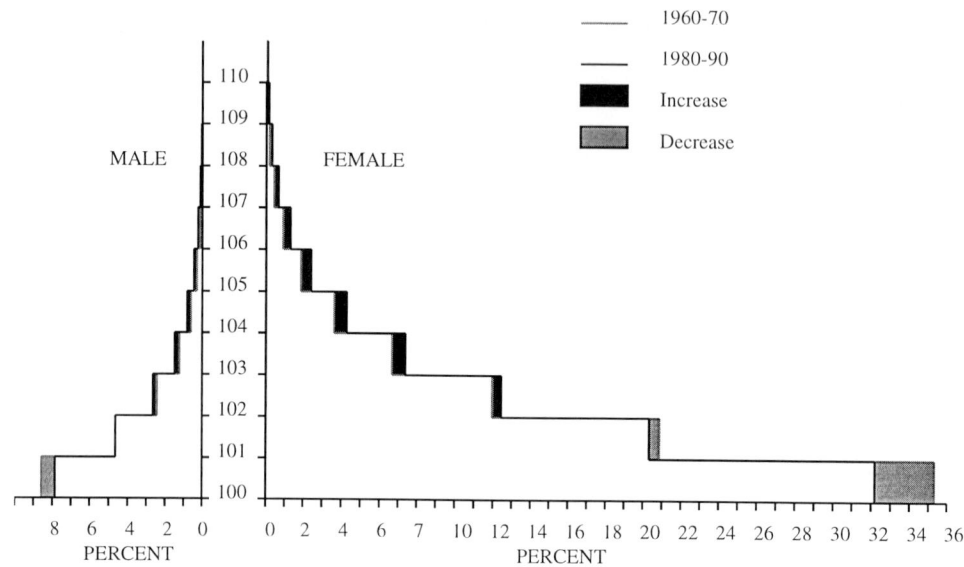

Figure 27. PROPORTIONATE AGE PYRAMID OF CENTENARIANS.
Thirteen countries with good data.

In the 1960s, as many as 44 percent of all centenarians were still in their first year in this category. Twenty years later, the proportion has fallen to 40 and corresponding increases have accrued to ages 102 and above. Also this pyramid has lost some of its extremely broad base and begun to fill up at higher ages.

It follows from declining centenarian mortality and thus comes as no surprise that even the centenarian population has a tendency to age and that, barring a mortality increase, only an ever-increasing influx of new centenarians can "rejuvenate" it.

The stationary oldest-old population of individual countries has been calculated on the sex ratio 35:65 and the mortality regime of 1980-90 in the country concerned. They are given in Annex Table 10. The total size is of course a direct result of life expectancy at 80 but what is of interest here is the age distribution which is obtained, not in its historical context but as function of the mortality of the period. The results are summarized in Table 29 and given in Figure 28.

Table 29. AGE DISTRIBUTION OF STATIONARY POPULATION.

Country, aggregate, period and sex			Age group				
			80-84	85-89	90-94	95-99	100-
13 countries:		both sexes:					
		1960-70	62.34	27.96	8.20	1.38	0.12
		1980-70	55.61	30.15	11.33	2.59	0.32
13 countries:		1980-90					
		Male	60.81	28.39	8.96	1.67	0.17
		Female	53.35	30.91	12.35	2.98	0.41
		1980-90:					
Both sexes:							
Iceland			51.43	30.76	13.41	3.74	0.66
Japan			53.91	30.66	12.13	2.89	0.41
Netherlands			54.26	30.31	12.05	2.95	0.42
Switzerland			54.48	30.73	11.80	2.67	0.32
Norway			54.57	30.41	11.83	2.80	0.40
France			54.60	30.56	11.78	2.71	0.35
Denmark			54.71	30.41	11.82	2.72	0.33
Sweden			54.76	30.47	11.72	2.70	0.34
England & Wales			55.62	29.78	11.43	2.77	0.40
Italy			56.86	29.96	10.69	2.24	0.25
Finland			57.21	29.62	10.60	2.27	0.31
Belgium			57.27	29.58	10.56	2.30	0.29
Scotland			57.57	29.22	10.44	2.39	0.38
Germany, West			57.69	29.53	10.31	2.20	0.27
Ireland			58.85	28.97	9.98	2.01	0.19
Luxembourg			58.87	29.21	9.74	1.94	0.25
Austria			59.45	29.21	9.45	1.72	0.17
Portugal			59.67	28.78	9.44	1.90	0.21
Hungary			63.65	27.36	7.66	1.23	0.10
Czechoslovakia			64.06	27.25	7.52	1.09	0.07
Germany, East			64.18	27.36	7.32	1.06	0.07

In all populations of the database, the majority of the people aged 80 and over are less than 85 years of age. Large differences, however, exist as can easily be noted. The percentage below 85 among all those above 80 varies from 51 in Iceland to 64 in Eastern Europe, and there is a clear tendency for decline. In the group of thirteen countries, the percentage dropped in 20 years from 62 to 55.

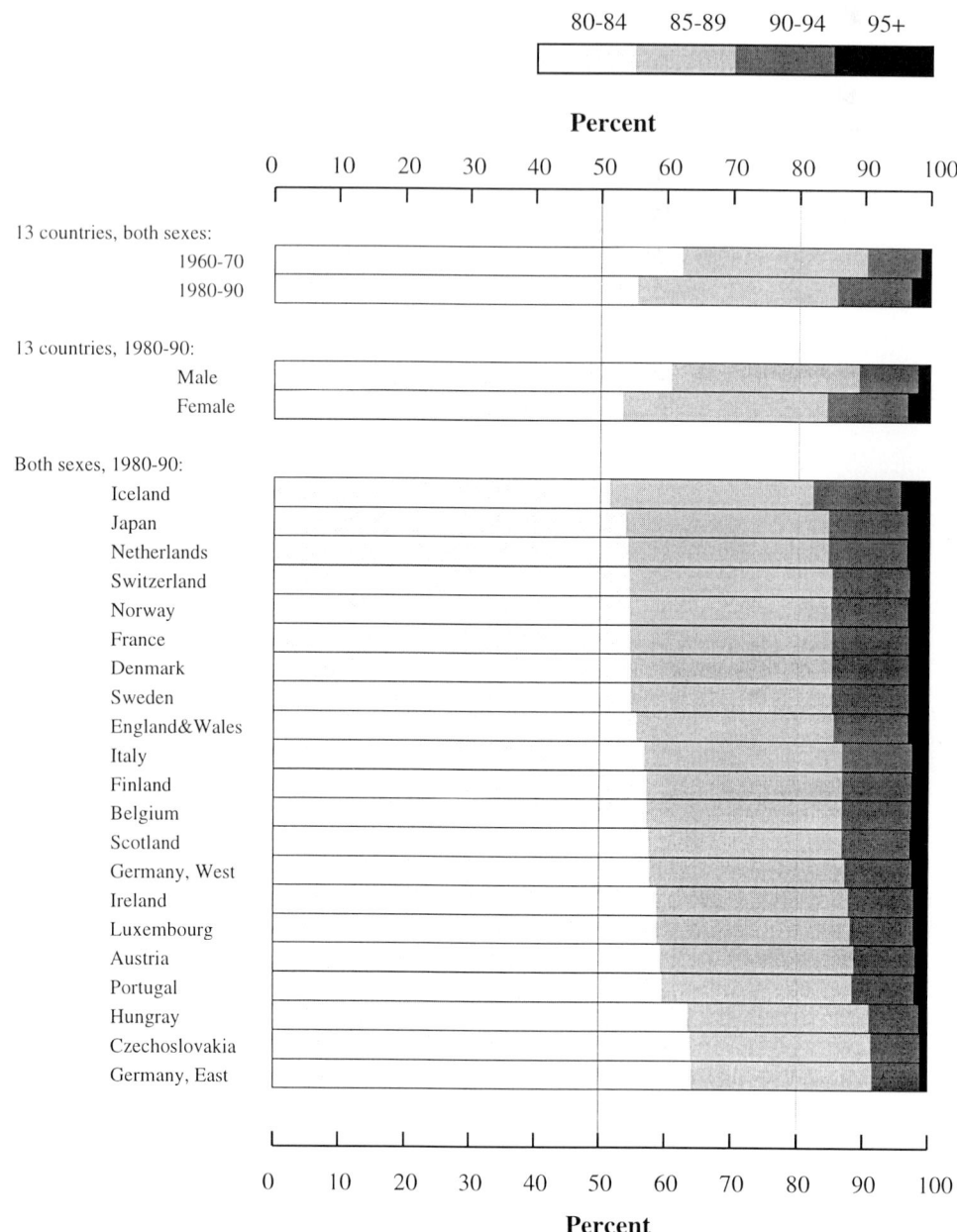

Figure 28. AGE DISTRIBUTION OF STATIONARY POPULATION.

14. The changing survival curve

Being of relatively short duration, survival in old age follows a rapidly falling line which in arithmetic scale slows down as it approaches zero but in logarithmic scale continues to fall ever more precipitously. The former case, a sweeping curve, is easily recognized as the last part of the survival function describing the entire human life. In a study limited to the oldest old, the starting level at age 80 is in all cases equal and this fact conditions all comparisons because we observe only the effects of mortality after this age.

The various survival curves in Figure 29, based on Annex Table 3, may at first sight look rather similar but at closer examination show that by age 90 or soon thereafter, the level of one curve may be twice that of another, and that this relative difference keeps growing even larger at still older ages. In fact, each of the decennial curves of the group of thirteen countries falls more slowly than the preceding one. Such differences are more marked among women, particularly between the last decades. The differences between the three groups of countries are also quite noticeable.

A closer look at the change is awarded when examining the first differences of the survival functions over time in Tables 30 and 31 and in Figure 30. Instead of the function l_x, these tables and figures are based on the life-year function L_x which gives virtually the same result and has the advantage of being additive, thus allowing a better appreciation of the age pattern. The sum of the increase in L_x by age equals the increase in life expectancy at 80.

In the group of thirteen (Table 30), 80-year-old men gained between the first two decades on the average 0.2 years of life-time, between the next two, 0.3 years, and between the last two, 0.5 years, all this adding up to just over one year (see bottom line). Among women, the total gain was 1.8 years and also in this case roughly half of it took place between the last two decades. The acceleration was thus considerable.

In all cases, the greatest benefits befell ages 86 or 87 and, more generally, the 85-89 group. The relative age distribution of the gains tended to move over time to higher ages. This shift, visible in Figure 30, was very pronounced among women: in the course of time, the 90-94-year-old became much greater beneficiaries of additional life-time than the 80-84-year-old. It must, however, be kept in mind that this is the case only regarding mortality decline above age 80. What happened at the same time below 80, probably affected the age groups in a different way. The gap in Figure 30 between age 80 and the peak would undoubtedly be filled if the gains were measured beginning with a younger age.

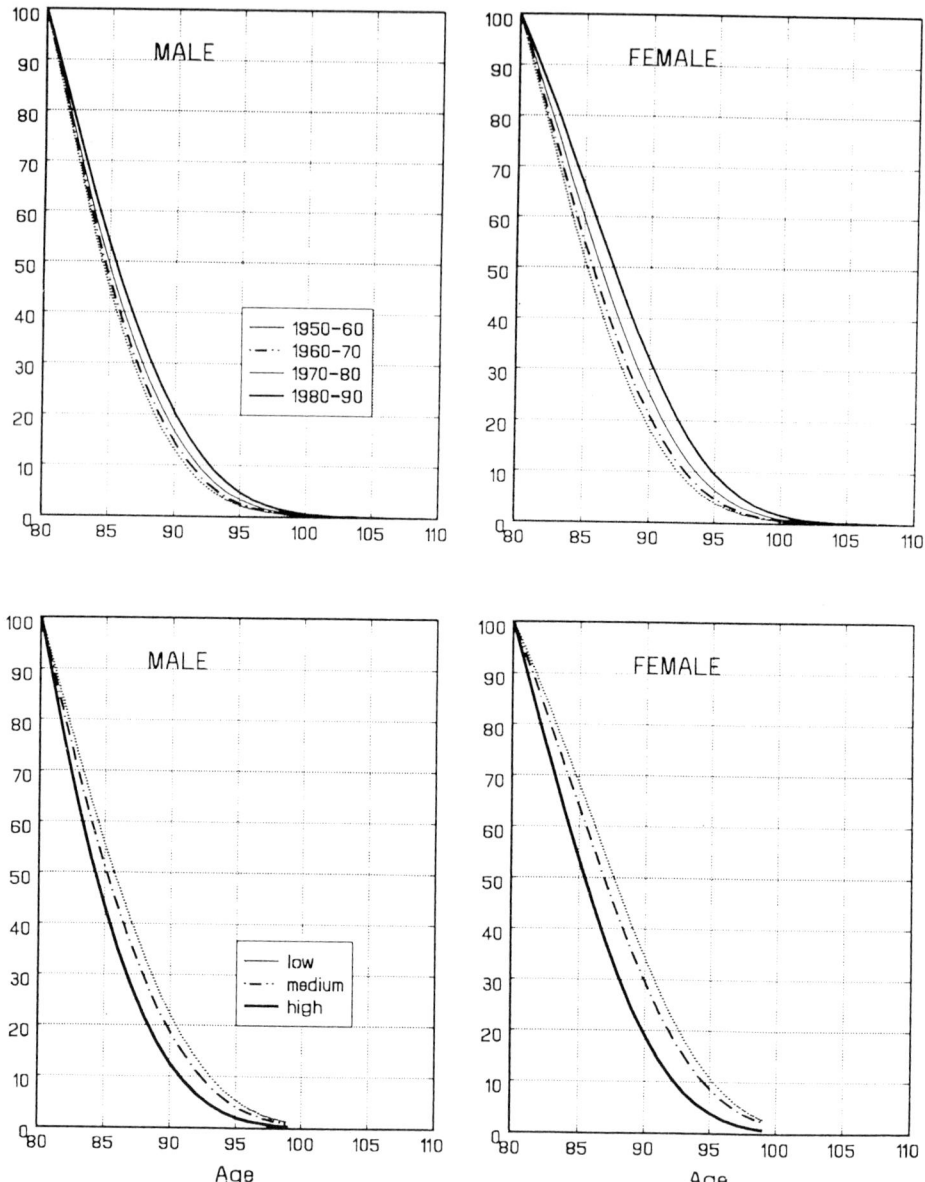

Figure 29. SURVIVORS OUT OF 100 PERSONS AGED 80.
Top: Thirteen countries, successive decades.
Bottom: Low, medium and high mortality countries, 1980-90.

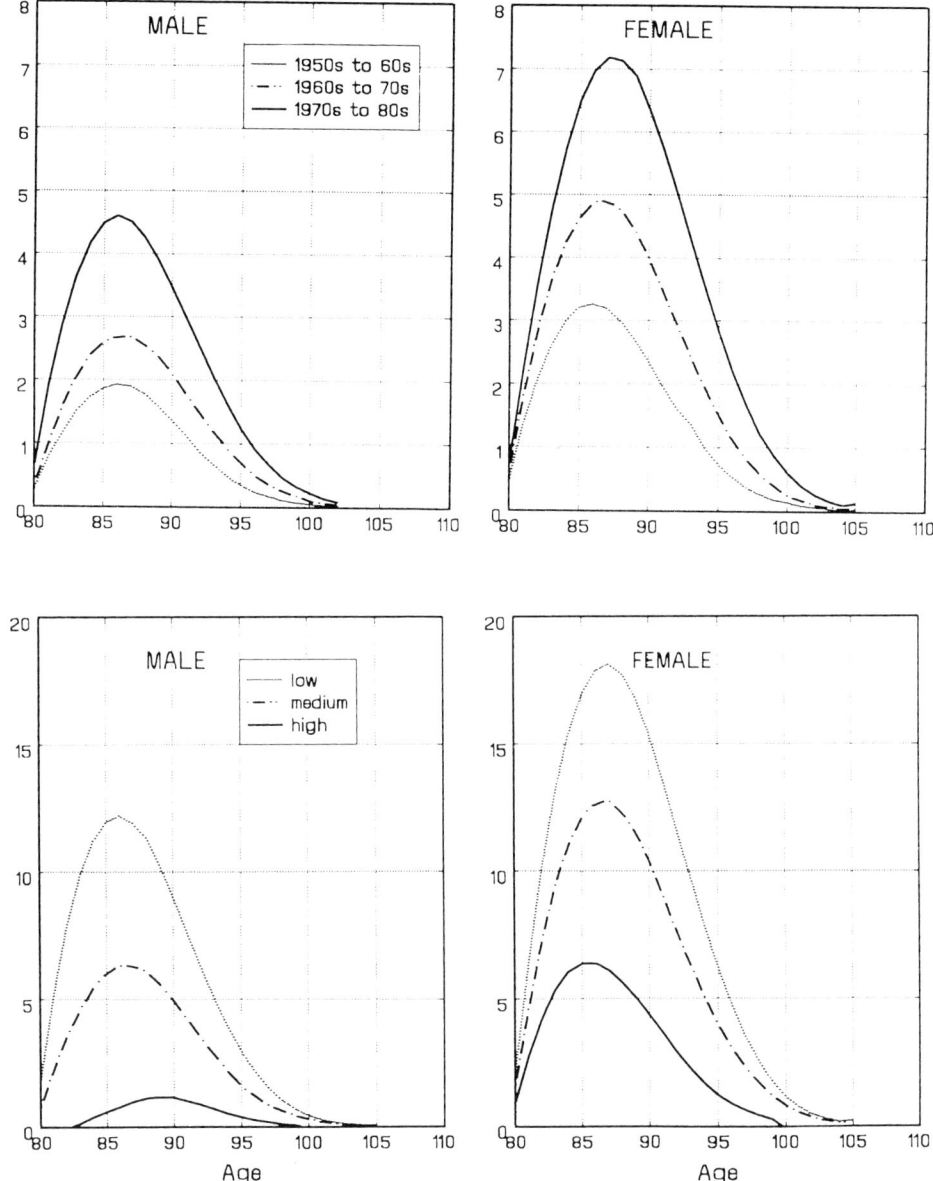

Figure 30. YEARS OF LIFE GAINED PER 100 PERSONS AGED 80.
Top: Thirteen countries, intervals between successive decades.
Bottom: Low, medium and high mortality countries, between 1950-60 and 1980-90.

Table 30. **YEARS GAINED PER 10.000 PERSONS AGED 80 THROUGH MORTALITY DECLINE BETWEEN SUCCESSIVE DECADES.**
Thirteen countries with good data.

Age	Male					Female				
	1950s to 1960s	1960s to 1970s	1970s to 1980s	Total		1950s to 1960s	1960s to 1970s	1970s to 1980s	Total	
				No.	%				No.	%
80	28	34	69	131	1.4	49	63	77	189	2.0
81	77	99	191	367	4.5	136	180	224	540	6.3
82	116	158	288	562	8.0	205	281	358	844	11.2
83	149	205	363	717	12.0	260	364	477	1101	16.7
84	172	238	417	827	16.7	299	425	576	1300	23.0
85	186	259	449	894	22.0	321	465	650	1486	29.9
86	192	268	460	920	28.1	326	488	697	1511	37.7
87	189	267	451	907	35.1	318	491	718	1527	46.5
88	178	256	426	860	43.2	298	475	713	1486	56.2
89	159	237	390	786	52.1	269	442	689	1395	66.7
90	137	210	347	694	62.2	235	399	635	1269	78.3
91	113	178	301	592	73.4	197	348	573	1118	90.9
92	87	148	253	488	85.6	161	294	501	956	104.7
93	67	118	206	391	100.0	128	240	427	795	120.3
94	48	92	162	302	115.3	98	191	352	641	137.3
95	34	69	123	226	132.2	72	148	281	501	155.6
96	23	50	91	164	151.9	53	110	219	382	177.7
97	16	35	66	117	177.3	37	81	166	284	204.3
98	10	25	46	81	207.7	26	58	121	205	235.6
99	6	17	32	55	250.0	17	40	87	144	271.7
100	4	9	22	35	291.7	13	25	60	98	326.7
101	2	6	13	21	350.0	8	16	39	63	370.6
102	1	3	8	12	400.0	5	10	25	40	444.4
103	-	2	5	7	350.0	3	6	15	24	480.0
104	-	1	3	4	400.0	1	4	9	14	466.7
105-	1	-	4	5	...	2	3	12	17	...
80-84	542	734	1328	2614	7.3	949	1313	1712	3974	10.5
85-89	904	1287	2176	4367	32.5	1532	2361	3462	7355	43.7
90-94	452	746	1269	2467	78.4	819	1472	2488	4779	97.7
95-99	89	196	358	643	158.3	205	437	874	1516	185.8
100-	8	21	55	84	350.0	32	64	160	256	382.1
Total	1995	2984	5186	10165	19.4	3537	5647	8696	17880	29.6

In relative terms, the gains increased extremely sharply with age. By early 90s, the number of survivors had doubled and after age 100 it had grown several times over.

Table 31 reveals wide differences between the three groups of countries: for men the total gain was in countries of low mortality 1.3 years, of medium mortality 0.7 years and in high mortality populations barely 0.1 year. This stark international contrast is present, though somewhat more subdued, among women.

Table 31. **YEARS GAINED PER 10.000 PERSONS AGED 80 BY MORTALITY DECLINE BETWEEN 1950-60 AND 1980-90 IN LOW, MEDIUM AND HIGH MORTALITY COUNTRIES.**[1]

Age	Male			Female		
	Low	Medium	High	Low	Medium	High
80	183	80	- 5	218	162	97
81	514	227	- 13	630	459	273
82	781	353	- 8	989	716	419
83	983	462	13	1292	932	532
84	1119	547	38	1529	1099	604
85	1194	604	58	1692	1212	635
86	1219	630	76	1787	1270	638
87	1190	631	97	1814	1278	610
88	1120	606	111	1776	1233	561
89	1023	557	116	1680	1149	501
90	899	495	113	1538	1038	435
91	765	423	99	1364	907	366
92	633	349	85	1175	770	294
93	506	280	68	983	636	227
94	392	215	51	795	509	169
95	295	160	36	624	397	121
96	214	118	24	475	303	87
97	150	85	15	350	227	62
98	102	61	8	250	167	41
99	68	43	5	173	120	26
100	43	28	...	116	81	...
101	25	17	...	75	53	...
102	15	9	...	47	33	...
103	9	5	...	29	20	...
104	5	3	...	17	12	...
105-	5	4	...	21	12	...
80-84	3580	1669	25	4658	3368	1925
85-89	5746	3028	458	8799	6142	2945
90-94	3195	1762	416	5855	3860	1491
95-99	829	467	88	1872	1214	337
100-	102	66	8	305	211	36
Total	13452	6992	985	21439	14795	6734

[1] For identification of the groups of countries, see Table 11.

It was seen in Chapter 5 that for women, mortality reductions were heavily concentrated at "younger" ages close to 80 years while for men they were more evenly distributed. This was the case with relative reductions. Here, in absolute terms, the situation is the opposite as can be ascertained by comparing age groups 80-84 and 90-94 either in Table 30 or in the top two frames of Figure 30 (areas below the bold line). Men have made greater gains at ages 80-84 than 90-94, women at ages 90-94 more than at 80-84. The reason is that the survival situation of female octogenarians is more "mature", survival ratios already much higher leaving less room for further gains.

The slight shift in the peak age of gain which was observed among females of the group of thirteen, is replicated in the international comparison (last frame in Figure 30). When we proceed from high to lower mortality, the gains move to older age where there still is more room for improvement.

The men in the high-mortality group were an exception to this rule for particular reasons. The survival conditions of middle-aged men in these countries actually deteriorated sending ripple effects which produced stagnation among octogenarians, and only still older men drew any benefit at all.

It can be concluded that the main impact of the decline in old age mortality is being felt between ages 85 and 90, and that there is a tendency for it to move slowly higher as the situation matures.

15. *Realized living potential*

With the term realized living potential (R.L.P.) we indicate the length of time actually lived compared with the length of the interval in question. We are using the words "living potential" and not "life potential" because the latter have other connotations while here the question is simply of survival.

Beginning at age 80 this indicator has been calculated for finite intervals and is shown in relation either to the number reaching age 80 or the number entering the interval in question. The realized living potential is given in Annex Table 11 by age group and sex for each country and period, expressed in years lived per each 80-year-old, and in Annex Table 12 per each person reaching the specified age interval. The former set of data is summarized in Table 32 for countries with acceptable data quality in the 1980-90 decade. If the ages 100 and over were included, the total of the years lived in all age intervals would equal life expectancy at age 80. However, the total for 80-100 comes very close to it.

TABLE 32. REALIZED LIVING POTENTIAL (PERCENT) AT AGES 80-100 AND
YEARS LIVED IN EACH 5-YEAR AGE INTERVAL PER EACH
PERSON REACHING AGE 80. LIFE TABLES 1980-90[1].

Sex and country	R.L.P. 80-100 %	Years lived per each 80-year-old			
		80-85	85-90	90-95	95-100
Male:					
Iceland	35.95	4.04	2.17	0.80	0.18
Japan	33.21	3.91	1.94	0.65	0.13
Switzerland	32.47	3.89	1.89	0.60	0.11
Norway	32.24	3.85	1.86	0.62	0.12
Netherlands	32.01	3.82	1.83	0.62	0.13
France	31.95	3.86	1.84	0.58	0.11
Sweden	31.89	3.86	1.84	0.58	0.11
Denmark	31.74	3.81	1.82	0.60	0.11
Italy	30.82	3.79	1.75	0.54	0.10
Finland	29.99	3.73	1.68	0.51	0.09
England & Wales	29.79	3.72	1.64	0.50	0.09
Germany, West	29.58	3.72	1.63	0.48	0.08
Belgium	29.55	3.71	1.63	0.48	0.09
Austria	29.26	3.71	1.61	0.46	0.07
Portugal	28.81	3.70	1.57	0.43	0.07
Ireland	28.36	3.67	1.53	0.41	0.06
Luxembourg	28.22	3.63	1.53	0.43	0.05
Scotland	28.14	3.63	1.51	0.42	0.07
Hungary	25.76	3.50	1.30	0.31	0.04
Germany, East	25.73	3.52	1.30	0.29	0.04
Czechoslovakia	25.44	3.47	1.28	0.30	0.04
Female:					
Iceland	43.16	4.30	2.70	1.26	0.37
Netherlands	40.97	4.24	2.57	1.10	0.29
Japan	40.85	4.25	2.57	1.08	0.27
Switzerland	40.53	4.25	2.56	1.05	0.25
France	40.47	4.24	2.55	1.05	0.26
Sweden	40.20	4.23	2.52	1.04	0.25
Norway	40.02	4.21	2.50	1.03	0.26
Denmark	39.84	4.20	2.49	1.03	0.25
England & Wales	39.08	4.15	2.41	0.99	0.26
Italy	37.48	4.13	2.31	0.87	0.19
Belgium	37.25	4.11	2.28	0.87	0.20
Finland	36.95	4.09	2.25	0.85	0.19
Scotland	36.92	4.06	2.24	0.87	0.21
Germany, West	36.77	4.09	2.24	0.83	0.19
Luxembourg	35.56	4.04	2.15	0.76	0.17
Ireland	35.53	4.01	2.12	0.79	0.18
Austria	34.87	4.03	2.10	0.71	0.13
Portugal	34.58	4.00	2.05	0.72	0.15
Hungary	30.90	3.82	1.75	0.52	0.09
Germany, East	30.78	3.84	1.74	0.50	0.08
Czechoslovakia	30.64	3.82	1.73	0.50	0.08

[1] The following life tables refer to 1980-89: Iceland, Ireland, Italy, Luxembourg and Netherlands.

104

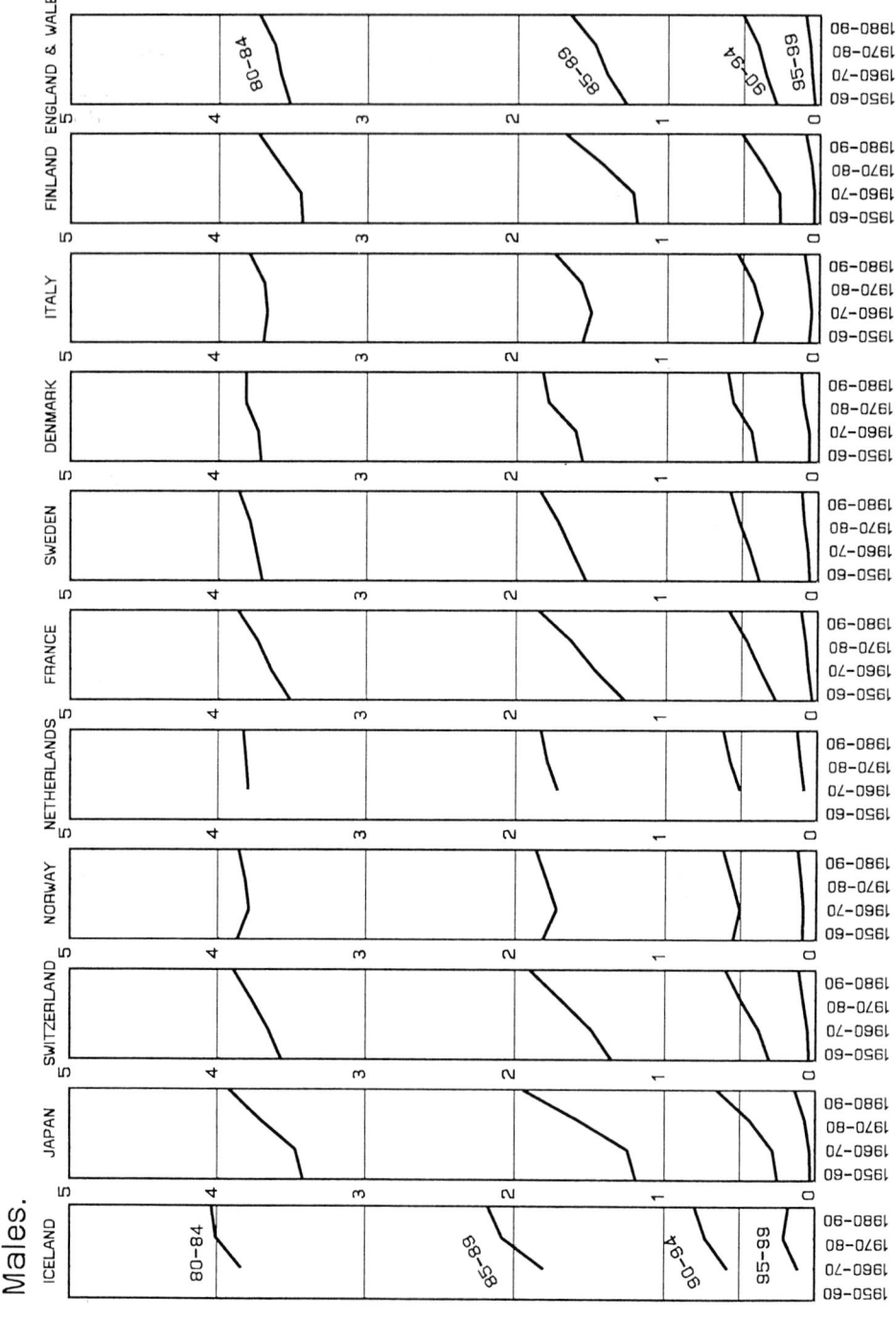

Figure 31. YEARS LIVED AT SPECIFIED AGE INTERVALS PER EACH PERSON REACHING AGE 80.

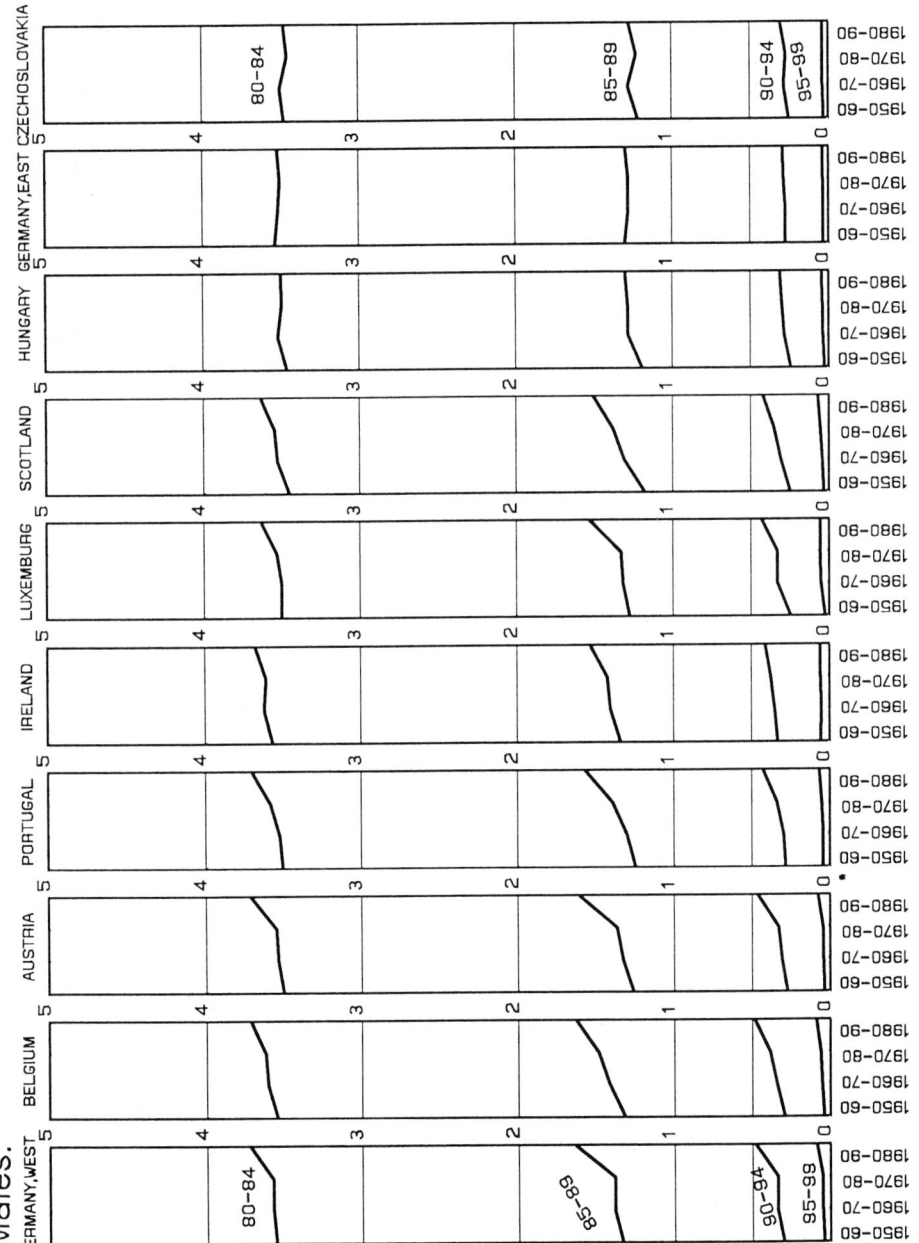

Figure 31 (cont.).

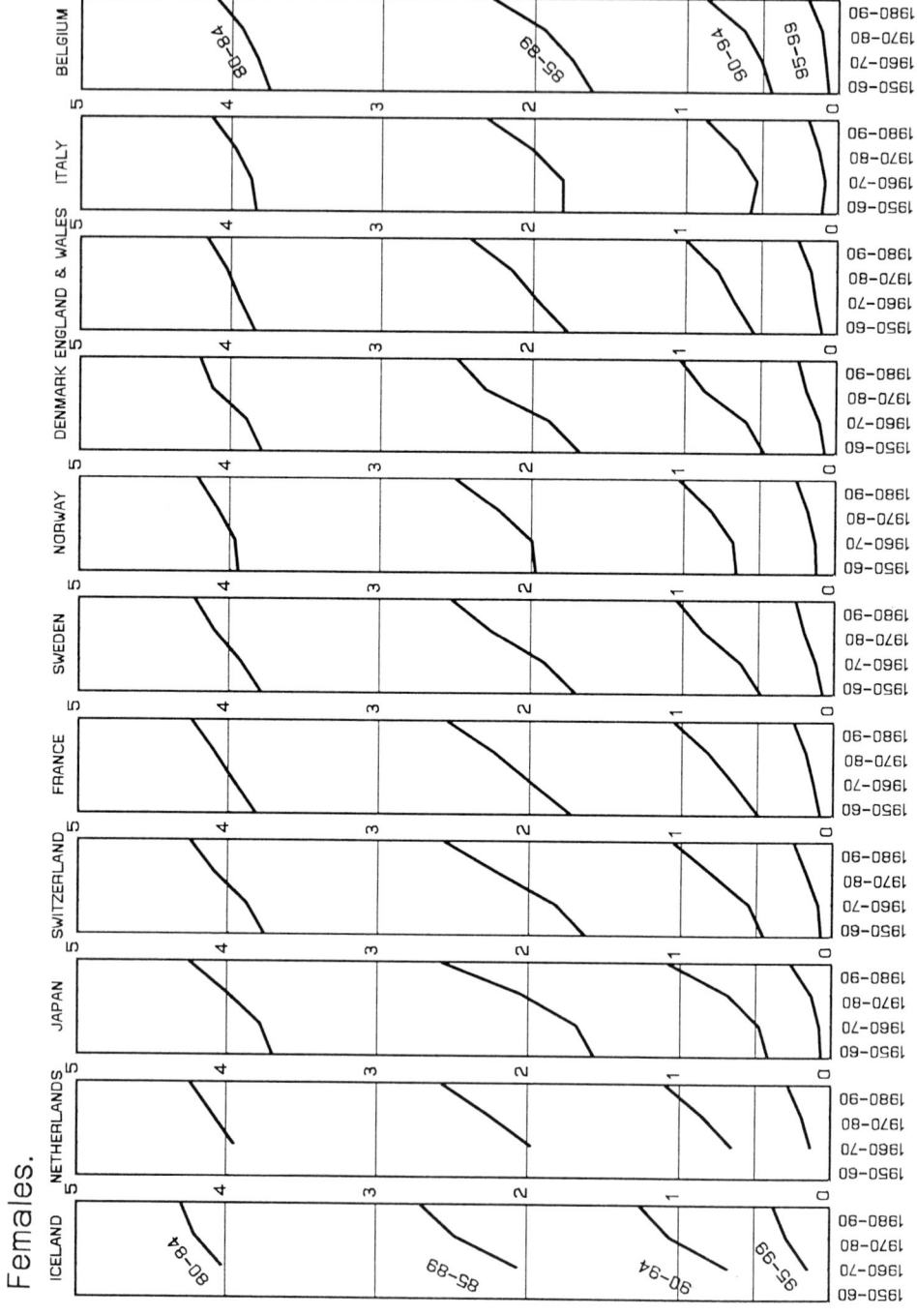

Figure 31. YEARS LIVED AT SPICIFIED AGE INTERVALS PER EACH PERSON REACHING AGE 80.

Females.

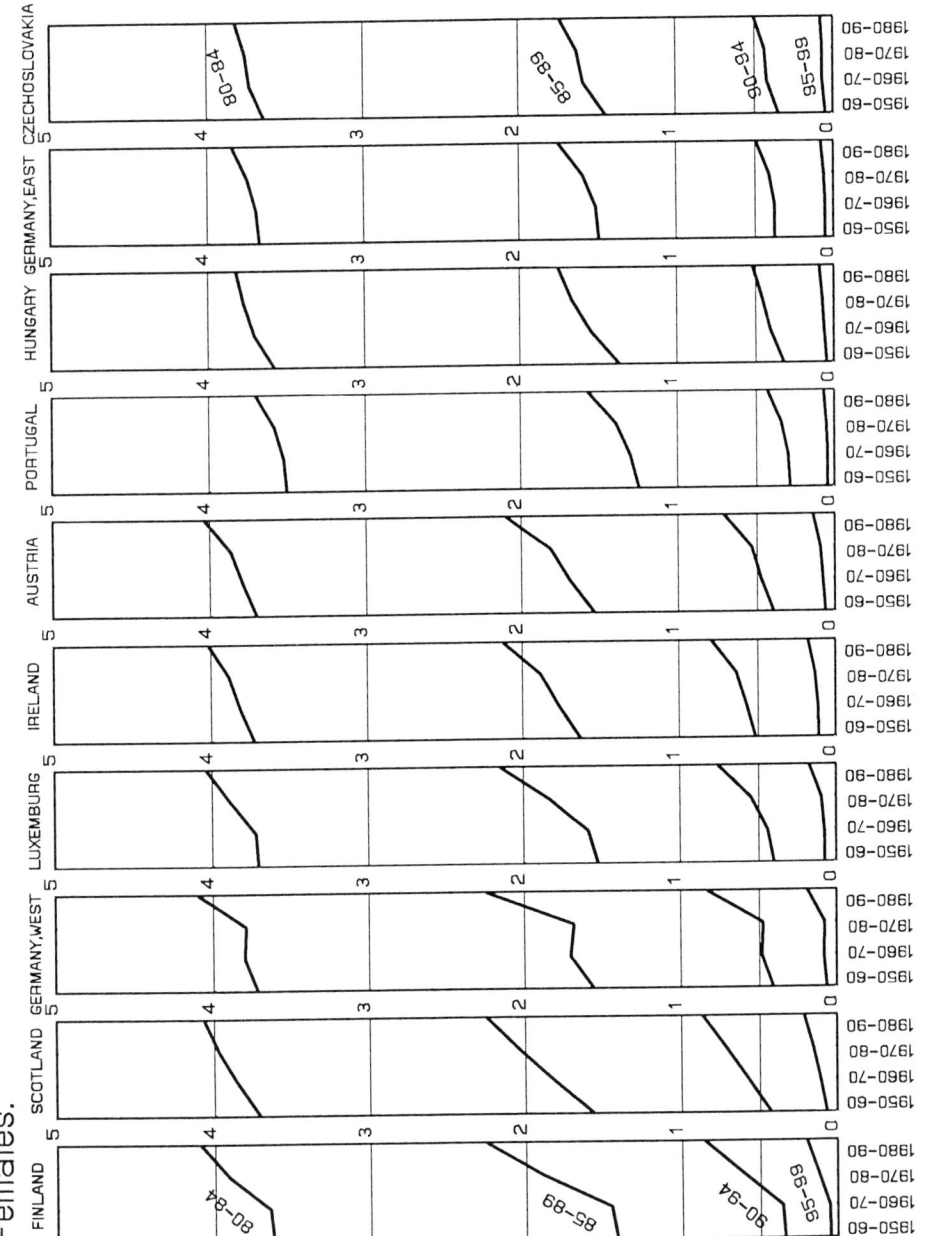

Figure 31 (cont.).

In the first column of Table 32, R.L.P. is expressed in percent of the 80-100 interval. For men, the highest value is about 36 percent for Iceland while most countries cluster in a narrow range around 30 percent, Eastern Europe around 25 percent. Women approach or reach the 40 percent mark in many countries but barely 30 percent in regimes of high mortality.

Both the levels and trends in survival can be compared internationally in Figure 31 where 21 countries are ranked in order of life expectancy at age 80. For males it shows the leading position of Iceland, rapid progress in Japan, Switzerland and France, almost no improvement in Norway and the Netherlands, sluggish in Sweden and Denmark, uncertain early data in Italy, rapid progress in Finland after 1970 and in West Germany and Austria after 1980. Several other countries show solid improvement, in some cases quite fast, but stagnation is evident in the former East bloc.

For women the progress is much more impressive throughout. The rise is particularly rapid at ages 85-90 and in many cases faster above than below this interval. Even at 95-100 the advance is often easily noticeable even in this scale. In Scandinavia and the Netherlands, where progress was slow for men, it has been rapid for women. Steady improvement can be seen even in Eastern Europe.

Men of 80-85 seem to meet resistance at the 4-year level almost as if it was an asymptote. This, of course, is not the explanation. The great international diversity in the male scene points to reasons specific to each country. In contrast, the development regarding women has been both very regular and widely uniform as has been pointed out earlier. One factor which could have caused mortality differences - smoking - was never prevalent in these female cohorts which reached adult age before or right after World War I.

16. Seven ways of looking at mortality change

In the following, an attempt is made to sort out some of the more important indicators of mortality change which have been discussed in earlier chapters and which are particularly relevant to old age. The list includes only parameters which can be calculated for each individual age and therefore excludes all summary measures and does not, of course, pretend to exhaust all points of view.

Seven indicators were selected for the review and are given here with a brief characterization which will be explained below.

Indicator	**Characterization**
1. Relative decrease/increase in age-specific mortality	The public health approach
2. Absolute decrease/increase in age-specific mortality per population at risk	An individual's chances between life and death
3. Relative increase/decrease in age-specific survival	The biological view
4. Lives saved/lost in stationary population	Point 2 related to a population model
5. Life-years gained/lost in stationary population	"Fall-out" of point 4. The end result
6. Relative gain/loss of life-years in stationary population	Expansion of survival
7. Age shift in mortality up/down	Delay/acceleration in the aging process

The seven indicators will be examined by age and sex in the light of a single set of data, the life tables for 1960-70 and 1980-90 in the group of thirteen countries with data of good quality. The calculations are based on the annual probability of dying q_x or its derivatives. Indicators 1 - 6 will be expressed in percent, indicator 7 in years.

Indicator 1, percentage decline in age-specific mortality is given in Table 33 and illustrated in Figure 32, Graph 1, for each sex. We call this the public health approach fully knowing that public health investigation does not necessarily end there. It is, however, as a rule, the first approach and often sufficient to describe epidemiological events and cycles and the response to preventive or curative measures. In this particular case, mortality has declined very substantially for both sexes, more for women than men. The decline has been age-selective in favour of the relatively young - and much more strongly so for women. Close to age 100, the decline has been equal for both sexes.

TABLE 33. MORTALITY CHANGE INDICATORS.
Thirteen countries with good data from 1960-70 to 1980-90.

Age	Decline of q_x percent		Decline of q_x per 100 pop.		Increase of p_x percent	
	Male	Female	Male	Female	Male	Female
80	17.4	31.0	2.05	2.79	2.32	3.07
81	17.2	29.8	2.22	2.98	2.55	3.31
82	16.9	28.8	2.28	3.19	2.77	3.59
83	17.0	27.8	2.59	3.41	3.06	3.89
84	16.7	26.7	2.76	3.60	3.31	4.16
85	16.6	25.6	2.99	3.80	3.64	4.46
86	16.2	24.5	3.15	3.98	3.91	4.75
87	16.1	23.4	3.38	4.07	4.28	5.02
88	15.7	21.9	3.54	4.19	4.57	5.18
89	15.3	20.6	3.70	4.27	4.88	5.39
90	14.9	19.3	3.86	4.30	5.21	5.54
91	14.7	18.2	4.06	4.28	5.62	5.78
92	14.3	17.2	4.24	4.44	6.02	5.98
93	13.8	16.3	4.33	4.50	6.32	6.22
94	13.2	15.4	4.42	4.54	6.63	6.43
95	13.0	14.8	4.56	4.65	7.04	6.78
96	12.9	14.3	4.77	4.78	7.57	7.13
97	13.3	14.3	5.18	5.04	8.47	7.78
98	14.5	13.2	6.01	4.86	10.28	7.70
99	12.8	12.6	5.64	4.92	10.06	8.08
100	11.2	10.6	5.06	4.27	9.21	7.16
101	9.6	9.3	4.47	3.92	8.41	6.76
102	10.8	8.8	5.31	3.85	10.41	6.85
103	11.2	7.9	5.56	3.60	11.08	6.58
104	14.5	8.2	7.60	3.84	16.02	7.23
105	11.8	11.2	6.16	5.62	12.94	11.29
106	2.2	9.1	1.06	4.74	2.09	9.90
107	-1.4	12.0	-0.78	6.94	-1.70	16.41
108	-15.5	6.3	-6.82	3.63	-12.18	8.61
98 - 100	12.8	12.1	5.57	4.68	9.86	7.64
101 - 103	10.5	8.7	5.11	3.79	9.93	6.73
104 - 106	9.5	9.5	4.94	4.74	10.16	9.43
80 - 84	17.0	28.6	2.40	3.19	2.79	3.60
85 - 89	16.0	23.0	3.35	4.07	4.24	4.95
90 - 94	14.1	17.1	4.18	4.43	5.94	5.98
95 - 99	13.3	13.8	5.23	4.85	8.62	7.47
100 - 104	11.5	8.9	5.60	3.90	10.91	6.92

[1] Ages 89 - 99 calculated from 3-year moving averages, ages 100 and over from 5-year moving averages.

TABLE 33. (cont.) MORTALITY CHANGE INDICATORS.
Thirteen countries from 1960-70 to 1980-90.

Age	Lives saved per 100 80-year-old		Years gained per 100 80-year-old		Years gained per-cent of 1960-70 level		Age shift, years	
	Male	Female	Male	Female	Male	Female	Male	Female
80	2.05	2.79	1.02	1.39	1.1	1.5	2.15	3.16
81	1.98	2.75	2.92	4.05	3.6	4.7	2.20	3.12
82	1.87	2.70	4.48	6.40	6.3	8.3	2.22	3.07
83	1.78	2.61	5.70	8.41	9.3	12.3	2.25	3.03
84	1.63	2.47	6.58	10.00	12.8	16.8	2.22	2.98
85	1.49	2.30	7.09	11.15	16.7	21.8	2.27	2.91
86	1.32	2.10	7.29	11.84	21.1	27.4	2.29	2.84
87	1.16	1.87	7.18	12.07	26.0	33.6	2.33	2.79
88	0.98	1.58	6.82	11.84	31.5	40.3	2.30	2.68
89	0.81	1.35	6.25	11.23	37.6	47.7	2.28	2.62
90	0.66	1.11	5.55	10.30	44.4	55.7	2.29	2.54
91	0.53	0.90	4.78	9.16	52.1	64.3	2.34	2.51
92	0.41	0.71	4.00	7.92	61.1	74.0	2.39	2.49
93	0.30	0.55	3.24	6.68	71.1	85.0	2.50	2.52
94	0.22	0.42	2.53	5.47	81.9	97.2	2.76	2.56
95	0.16	0.31	1.92	4.32	94.1	109.9	2.83	2.65
96	0.11	0.23	1.42	3.31	109.2	124.0	2.54	2.56
97	0.07	0.17	1.01	2.48	123.2	140.9	2.33	2.56
98	0.06	0.11	0.71	1.78	144.9	156.1	2.64	2.40
99	0.03	0.07	0.48	1.25	171.4	176.1	3.40	2.55
100	0.02	0.04	0.30	0.85	187.5	197.7		
101	0.01	0.02	0.20	0.55	250.0	211.5		
102	0.01	0.01	0.12	0.35	300.0	233.3		
103	-	0.01	0.06	0.22	300.0	275.0		
104	-	-	0.02	0.14	100.0	350.0		
105	-	-	0.02	0.08				
106	-	-	0.02	0.06				
107	-	-	-	0.03				
108	-	-	-	0.02				
98-100	0.04	0.07	0.50	1.29	167.5	176.6		
101-103	0.01	0.01	0.13	0.37	283.3	239.9		
104-106	-	-	0.02	0.09				
80- 84	9.31	13.32	20.70	30.25	5.7	7.8		
85- 89	5.76	9.20	34.63	58.13	24.2	31.7		
90- 94	2.12	3.69	20.10	39.53	56.0	69.4		
95- 99	0.43	0.89	5.54	13.14	112.4	128.7		
100-	0.04	0.08	0.74	2.30	231.2	234.7		
Total	17.66	27.18	81.71	143.35	15.0	22.4		

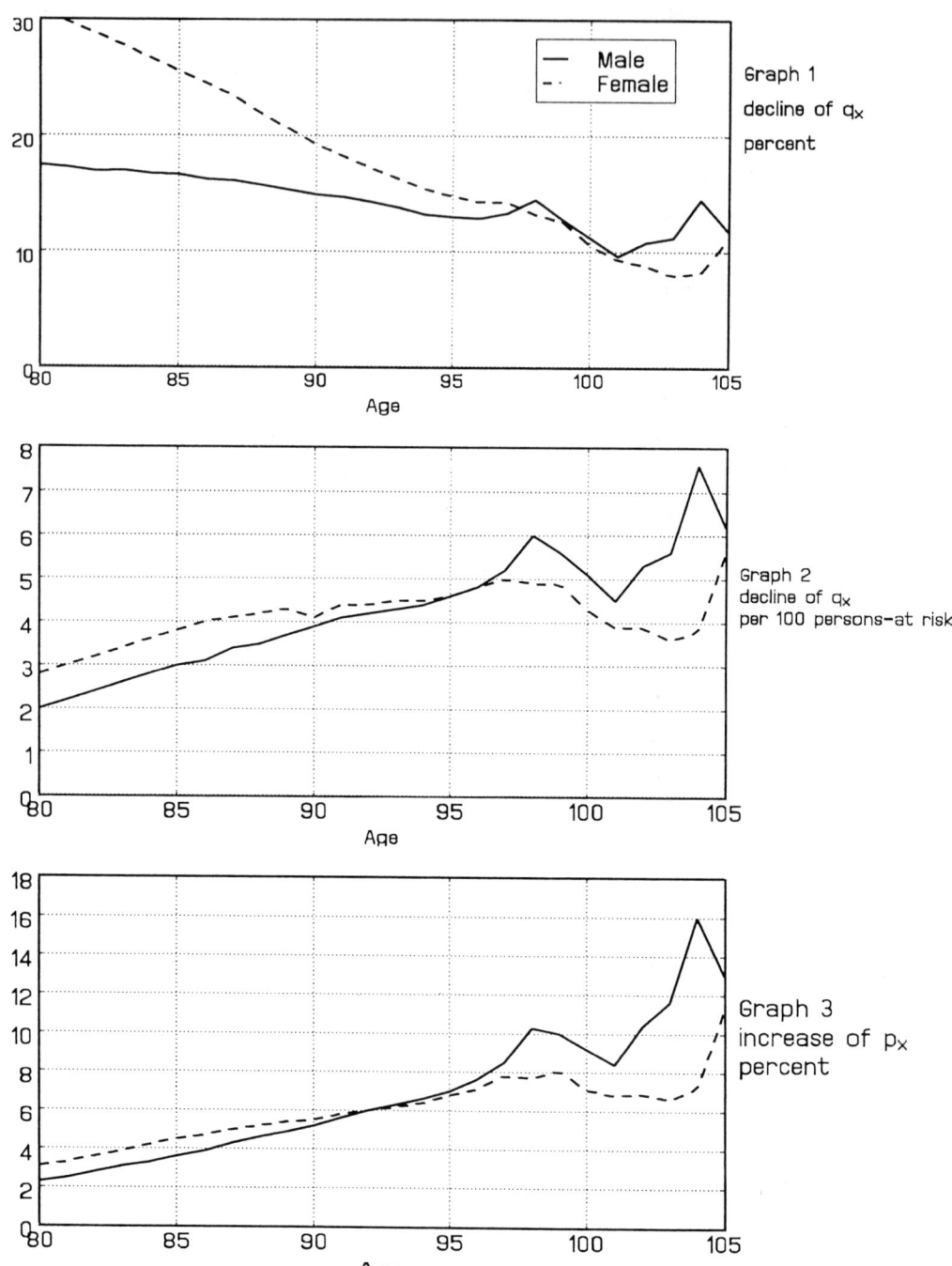

**Figure 32. MORTALITY CHANGE INDICATORS.
CHANGE IN MORTALITY FROM 1960-70 TO 1980-90.
Thirteen countries.**

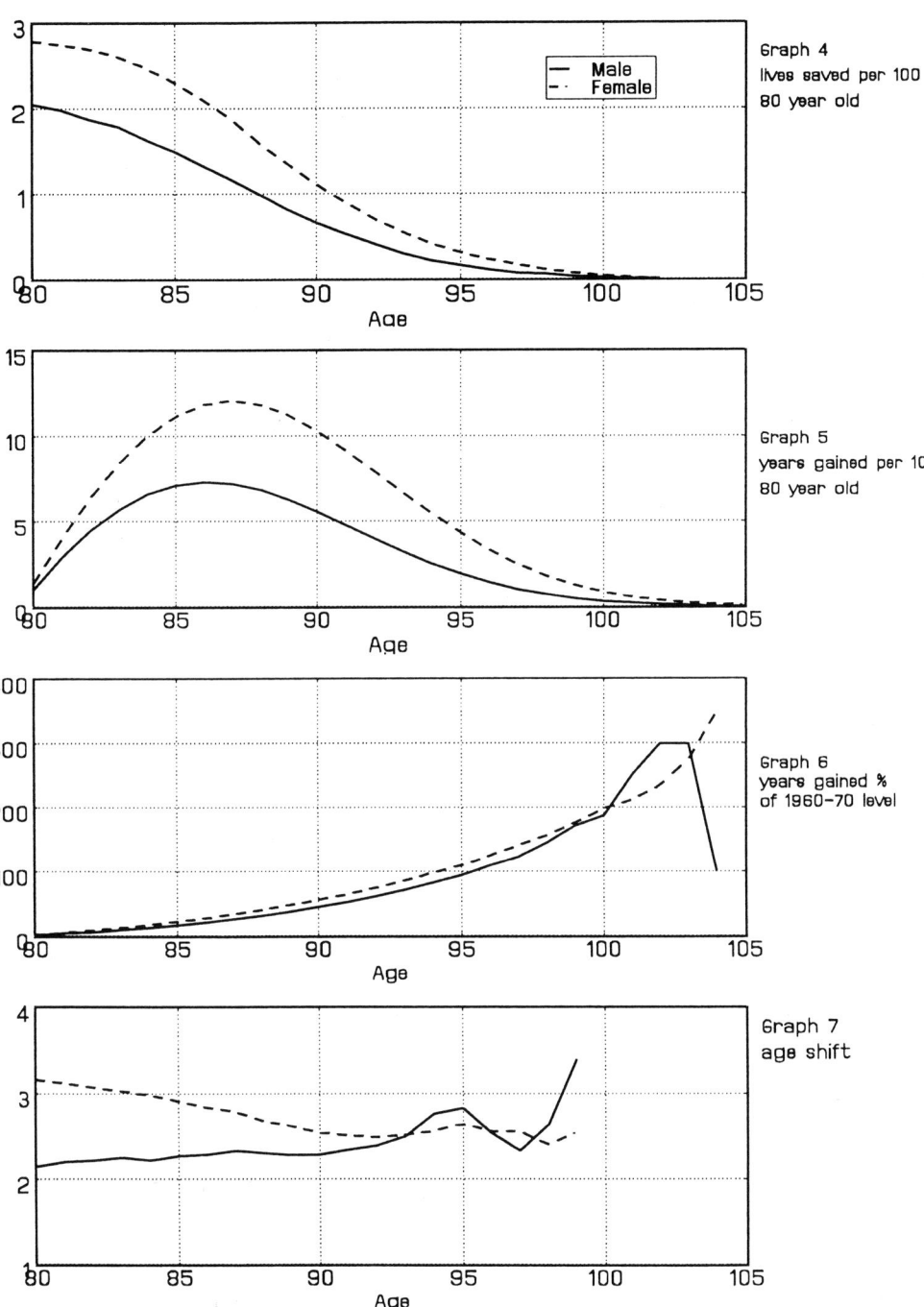

Figure 32 (cont.).

Graph 2 shows the same data per population-at-risk and thereby also for a single individual. The striking difference from Graph 1 is that in these terms the change has been greater for older persons. This means that an individual's chances to survive have improved more around age 100 than at 80. The female advantage in the recent development is confirmed here for ages below 95 but with a narrower margin. This demonstration may be taken to show that when probabilities are high, Indicator 2 suitably complements the evidence of Indicator 1.

At high ages, death is less and less often the result of an external agent and increasingly that of the failure of a vital organ, its endurance exhausted. It may therefore be more appropriate to speak of the ebbing force of life than the growing force of mortality. It is perhaps not pure semantics to say that it is the likelihood of further survival which then becomes the centrepiece of observation and speculation.

We call this the biological point of view and it is demonstrated in Graph 3 by the survival probability p_x. Around age 80 where p is high, there is little difference between indicators 2 and 3 but when p grows smaller, a change in it becomes relatively larger. When the chances of survival are 50:50, indicators 1 and 3 are equal. In the history depicted here, indicator 3 has a steeply ascending slope meaning that the chances of survival have improved most for the centenarians. The females have further improved their relative position in the age range 80-90 but at still higher ages the likelihood of survival has increased equally for both sexes and finally more for men.

When mortality declines, lives are saved, and Graph 4 is an attempt to quantify them by applying the change in q_x to a population standard. This raises the question to which population it should be applied when the changing q_x constantly modifies l_x and when d_x is the product of the two. Actually, a life saved is not an unambiguous concept. However, the choice of the standard does not radically affect the result and hardly at all its age pattern which is of primary interest here. We have used as the standard the stationary population which corresponds to the mean of the two lifetables. According to this estimate, or any other made along the same lines, lives were saved mostly in the lower eighties but a measurable number much later, even around age 100.

In old age, a more meaningful indicator than the number of lives saved is the length of time added to life. This is obtained directly as the difference in parameter L_x in the mortality regimes which are compared. In our example, they are given in Table 33 as "Years gained per 100 80-year-old" and illustrated in Graph 5 of Figure 32. This equals the increase in life expectancy at age 80 and gives its distribution to different ages. While Graph 4 shows where the lives are saved, Graph 5 shows where they are lived. The total gain in life-years was for each sex slightly more than four per each life saved.

The age distribution of indicators 4 and 5 is radically different from the relative gain in life-years by age in Graph 6. While the gains are mostly made at ages 80 to 85 and spent at ages 85 to 90 or 95, their relative impact is greatest well above these ages. In our example, the gain in years lived was about 50 percent at age 90, 100 percent at 95, 200 percent at 100 and about 250 percent at age 105.

Our last indicator is the age shift of mortality, developed in Chapter 8. It measures a different dimension of mortality change, one closer to the aging process. It has the property of being adapted to the particular age pattern of mortality of the population in question. Presented in Graph 7, it is the composite of thirteen different patterns which, as was shown, do diverge a great deal. As an average, mortality has shifted among the oldest-old about 2.5 - 3 years for women and 2 - 2.5 years for men.

For a final comparison the indicators are brought together in Figure 33. Only the female indicators are shown because the pattern is closely similar for men but the development has been more regular and more uniform for women and, we believe, more indicative of the broad background factors which have caused the recent extraordinary mortality decline in old age. It is believed that, as discussed above, each of the seven indicators has a story to tell. It is felt that, in particular, indicator 1 (relative decline of mortality) is in old age usefully supplemented by indicator 2 (absolute decline) and by a measure of the desired end result, indicator 5 (years of life gained). When studying the fundamentals of longevity, life expectancy can be complemented by indicators 3 (age-specific survival) and 7 (age shift).

We should be aware that the study of life and death needs to be complemented by study of healthy, or disease-free, life. A prime promoter of this emerging branch of science is the project REVES, acronym of the French initials of Network on Health Expectancy (see Robine et al. 1993). This becomes more and more compelling as survival is extended to ever higher ages. As also this branch of study uses life table techniques, the seven indicators may find applications in it.

females.

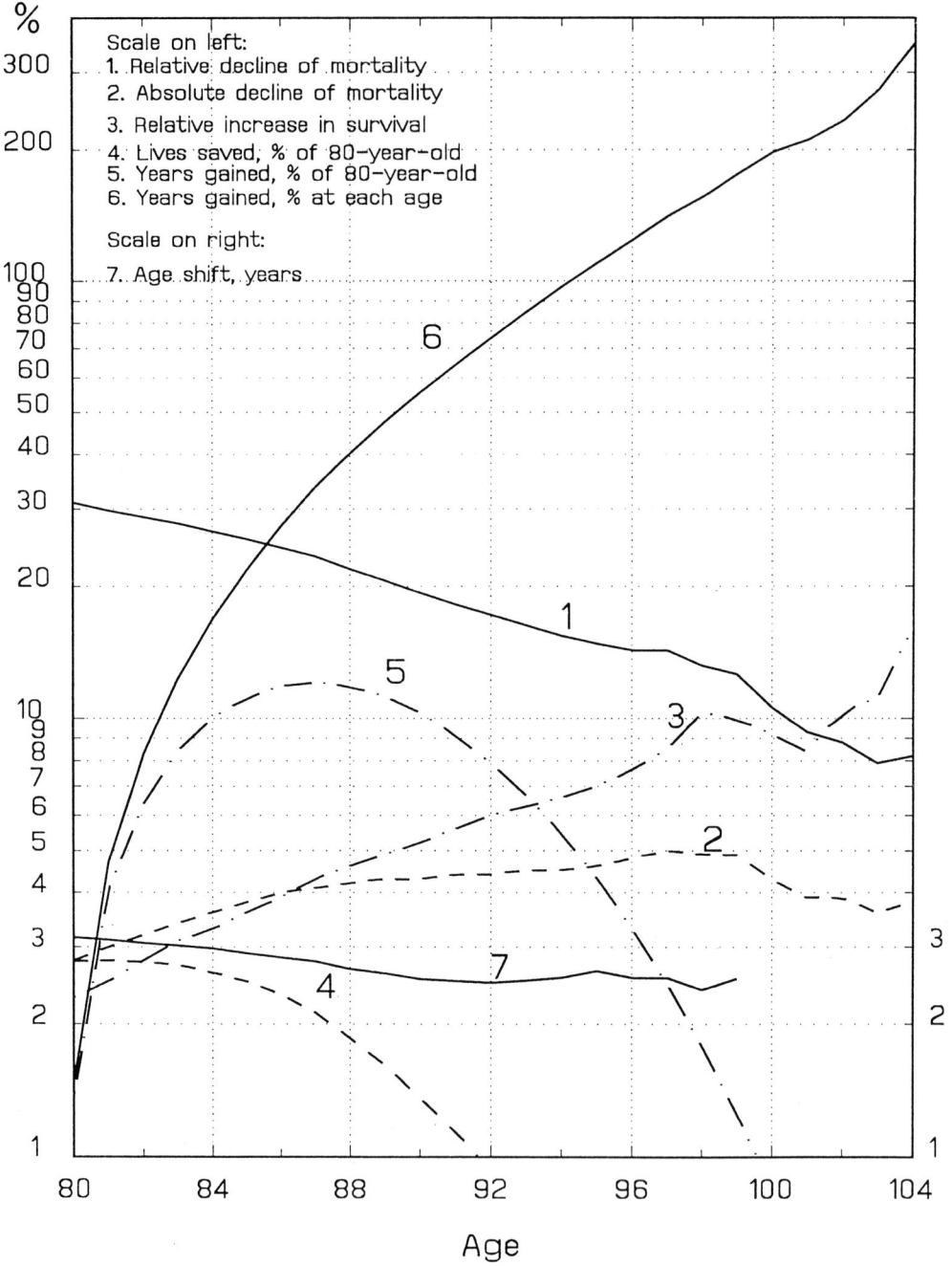

Figure 33. SEVEN INDICATORS OF MORTALITY CHANGE, FROM 1960-70 TO 1980-90. Thirteen countries.

17. Growing numbers of old people

The aging of Western populations during this century was brought about by the great demographic transition in which both fertility and mortality fell sharply. Mortality was reduced most importantly in infancy and childhood but considerably also in youth and middle age with the result that increasing numbers of people lived to retirement age. These swelling numbers ensured that, though mortality in old age declined only slowly if at all, more people reached high ages than before.

The increase in the numbers of oldest-old was, however, quite moderate until a new factor came into play in the post-1950 era: a decisive decline in age-specific mortality even at oldest ages, a development as unprecedented as it was unexpected. Not only were more people reaching ages 65 and 80 but those who did were surviviving considerably longer than their predecessors. This caused an acceleration in aging and a situation where the growth rate is the faster, the higher the age. The annual rate of increase of the oldest-old contrasted sharply with that of the population as a whole (absolute numbers given in Annex Table 16):

	Western Europe (12 countries)	Eastern Europe (5 countries)	Japan
Ages 80 and over:			
1960 to 1970	2.4%	2.4%	3.7%
1970 to 1980	2.7%	2.4%	5.3%
1980 to 1990	3.7%	2.3%	6.2%
Total population:			
1960 to 1990	0.6%	0.1%	0.9%

In all three regions, the growth of the old age population was many times as fast as that of the general population leading to a rapid process of extreme aging. In Eastern Europe, the growth was caused mainly by past decline in death rates at younger ages which allowed constantly growing numbers to survive to retirement age and beyond but, lacking the additional impetus of declining old age mortality, the growth did not accelerate. In Western Europe and still more in Japan, this new phenomenon led to considerable acceleration.

A wide diversity can be observed between individual countries. This is shown in Table 34 for 28 countries (absolute numbers in Annex Table 15), including some where data quality is not very good but considered sufficient to give an approximate idea of the overall growth. Japan is far ahead of the field with a 30-year growth factor of 4.42 while in most countries it varies between 2 and 3. The development of the growth rates over time reflects trends in population size, mortality decline and past historical events. A major factor to be taken into account are war losses which, once suffered, will mark the cohorts in question until their extinction.

Table 34. GROWTH OF THE OLDEST-OLD POPULATION, BY COUNTRY.

Country	Annual rate of growth, %			Growth factor 1960-90
	1960-70	1970-80	1980-90	
Australia	...	2.7	4.1	...
Austria	2.5	2.4	3.5	2.29
Belgium	1.8	2.5	3.0	2.05
Canada	3.9	2.6	3.7	2.63
Czechoslovakia	2.6	3.0	3.1	2.36
Denmark	3.1	3.6	3.2	2.57
England & Wales	2.2	1.9	3.3	2.08
Estonia	3.1	2.1	2.3	2.10
Finland	2.3	4.8	5.4	3.41
France	2.4	2.6	3.4	2.29
Germany, East	1.9	1.7	1.9	1.72
Germany, West	3.0	3.3	4.4	2.86
Hungary	3.5	3.1	2.3	2.40
Iceland	1.9	5.3	2.4	2.50
Ireland	0.3	0.8	1.7	1.33
Italy	1.9	2.6	3.7	2.25
Japan	3.7	5.3	6.2	4.42
Latvia	2.8	1.6	2.3	1.93
Luxembourg	2.1	3.0	3.9	2.42
Netherlands	3.7	3.4	3.3	2.76
New Zealand	2.5	1.4	3.4	2.04
Norway	1.8	3.4	2.9	2.23
Poland	...	4.8	4.1	...
Portugal	2.4	2.3	3.7	2.31
Scotland	1.7	2.1	3.0	1.96
Spain	3.2	3.1	4.9	2.61
Sweden	2.9	3.3	3.5	2.60
Switzerland	2.9	4.1	4.3	3.02

Figure 34, based on data in Annex Table 13, demonstrates how the increase of the male population at specific ages was in recent years affected by casualties in World War I. At the present time and during the next 10 - 12 years, the number of men to reach age 80 is reduced in countries which participated in World War II. In addition, the cohorts of both sexes are affected by temporary fluctuations in the birth rate during crisis periods.

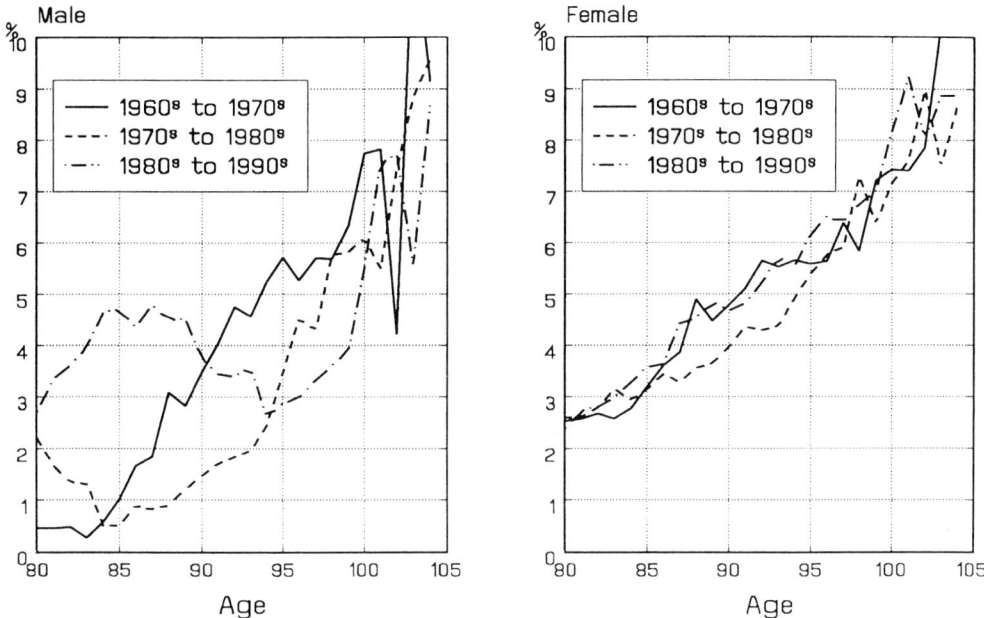

Figure 34 ANNUAL GROWTH RATE OF OLDEST-OLD POPULATION.
   In 10 countries involved in World War I.

The proportion of oldest-old in total population has naturally increased substantially in the same 30-year period (see Table 35). In the 25 countries, for which data are available for both 1960 and 1990, the proportion of oldest-old has doubled from 1.42 to 3.00 percent and everyone of them had in 1990 a higher percentage of oldest-old than the highest observed in 1960.

Table 35. PROPORTION AGED 80 AND OVER IN TOTAL POPULATION, PERCENT

1 January 1960		1 January 1990	
France	2.00	Sweden	4.19
Norway	1.96	Germany, West	3.79
England & Wales	1.95	Norway	3.68
Belgium	1.85	France	3.67
Sweden	1.84	Denmark	3.67
Germany, East	1.83	England & Wales	3.66
Latvia	1.78	Switzerland	3.63
Austria	1.71	Austria	3.57
Scotland	1.62	Belgium	3.53
Estonia	1.61	Scotland	3.35
Denmark	1.60	Germany, East	3.33
Germany, West	1.57	Italy	3.03
Italy	1.57	Luxembourg	2.98
Switzerland	1.51	Netherlands	2.86
New Zealand	1.50	Finland	2.77
Luxembourg	1.49	Latvia	2.69
Iceland	1.44	Estonia	2.57
Netherlands	1.35	Portugal	2.53
Canada	1.26	Hungary	2.50
Spain	1.22	Iceland	2.48
Portugal	1.21	Spain	2.47
Czechoslovakia	1.10	Japan	2.29
Hungary	1.08	Czechoslovakia	2.26
Finland	0.92	Canada	2.22
Japan	0.69	Ireland	2.20
		New Zealand	2.17
		Australia	2.12
		Poland	1.92
		Chile	0.88
		Singapore	0.87
25 countries	1.42	25 countries	3.00

From: Kannisto, 1994, p. 24.

The diverging trends and the past history have caused wide-spread changes in the ranking of countries. Nevertheless, France, Norway and Sweden have remained in the group of top five. East and West Germany, both aging but at different speeds, have moved in opposite directions in ranking. Japan and Finland, the last two in 1960, have moved much higher. Countries outside of Europe are among the least aged.

Besides growing rapidly in size, the oldest-old population itself is aging. For the group of thirteen countries as a whole, the following aging indicators in successive age groups describe the development.

1) Population aged 80 and over:

	Growth factor 1960 - 1990	Percent aged 90 and over 1960	1990
Males	2.3	5.0	7.6
Females	2.9	6.7	11.6

2) Population aged 90 and over:

	Growth factor 1960-1990	Percent aged 100 and over 1960	1990
Males	3.4	0.4	1.0
Females	5.0	0.7	1.5

3) Population aged 100 and over:

	Growth factor 1960-1990	Percent aged 105 and over 1960	1990
Males	8.6	2.5	3.6
Females	11.1	2.6	4.1

4) Population aged 105 and over:

	Growth factor 1960-1990	Mean age 1960	1990
Males	12.4	106.1	106.5
Females	17.2	106.0	106.4

The growth factor has been ever higher at successive ages, and always higher for women than men. The proportion of those in the next higher age group has also regularly grown and has been higher for women than men. The mean age of persons 105 years or older grew very slightly and, being based on small numbers, was marginally higher for men.

The age pyramid in absolute numbers in Figure 35 demonstrates the magnitude of the increase in numbers, very substantial, particularly among women, up to ages around 90. The highest ages require a presentation in larger scale (in the upper right corner) to show the explosive growth of the centenarian population.

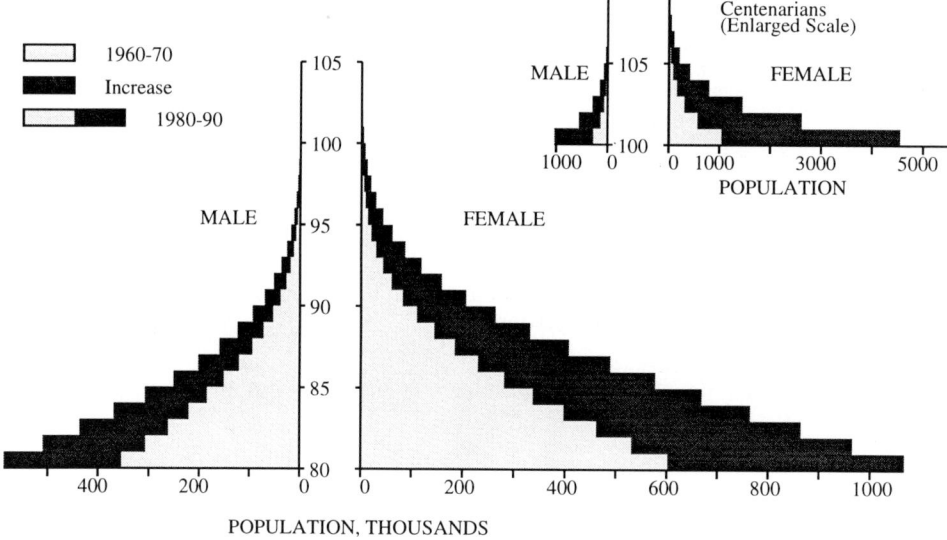

Figure 35. GROWTH OF THE OLDEST-OLD POPULATION.
Thirteen countries with good data.

Contribution of recent mortality decline to the growing numbers.

The following is an assessment of the contribution of the decline in oldest-old mortality after 1960 to the growing numbers of oldest-old in each country. For the purpose, the actual cohorts as they reached age 80 were projected up to 1 January 1990 according to the national life table of 1950-60 (in case of the Netherlands, 1960-70), available in Annex Table 2, and then compared with the actual population of 1 January 1990. Divided by the population on 1 January 1960, this gives two sets of growth factors: projected and actual. The results are given in Annex Table 16 by country, age group and sex and illustrated in Figure 36 with bar charts in which the lower, blue part shows the growth factor as projected, i.e. if mortality had remained unchanged at the 1950-60 level. The entire bar shows the actual growth factor, and the red part the contribution of the decline of oldest-old mortality.

In most cases, the existing momentum would have increased the old age population by about 50 percent, or, at most, doubled it. In most countries, furthermore, the lower part of the bar does not increase with age, indicating that the cumulative nature of survival by age was still largely absent in the 1950s. In several countries, shown among the first in Figure 36, the subsequent mortality decline was so slight as to have relatively little effect. In the majority of the countries, however, its effect was decisive. Without it, the oldest-old population would have grown only modestly, and the phenomenon of faster growth at older ages would have been largely absent. As it was, the oldest groups grew in many countries by a factor of 10 or 20.

Most spectacular are the growth factors of the centenarians. VAUPEL and JEUNE (1994) found in a study of Scandinavian cohorts born between 1860 and 1890 that the contribution of mortality decline above age 80 to the increase in the number of centenarians varied as follows between groups of cohorts:

> Denmark   65 - 68 percent
> Norway   51 - 65   "
> Sweden   65 - 75   "

amounting thus to about two thirds of it. The remainder was mostly due to mortality decline at younger ages leaving only a marginal importance to the increase in births.

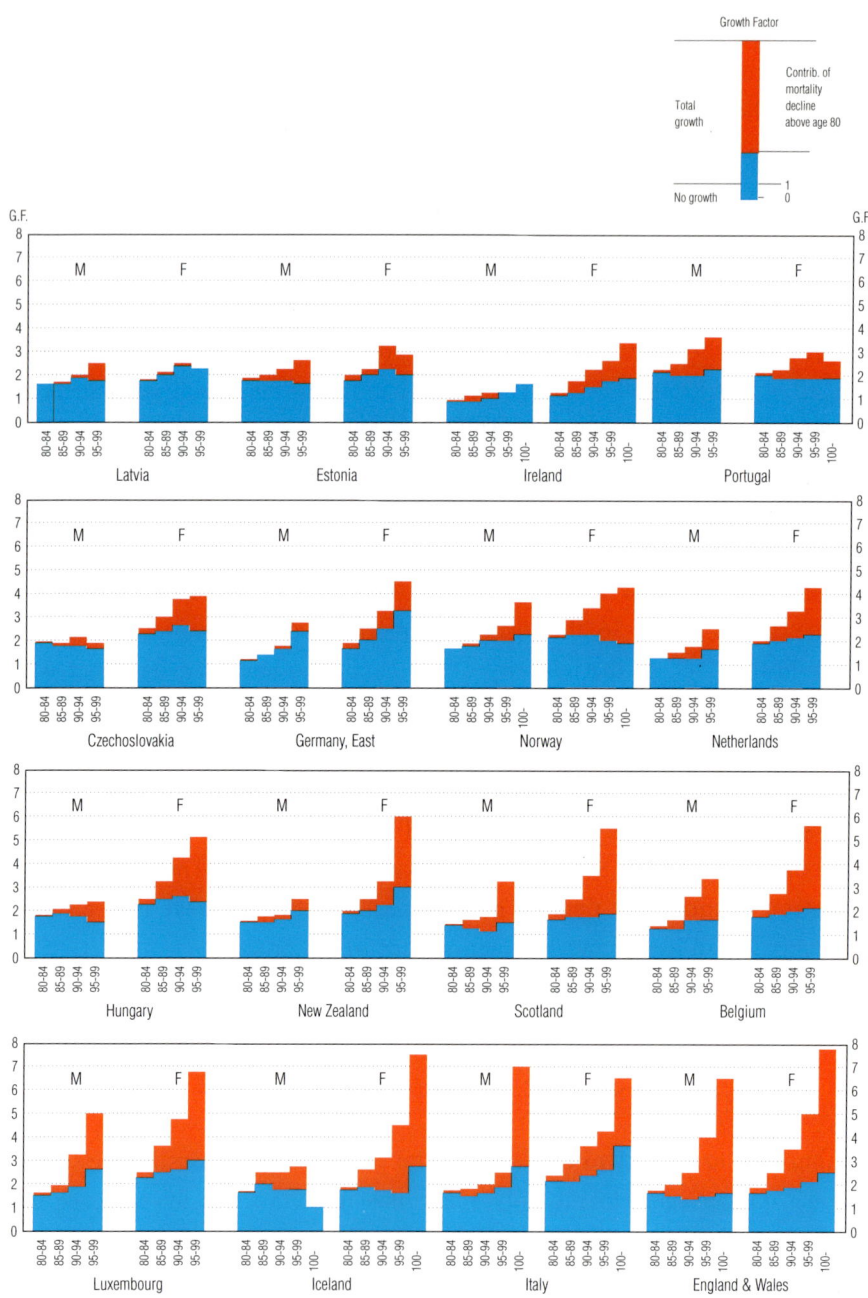

Figure 36. **GROWTH FACTOR OF OLDEST-OLD POPULATION FROM 1960 TO 1990 AND CONTRIBUTION OF MORTALITY DECLINE ABOVE AGE 80 TO IT.**

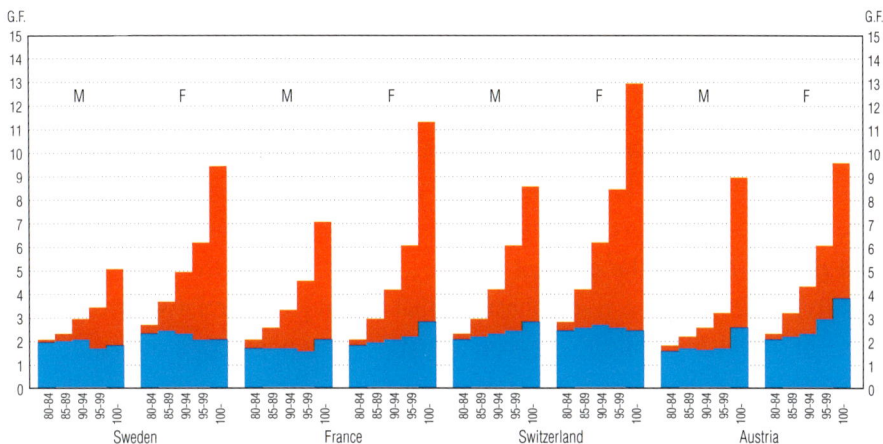

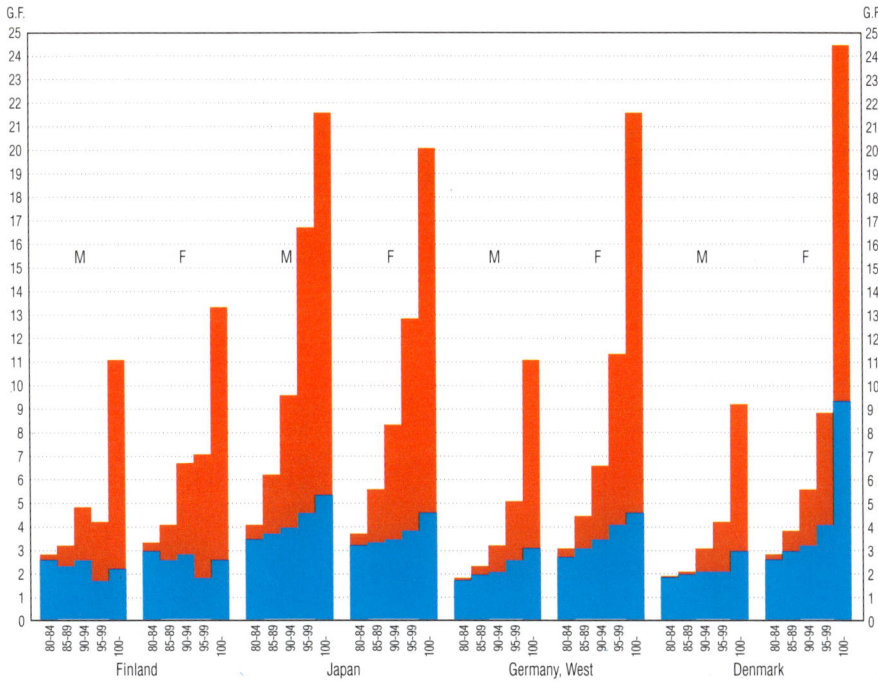

Figure 36 (cont.)

With our material we cannot trace cohorts from birth and so separate the two last-mentioned components but we can show the contribution of mortality decline above age 80 since 1960. Table 36 shows the results regarding centenarians in 1990 in ten countries with reliable information. The methodology is different and our data apply to all living centenarians instead of those who reached age 100, and consequently, the figures are not strictly comparable. They measure, however, essentially the same thing, and our data corroborate the findings of Vaupel and Jeune that the increase in the number of centenarians is overwhelmingly due to the recent decline in the mortality of the oldest-old: an average of 78 percent with a range from 63 to 88. This decline increased the growth factor from a projected 2.9 to the actual 9.7 and thus the growth portion (where the original population is excluded) from 1.9 to 8.7.

Finally, it needs to be re-emphasized that although the relative growth has been most rapid at the highest ages, the great bulk of the population increase among the oldest-old - 85 to 90 percent - has taken place at ages between 80 and 90 years. The spectacular surge in the number of centenarians is a salient feature of the recent development and as such of great significance but very small in terms of population.

Table 36. INCREASE IN THE NUMBER OF CENTENARIANS AND CONTRIBUTION OF MORTALITY DECLINE ABOVE AGE 80 TO IT, 1960-1990.
(Both sexes)

Country	Centenarians 1960	Centenarians 1990		Contribution %	Growth factor	
		Projected[1]	Actually		Projected	Actual
Austria	25	85	232	71.0	3.4	9.4
Denmark	19	68	325	84.0	3.6	17.1
England & Wales	531	1284	4042	78.6	2.4	7.6
Finland	11	26	141	88.5	2.4	12.8
France	371	966	3853	82.9	2.6	10.4
Italy	265	929	2047	62.7	3.5	7.7
Japan	154	729	3126	80.7	4.7	20.3
Norway	73	147	300	67.4	2.0	4.1
Sweden	73	148	579	85.2	2.0	7.9
Switzerland	29	81	338	83.2	2.8	11.7
Total	1551	4463	14983	78.3	2.9	9.7
Male	301	752	2456	79.1	2.5	8.2
Female	1250	3711	12527	78.2	3.0	10.0

1) Assuming constant mortality above age 80.

Table 37. CONTRIBUTION OF MORTALITY DECLINE AT AGES 80 AND OVER TO POPULATION GROWTH FROM 1960 TO 1990, PERCENT.

Country	AGE					
	80-84	85-89	90-94	95-99	100-	Total
MALE						
Austria	18.9	43.9	60.6	66.9	81.5	30.6
Belgium	20.3	47.3	62.7	74.7	...	35.5
Czechoslovakia	2.5	11.9	36.1	20.5	...	6.4
Denmark	7.6	29.6	47.8	66.5	76.9	20.7
England & Wales	15.0	46.2	70.2	80.9	88.5	29.1
Estonia	10.1	27.5	40.7	56.5	...	17.4
Finland	13.0	41.1	60.8	77.9	88.6	24.2
France	21.3	52.4	70.7	82.3	83.6	36.4
Germany, East	8.8	1.4	9.4	18.4	...	5.8
Germany, West	13.5	33.4	50.9	63.7	...	23.6
Hungary	5.4	18.5	37.0	60.5	...	11.4
Iceland	10.9	30.1	50.5	58.9	...	24.5
Italy	9.1	29.9	36.0	39.5	69.7	17.2
Japan	17.2	46.6	65.8	77.1	79.0	30.1
Latvia	0.7	7.2	7.7	48.3	...	3.8
Luxembourg	12.6	37.9	60.7	57.0	...	26.3
Netherlands	2.3	16.5	42.0	57.8	...	13.2
New Zealand	6.0	23.6	25.5	27.0	...	12.6
Norway	-0.8	6.2	20.8	39.6	51.6	4.6
Portugal	22.0	31.6	48.9	50.6	...	19.0
Scotland	18.9	56.6	78.6	76.5	...	34.5
Sweden	9.9	30.4	47.2	69.5	80.1	20.2
Switzerland	16.2	43.7	60.9	70.6	68.3	29.4
FEMALE						
Austria	17.1	41.6	53.4	61.3	68.6	29.8
Belgium	19.1	46.1	63.1	75.7	...	35.0
Czechoslovakia	9.3	26.6	40.3	48.1	...	17.2
Denmark	16.1	44.2	64.3	77.7	86.4	33.3
England & Wales	17.5	44.6	60.7	70.4	77.3	34.8
Estonia	9.3	26.3	40.5	48.9	...	18.8
Finland	16.6	48.9	68.5	86.6	87.8	32.1
France	22.4	51.2	67.0	77.4	82.8	40.8
Germany, East	12.2	26.1	33.1	36.1	...	18.9
Germany, West	15.5	40.5	56.1	70.0	...	28.6
Hungary	12.2	33.0	47.6	65.1	...	22.1
Iceland	13.3	40.3	61.7	79.0	79.3	33.9
Italy	14.1	36.9	44.3	48.0	60.8	25.2
Japan	18.3	48.6	66.4	75.6	81.1	33.7
Latvia	4.4	12.5	3.7	-9.9	...	6.6
Luxembourg	16.3	42.3	58.6	64.1	...	29.6
Netherlands	13.9	38.0	54.5	64.7	...	·28.5
New Zealand	10.2	30.2	42.7	58.5	...	22.2
Norway	12.0	32.8	48.5	64.7	72.5	24.9
Portugal	12.5	29.0	43.8	49.0	...	21.0
Scotland	19.7	49.5	67.1	79.7	...	37.6
Sweden	17.6	45.4	64.3	78.8	86.3	34.0
Switzerland	19.6	49.5	65.7	77.1	86.8	36.7

18. The expanding frontier of survival

The maximal age attainable by man is naturally a matter of great interest and has been the subject of speculation ever since the classical era. Without entering this time-honoured and extremely wide field of literature we shall mention only a few carefully reasoned estimates based on reliable cases. Extrapolating his data on four European countries with reliable information, the French demographer Paul VINCENT (1951) set the maximal age under the circumstances then present, at 110, and Françoise DEPOID (1973), using the same method but newer data, at 117 for men and 119 for women. OLSHANSKY et al. (1993) considered that there is no indication that humans are capable of living much past the age of 110. DUCHENE and WUNSCH (1988) considered that the intrinsic aging process leads to a maximal life span of 115 years. Other, equally serious estimates have arrived at ages 125 - 130. The maximal age attainable depends closely on the trajectory of the mortality curve at extremely high ages which is the subject of another monograph in this series by THATCHER et al. (forthcoming).

The highest so far known and properly verified case of longevity is that of Jeanne Calment (subject of a book by ALLARD et al., 1994) who was born on 21 February 1975 in Arles, France. Her age was verified from official documentation *in loco* on her 120th birthday by B. Jeune, J. Vaupel and this author.

The remarkable decline in old age mortality inevitably raises the question of what can be expected in the future. Answers will be sought in the following by calculating what effects a continuing mortality decline would have on the oldest-old populations. The effects will be measured in terms of stationary population and the calculations do not constitute actual population projections which would have to be geared to observed age distributions which are historical results of events and influences which the populations in question have lived through in the past 100 years or so. In the countries of our database, the history has by no means been uniform.

An actual projection would require assumptions regarding the annual inflow of 80-year-old to the oldest-old population. The application of the stationary population concept assumes this flow to be constant. In the actual countries, it will tend to rise for some time though with fluctuations due to shortfall of births during World War I and losses in male cohorts incurred in World War II. In the longer run, the increases will generally slow down or stop, different countries evolving in their separate ways. It was, however, demonstrated in Chapter 17 that at ages 100 and over - the true frontier of survival - the growth in numbers does not depend to any great extent on what happens before age 80.

The basic assumption for the forward calculations which will follow is that the recent decline in oldest-old mortality will continue. Using the mortality decline observed between 1960-70 and 1980-90 in the thirteen countries with best information as standard, we measure the changes in stationary population which will result if this decline is repeated one, two or three more times. These shall be called Scenarios 1,2 and 3. With mortality change we shall understand the *relative change in annual age-specific probability of dying* (No. 1 of the seven mortality change indicators in Chapter 16) because a *constant decline per population-at-risk* would soon lead to negative mortality. The resulting q values are given in Table 38.

The mortality decline of the last two decades which is used as standard, accounted among men to an annual reduction of 0.95 percent at age 80, gradually slowing to 0.64 percent at age 100. Among women, the progress at 80 was twice as fast, 1.84 percent and slowed down by age 100 to approximately the same 0.64 as for men.

No time frame is imposed for the scenarios. If the development continues at the same pace as during the last two decades, the scenarios will take 20, 40 and 60 years respectively to unfold. If the decline accelerates or slows down, they will simply be realized in either less or more time.

Projection of past change into the future ignores the possibility of fundamental breakthroughs in science which might profoundly reduce the mortality from specific causes or slow the process of senescence. It also ignores the possibility of deteriorating environment with adverse effects on health as well as that of possible appearances of new diseases or more virulent strains of existing ones.

It is very common in population projections to give pride of place to alternatives where ongoing changes in demographic parameters will run their course in a short period and give way to constant rates. Such caution does not seem to be called for regarding the oldest-old today. The decline has gathered strong momentum, the considerable international differences have so far not narrowed and large inequalities in death rates have been found to exist between social groups in the same country. In a modern state, there is no excuse for the existence of large social inequalities in health and survival which to an increasing extent depend on health-related behaviour: smoking, diet, physical exercise etc. The expectation is that people will continue to improve their chances of survival by modifying their lifestyle accordingly and by taking advantage of improvements in medical and public health practices. There is of course no certainty that they will do so and powerful special interests are at work to prevent some aspects of it.

Table 38. PROBABILITY OF DYING PER 10.000 ACCORDING TO THREE SCENARIOS.

	Male					Female				
X	q ratio	1980-90	S 1	S 2	S 3	q ratio	1980-90	S 1	S 2	S 3
80	.8264	976	807	667	551	.6907	623	430	297	205
81	.8281	1069	885	733	607	.7024	704	494	347	244
82	.8298	1170	971	806	669	.7132	796	568	405	289
83	.8317	1273	1059	881	733	.7240	891	645	467	338
84	.8335	1384	1154	962	802	.7350	995	731	537	395
85	.8356	1503	1256	1050	877	.7461	1107	826	616	460
86	.8379	1628	1364	1143	958	.7575	1229	931	705	534
87	.8408	1761	1481	1245	1047	.7696	1360	1047	806	620
88	.8436	1903	1605	1354	1142	.7820	1500	1173	917	717
89	.8471	2051	1737	1471	1246	.7942	1649	1310	1040	826
90	.8508	2206	1877	1597	1359	.8059	1806	1455	1173	945
91	.8545	2369	2024	1730	1478	.8172	1970	1610	1316	1075
92	.8583	2540	2180	1871	1606	.8270	2140	1770	1464	1211
93	.8622	2713	2339	2017	1739	.8359	2313	1933	1616	1351
94	.8649	2887	2497	2160	1868	.8433	2492	2102	1773	1495
95	.8653	3056	2644	2288	1980	.8502	2669	2269	1929	1640
96	.8672	3212	2785	2415	2094	.8563	2844	2435	2085	1785
97	.8696	3392	2950	2565	2231	.8635	3025	2612	2255	1947
98	.8727	3618	3157	2755	2404	.8721	3226	2813	2453	2129
99	.8762	3817	3345	2931	2568	.8800	3419	3009	2648	2330
100	.8800	4002	3522	3099	2727	.8800	3607	3174	2793	2458
101	.8850	4238	3751	3320	2938	.8850	3809	3371	2983	2640
102	.8900	4368	3888	3460	3079	.8900	3991	3552	3161	2813
103	.8950	4425	3960	3544	3172	.8950	4173	3735	3343	2992
104	.9000	4495	4045	3640	3276	.9000	4307	3876	3488	3139

q ratio = q (1980-90) / q (1960-70)
q in 1980-90 and q ratio have been smoothed with 5-age moving averages,
q ratio for ages 100 and over has been extrapolated.

Of the successive scenarios, No. 1 can be considered very likely, in fact almost assured since it is already well underway from its central point 1985 and, according to all indications, mortality decline is continuing. Scenario 2 may also be considered realistic while Scenario 3 is more uncertain based as it is on age-specific death rates so low that their plausibility may be questioned.

The depth of the mortality transformation under the various scenarios can be seen in the first lines in Table 39. Scenario 1 implies mortality reductions of 12 - 17 percent for men and 12 - 31 percent for women which translate into mortality shifts of 2.1 and 2.7 years respectively. Thus, while the scheduled mortality reductions are much larger for women than men, they cause age shifts of more equal size and are, therefore, in a sense, equally deep-going.

A second repetition of the last 20 years' development would lead to death rates up to one-third lower for men and one-half lower for women than the most recent ones. The third scenario would reduce the death rates of 80-year-old women to only one-third of the present level - the likelihood of this to happen may be questioned. In the same scenario, persons of 86-87 years of age would be subject to the mortality of today's 80-year-old. So large an age shift which would be an expression of a commensurate delay in aging would be easily noticeable by people in their daily lives.

Another indicator, the modal length of life, i.e. the most common age at death would increase almost exactly in step with the age shift and, in females, would surpass 90 years.

The probability of surviving from age 80 to 100, at present still very small, would grow for each sex by a factor of 7 or 8, thereby approaching 5 percent for men and surpassing 10 percent for women.

Life expectancy at age 80 would increase under these conditions but less than spectacularly, for males from 6.25 to 9.05 and for females from 7.80 to 12.14 according to Scenario 3. How much would this increase contribute to life expectancy at birth, would depend on what proportion of the newborn survive to age 80. In 1986-88, these proportions were in France 0.37 for males and 0.63 for females. If we apply the ratio 0.5 to males and 0.7 to females - levels that may be reached in some countries early in the next century - the benefits are modest: in the last scenario 1.40 and 3.04 years would be added to the life expectancy of newborn boys and girls respectively.

If and when survival to age 80 increases, the gains are compounded. Under the quite extreme assumption that the last 20 years' decline is repeated no less than five times - corresponding to 100 years of mortality decline at present speed - the female life expectancy at age 80 would increase to 14.84 years or a full 7 years more than at present. The eradication of all mortality before age 80 would give to newborn girls a life expectancy of 94.8 years.

TABLE 39. SOME DEMOGRAPHIC EFFECTS IF THE DECLINE IN OLDEST-OLD MORTALITY IN THE LAST 20 YEARS IS REPEATED ONE, TWO OR THREE MORE TIMES. Thirteen countries with good data.

Item	Males				Females			
	No repeat	Once	Twice	Three times	No repeat	Once	Twice	Three times
Percent decline in mortality at age 80	-	17.4	31.7	43.5	-	31.0	52.3	67.1
90	-	14.9	27.6	38.4	-	19.4	35.0	47.7
100	-	12.0	22.6	31.9	-	12.0	22.6	31.9
Death rate at age 80 shifts to age	80.0	82.1	84.2	86.2	80.0	82.7	85.1	87.0
Modal length of life	80	82	83	85	85	88	90	92
Probability of survival from 80 to 100, percent	0.6	1.3	2.6	4.7	1.5	3.5	6.6	10.8
Life expectancy at age 80	6.25	7.13	8.06	9.05	7.80	9.25	10.71	12.14
Years added to life expectancy at birth[1]	-	0.44	0.90	1.40	-	1.01	2.04	3.04
Percent gain in life-years at age 80-84	-	4.7	8.9	12.4	-	5.5	9.5	12.4
85-89	-	19.4	38.3	56.2	-	21.8	40.5	55.8
90-94	-	44.0	94.6	149.8	-	47.7	97.8	146.6
95-99	-	85.6	209.7	375.4	-	88.2	206.8	348.7
100-	-	171.2	508.7	1095.2	-	153.5	434.9	874.5
80 and over	-	14.0	29.0	44.8	-	18.7	37.4	55.7
Life-years gained per each 80-year-old at age 80-84	-	0.18	0.34	0.47	-	0.23	0.40	0.52
85-89	-	0.34	0.68	0.99	-	0.52	0.97	1.34
90-94	-	0.24	0.53	0.83	-	0.45	0.94	1.40
95-99	-	0.09	0.22	0.39	-	0.20	0.48	0.80
100-	-	0.02	0.05	0.11	-	0.05	0.14	0.28
80 and over	-	0.88	1.81	2.80	-	1.46	2.92	4.34

[1] Assuming a survival ratio of 0.5 for males, 0.7 for females from birth to age 80.

Next in Table 39, we give the prospective percentage gains in years to be lived at various ages in a stationary population. The relative gain in life-years that can be expected from further mortality decline is quite modest in low eighties but progressively greater in the older age groups reaching a tenfold growth in centenarians - and this without any increase in numbers reaching 80. The overall gain would be larger for females because of their older age distribution.

A striking similarity between male and female growth percentages may be noted at all ages in all scenarios.

The last group of numbers in Table 39 gives the actual years of life to be gained under the different scenarios. In contrast to the relative gains which rise exponentially with age, the absolute gains accrue mostly to ages between 85 and 95 and are much larger for women than men. The phenomenally high growth rates of the oldest have a relatively modest impact because of the low base values. The number of centenarians might be multiplied by ten but it still would not make them a large population group. Even according to Scenario 3 they would make up only 1.4 percent of the males and 2.5 percent of the females at ages 80 and over (figures not shown in the table). They would constitute less than one percent of the total population but they would not be rare cases as they are today.

The message of these conditional results is that further decline in oldest-old mortality would profoundly affect not only the size but also the characteristics of the aged population. Aging, as reflected in mortality, would be significantly delayed.

Gains to be made in life-years would be differential by age so that (a) measured against lives now lost they would be greatest among the youngest but (b) measured against present lifetimes they would be largest among the oldest while (c) measured against an individual's life course or in a stationary population, they would be greatest between ages 85 and 95. It must be added, though, that any reduction of death rates *before* age 80 would be felt more at age 80 than later and would thus possibly alter the balance of the gains.

For a closer look at what might be called the dominion of death, in Figure 37, the survival curve has been inverted so that years lived are counted from the top. It constitutes the dividing line between life and death for those who reached age 80. If the corresponding lines for the three scenarios were shown, each one would be a little farther to the right but other differences would not be very obvious. We have therefore shown the putative gains in life-years at the bottom. The largest gains for both sexes (of which only the female is shown) always fall to ages slightly below 90. The present dominion of death would be quite significantly reduced at ages 80 to 85 but the inroads to be made into it at highest ages would be minor indeed. Decline of mortality before age 80 would accentuate this feature. A corresponding figure for males would be essentially similar.

Regarding methodology, a note may be appropriate here. The exercise seems to justify the most commonly used approach in projections, namely that of observed relative sex-age-specific change - which may be modified so as to alter the speed or gradually to stop it - as a valid and reasonable way to project future mortality. A time frame is not essential when dealing with a stationary population. In this case, the repetition of an observed 20-year change one, two and three times gave results which were internally consistent.

A further mortality decline from the present level would produce a large age shift but this would not be matched by an equal increase in life expectancy. In the third scenario, the age shift for males would be 6.2 years but the gain in life expectancy only 2.8 years. For females the corresponding figures would be 7.0 and 4.3 years.

Unless scientific breakthroughs occur, the extension of human life will meet resistance in the aging process which, even when pushed back, ultimately prevails.

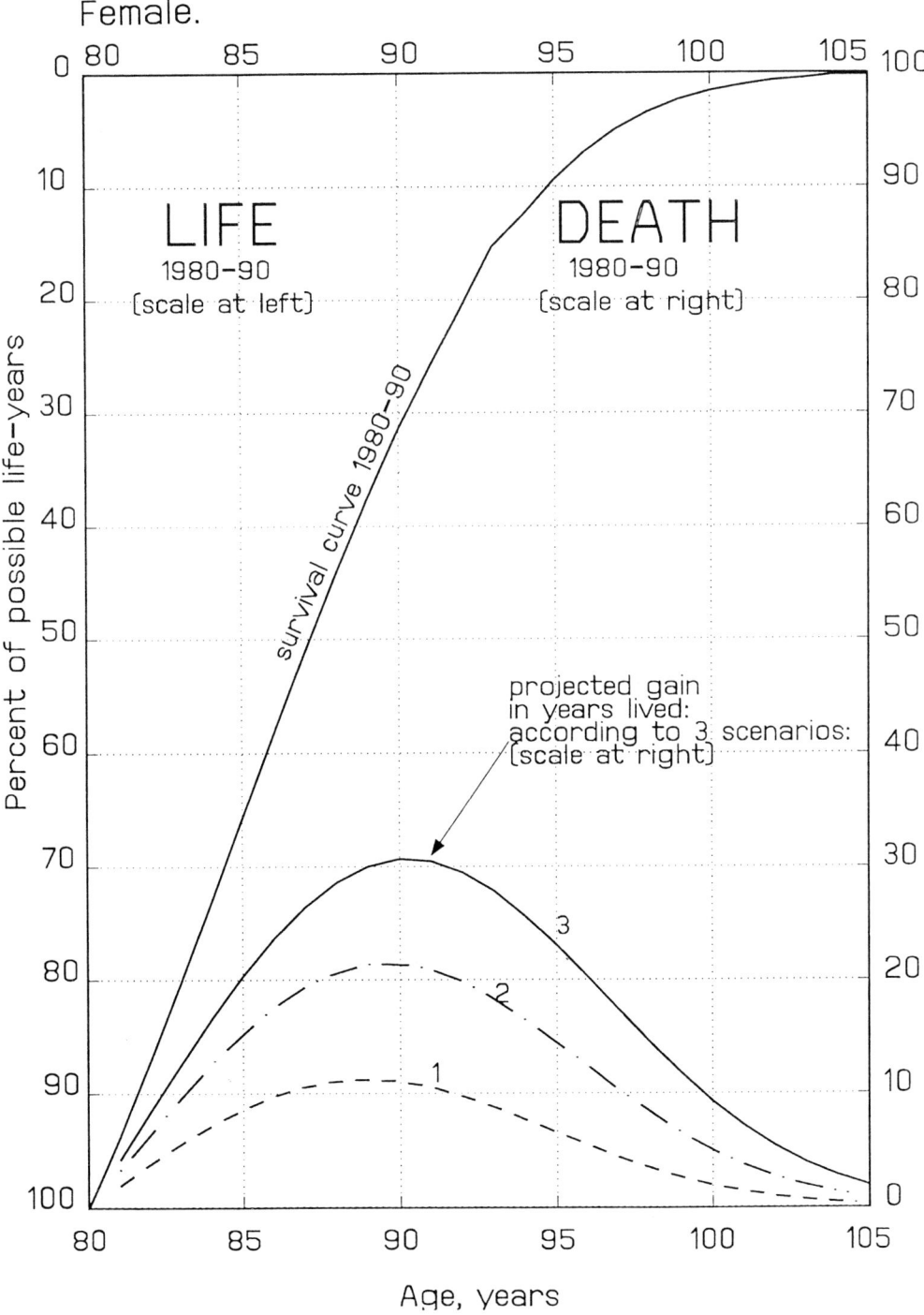

Figure 37. LIFE AND DEATH AT AGES 80 AND OVER.

19. Conclusions

Mortality in old age has in recent decades declined in a manner so unprecedented that it can rightly be called a new stage in epidemiological transition (Olshansky and Ault 1986; Rogers and Hackenberg 1987) causing a shift from fertility-dominated to mortality-dominated population aging (Yu and Horiuchi 1987; Horiuchi 1991). This unexpected but by now well-known decline encompasses all elderly age groups as high up as can today be reliably measured, that is to say around ages 106-108. The best available data on the oldest-old in the Odense database show that the characteristic pattern of this decline is one of larger relative gains around age 80 which then gradually diminish towards ages 100 and over. This is in line with the contention of BOURGEOIS-PICHAT (1952, 1978) that the causes of death prevalent in older ages are more resistant to reduction. Our own data do not reach below age 80 but the death rates published by the United Nations show a widespread decline among the elderly in general and, in many cases, larger reductions among people in their late sixties or seventies than above it. (Kannisto 1994, p. 48). Exceptions to this pattern of diminishing progress with advancing age which have been observed among men in some countries are clearly associated with unfavourable development in the mortality of middle-aged men and thus alien to the new transition.

The decline so far observed has varied between countries as to time of onset, speed, depth and acceleration or slow-down but has reached virtually all low-mortality countries and is going on unabated. A sustained decline in old age mortality began earlier for women than men (the average year of onset in 25 countries was for women 1968, for men 1976; Kannisto 1994, p. 42) and has been, in percentage terms, deeper for women than men in virtually every country.

We are not able to measure the mortality of the oldest-old in the U.S. or Canada with the extinct-cohort method from available data because of age overstatement. At ages below 75, however, the official data are undoubtedly reliable and show that the mortality of middle-aged and elderly U.S. and Canadian men began declining rapidly in late 1960s, and among women somewhat earlier. (U.N. Demographic Yearbook). There is hardly any doubt that this decline extended to the oldest-old. North America therefore entered the new stage of epidemiological transition earlier than most of Western Europe. Only in France, did a sustained decline begin for both sexes - and in some others for women - already in the 1950s.

All data of good quality indicate a monotonic, though less than exponential, rise in mortality with advancing age and no evidence of a plateau or peak is seen before age 110 at least.

The often assumed convergence of male and female death rates in old age is revealed as only apparent. Although the sex ratio of mortality falls, the difference per population-at-risk remains roughly constant at least some years past age 100.

Data which are based on accurate age information have not produced any significant mortality crossover by age either over time or between populations. Trajectories calculated from unreliable data, however, have a very strong tendency to flatten out and intersect more reliable curves.

We suggest that change in old age mortality may be better understood if it is observed through an array of indicators selected for their relevance at high ages. Thus, the relative reduction in the death rate is usefully complemented by the absolute (per population) reduction which has a different age pattern and possibly a different gender relationship. At highest ages the ebbing force of life may be more appropriately measured by the probability of survival than that of dying. The relative increase in the former describes the expanding frontier of survival. Since the desired end result in combatting death is increase in lifetime, the gain in years lived per person, broken down by age in which it is lived, is perhaps the most significant parameter of change. Finally, the age shift is another meaningful and easily conceptualized indicator which can be taken to reflect delay in individual aging.

It has been, we believe, conclusively demonstrated that the recent decline in old age mortality has been caused by period factors with simultaneous and apparently immediate effect at all old age groups (Kannisto 1994, pp. 55-59). It is manifestly not the result of supposedly healthier cohorts growing older and gives no support to BARKER's fetal origins hypothesis of adult disease (Barker 1992). As deaths are often the result of long term morbid processes, the past has certainly an effect on today's mortality and cohorts may differ regarding their frailty. Yet, factors "here and now" seem to have affected these processes sufficiently to make an immediate difference and to submerge possible cohort effects.

This is not necessarily always the case. Smoking by women, for example, is reported to have increased in many countries. If this tendency persists, its adverse effects will be felt with a considerable time lag. If the increased smoking is cohort-related, the habit being acquired when young, the eventual mortality effect will also be cohort-dependent.

Regarding the causes of the mortality decline no unanimity exists and could hardly be expected but among researchers who have worked extensively on the subject, and many of whom have carried out representative, large-scale follow-up studies, a wide body of opinion emphasizes the role of such lifestyle factors as improved diet, less smoking, and physical exercise while many include as additional factors new or more widely available medical practices such as control of hypertension (Al-Roomi et al. 1989; Bah and Rajulton 1991; Epstein 1989; Valkonen et al. 1993). Utilization of some medical improvements is cited (La Vecchia et al. 1991) while some others see no impact by new hospital facilities (Mackenbach et al. 1988, 1989; Wing et al. 1986) or by intervention projects (Aase 1989). A follow-up study in the Finnish provinces of highest mortality from ischaemic heart disease showed that the rapid decline in the mortality was mostly due to change in three major risk factors: serum cholesterol, hypertension and smoking (Vartiainen et al. 1994).

Our own data do not provide direct evidence on the causes of the decline but the results are compatible with the existence of a major lifestyle factor. Advances in medical science and availability of new preventive or curative practices have certainly played a role but do not explain the 15 year time lag of Western Germany behind France and Belgium nor the lack of progress for Dutch and Norwegian men. The adverse development regarding men in Eastern Europe is usually ascribed to environmental pollution and deterioration of medical services but even here, lifestyle factors may have played a role and contributed to the divergent trends for men and women.

The existence of spatial differences needs to be carefully considered as they may be due to more permanent factors such as genetic heritage (Koskinen 1992) or the mineral composition of the soil (Gavrilov and Gavrilova 1991).

The new stage in mortality transition has spread to most of the advanced countries and possibly to elites in others. It has gathered considerable momentum and further acceleration is noticeable at least in some of the latest data. As, furthermore, mortality differences between countries, as shown in the relevant chapters, have not narrowed and as such differences are found to persist also between social groups in a given country despite continuous decline in all groups (Valkonen et al. 1993; Martelin 1994), ample scope for further decline in old age mortality clearly exists.

If this potential can and will be taken advantage of, and the progress of the last 20 years is repeated three more times, death rates of 80-year-old men will be reduced by nearly a half and of women by two-thirds. Even the mortality of centenarians would decline by one third. The present death rate of 80-year-old men would shift to age 86 and that of women to 87. The probability of surviving from 80 to 100 would increase for both sexes by a factor of 7 or 8 and approach 5 percent for men and exceed 10 percent for women. As a consequence, the numbers of very old people would continue to grow very rapidly - and the faster, the higher the age.

The bulk of the absolute increase, however, would be below age 100. If mortality declines only above age 80 and not below it, the greatest increase would be at ages 85-94. Considering also the probable decline below 80, very large gains can be expected at all ages from 80 to 94 and quite substantial ones at 95-99.

This development would change the modal (most common) age at death of men from the present 80 years to 85 and that of women from 85 to 92. Life expectancy at age 80 would increase for men by 2.8 years and for women by 4.3 years. The contribution to life expectancy at birth would be somewhat less than this. Under the rather extreme assumption that the present mortality decline would continue at the same speed for one hundred years and all mortality below age 80 is eliminated, female life expectancy at birth would still not reach more than 94.8 years. The extension of the length of life will ultimately meet strong resistance near age 100 unless mortality at these very highest ages will in the future decline faster than has been the case so far.

Barring unexpected adverse developments on one hand, and unforeseen scientific breakthroughs on the other, the new stage of mortality transition is likely to continue for some time to come, possibly for an extended period. This could be construed as better preservation of an individual's life potential and, therefore, the scope for improvement would be finite. The forward scenarios based on recent change describe how the continuation of the trend would increase and modify the oldest sector of modern populations but would not cause a revolutionary increase in the length of life of man.

References

AASE, Asbjørn (1989), Regionalizing mortality data: Ischemic Heart Disease in Norway. *Soc. Sci. Med.*, 29 (8), pp. 907-911.

ALLARD, Michel, LEBRE, Victor and ROBINE, Jean-Marie (1994), *Les 120 ans de Jeanne Calment*. Le Cherche-Midi Editeur, Paris.

AL-ROOMI, K.A., DOBSON, A.J., HALL, E., HELLER, R.F. and MAGNUS, P. (1989), Declining mortality from ischemic heart disease and cerebrovascular disease in Australia. *American Journal of Epidemiology*, 129 (3), pp. 503-510.

BAH, Sulaiman and RAJULTON, Fernando (1991), Has Canadian Mortality Entered the Fourth Stage of the Epidemiological Transition?. *Canadian Studies in Population*, 18 (2), pp. 18-41.

BARKER, D.J.P. (1992), Fetal and infant origin of adult disease. *British Medical Journal*, London.

BOURGEOIS-PICHAT, J. (1952), Essai sur la mortalité "biologique" de l'homme. *Population*, 7 (3), pp. 381-394.

BOURGEOIS-PICHAT, J. (1978), Future outlook for mortality decline in the world. *Population Bulletin of the United Nations*, 11, pp. 12-41.

BOURGEOIS-PICHAT, J. (1988), Du XXe au XXIe siècle: l'Europe et sa population après l'an 2000. *Population*, 43 (1), pp. 9-44.

DEPOID, Françoise (1973), La mortalité des grands vieillards. *Population*, 28, pp. 755-792.

DUCHENE, Josianne and WUNSCH, Guillaume (1988), *Population Aging and the Limits to Human Life*. Département de Démographie. Université Catholique de Louvain. Working Paper no. 146.

EPSTEIN, Frederick H. (1989), The Relationship of Lifestyle to International Trends in CHD. *International Journal of Epidemiology*, 18 (3) Suppl. 1, pp. 203-209.

GAVRILOV, L.A. and GAVRILOVA, N.S. (1991), *The Biology of Life Span: A Quantitative Approach*. Harwood Academic Publishers. New York.

HORIUCHI, Shiro (1991), Assessing the effects of mortality reduction on population aging. *Population Bulletin of the United Nations*, Nos. 31/32.

HORIUCHI, Shiro and COALE, Ansley J. (1990), Age patterns of mortality for older women: an analysis using the age-specific rate of mortality change with age. *Mathematical Population Studies*, 2 (4), pp. 245-267.

HUMPHREY, G.T. (1970), Mortality at the oldest ages. *Journal of the Institute of Actuaries*, 96, pp. 105-119.

JEUNE, B. (1994a), Centenarians - tail or tale? (in Danish). *Gerontology and Society*, 10 (1), pp. 4-6.

JEUNE, B. (1994b), *Morbus centenarius or sanitas longaevorum?* A critical review of centenarian studies. Population Studies of Aging no. 15. Centre for Health & Social Policy, Odense University.

KANNISTO, Väinö (1988), On the Survival of Centenarians and the Span of Life. *Population Studies*, 42, pp. 389-406.

KANNISTO, Väinö (1990), *Mortality of the elderly in late 19th and early 20th century Finland*. Tilastokeskus, Studies 175, Helsinki.

KANNISTO, Väinö (1994), *Development of Oldest-Old Mortality, 1950-1990*. Odense Monographs on Population Aging, 1. Odense University Press. Odense.

KOSKINEN, Seppo (1992), The explanation of regional differences in mortality from ischaemic heart disease in Finland. Paper presented at *IUSSP Seminar on Premature Adult Mortality in Developed Countries*, 1-5 June 1992, Taormina.

LA VECCHIA, Carlo, LEVI, Fabio, LUCCHINI, Franca and NEGRI, Eva (1993), Trends in mortality from cardiovascular and cerebrovascular disease. *Sozial- und Präventivmedizin*, 38, Suppl. 1. Basel.

LOUHIJA, Jukka (1994), *Finnish Centenarians*. A clinical epidemiological study. Helsinki.

MACKENBACH, J.P., LOOMAN, C.W.N., KUNST, A.E., HABBEMA, J.D.F. and VAN DER MAAS, P.J. (1988), Regional differences in decline of mortality from selected conditions: The Netherlands, 1969-1984. *International Journal of Epidemiology*, 17 (4), pp. 821-829.

MACKENBACH, J. P., LOOMAN, Casper W.N. and KUNST, Anton E. (1989), Geographic variation in the onset of decline of male ischemic heart disease mortality in the Netherlands. *American Journal of Public Health*, 79 (12), pp. 1621-1627.

MARTELIN, Tuija (1994), *Differential mortality at older ages*. Publications of the Finnish Demographic Society, 16. Helsinki.

MONTAGU, J.D. (1994), Length of life in the ancient world: a controlled study. *Journal of the Royal Society of Medicine*, 87 (1), pp. 25-26.

OLSHANSKY, S. Jay, CARNES, Bruce A. and CASSEL, Christine (1993), The aging of the human species. *Scientific American*, April 1993, pp. 18-24.

POPULATION REFERENCE BUREAU (1994), *1994 World Population Data Sheet*. Washington, D.C.

ROBINE, Jean-Marie (1993), Allongement de la vie et l'éspérance de vie sans incapacité. In: Jacques VALLIN (ed.), *L'avenir de l'éspérance de vie*. INED, Paris.

ROBINE, Jean-Marie, MATHERS, Colin D., BONE, Margaret and ROMIEU, Isabelle (eds., 1993), *Calculation of health expectancies; harmonization, consensus achieved and future perspectives*. Editions John Libbey Eurotext, Montrouge, France.

SMITH, David, W.E. (1993), *Human Longevity*. Oxford University Press.

THATCHER, A.R. (1987), Mortality at the highest ages. *Journal of the Institute of Actuaries*, 114, pp. 327-338.

THATCHER, A.R. (1992), Trends in numbers and mortality at high ages in England and Wales. *Population Studies*, 46, pp. 411-426.

THATCHER, A.R., VAUPEL, J., KANNISTO, V. (forthcoming), The force of mortality at ages 80-120. Odense Monographs on Population Aging.

U.S. BUREAU OF THE CENSUS (1991), *Global Aging*. Comparative Indicators and Future Trends. Washington, D.C.

VALKONEN, Tapani, MARTELIN, Tuija, RIMPELA, Arja, NOTKOLA, Veijo and SAVELA, Soili (1993), *Socio-economic mortality differences in Finland 1981-90*. Statistics Finland. Helsinki.

VALLIN, Jacques, (ed. 1993), *L'avenir de l'espérance de vie*. Acts of seminar of Société Internationale de Démographie, Economie et Sociologie Médicales, Paris 13. Sept. 1991. Presses Universitaires de France.

VARTIAINEN, Erkki, PUSKA, Pekka, PEKKANEN, Juha, TUOMILEHTO, Jaakko, JOUSILAHTI, Pekka (1994), Changes in risk factors explain changes in mortality from ischaemic heart disease in Finland. *British Medical Journal*, 2nd July 1994, 309:23-27.

VAUPEL, James W. and JEUNE, Bernard (1994), *The emergence and proliferation of centenarians*. Odense University. Population Studies of Aging No. 12. Odense.

VAUPEL, James W. and LUNDSTROM, Hans (1994), The future of mortality at older ages in developed countries. In: LUTZ, Wolfgang (ed.), *The Future Population of the World. What Can We Assume Today*. Earthscan Publications, London.

VINCENT, Paul (1951), La mortalité des vieillards. *Population*, 6 (2), pp. 181-204.

WALDRON, Ingrid (1993), Recent trends in sex mortality ratios for adults in developed countries. *Social Science and Medicine*, 36 (4), pp. 451-462.

WILMOTH, John (1995), The earliest centenarians. In: Jeune, B. and Vaupel, J.W. (eds.). *Exceptional Longevity*. Odense Monographs on Population Aging, no. 2. Odense University Press.

WING, Steve, HAYES, Carl, HEISS, Gerardo, JOHN, Esther, KNOWLES, Marilyn, RIGGAN, Wilson and TYROLER, R.A. (1986), Geographic Variation in the Onset of Decline of Ischemic Heart Disease Mortality in the United States. *American Journal of Public Health*, 76 (12), pp. 1404-1408.

WING, Steve, CASPER, Michele, RIGGAN, Wilson, HAYES, Carl, and TYROLER, R.A. (1988), Socioenvironmental Characteristics Associated with the Onset of Decline of Ischemic Heart Disease Mortality in the United States. *American Journal of Public Health*, 78 (8), pp. 923-926.

YU, Y.C., HORIUCHI, S. (1987), Population aging and juvenation in major regions of the world. Paper presented at the annual meeting of Population Association of America, Chicago, 30 April - 2 May 1987.

Annex tables
Väinö Kannisto, Zhenglian Wang, Kirill Andreev

List of Annex Tables on p.10

Annex Table 1. POPULATION AGED 80 AND OVER BY AGE AND SEX, 1950-1990, BY COUNTRY.

Australia

Sex and age	Population 1 January				
	1950	1960	1970	1980	1990
Male					
80 - 84	...	38 349	44 374	48 186	79 302
85 - 89	...	13 728	15 899	20 002	30 969
90 - 94	...	3 425	3 792	5 851	8 147
95 - 99	...	382	536	865	1 366
100 -	...	...	33	72	...
Total	...	55 884	64 634	74 976	119 784
Female					
80 - 84	...	64 075	77 800	97 555	137 123
85 - 89	...	26 580	33 067	50 361	72 047
90 - 94	...	7 657	9 594	16 994	27 153
95 - 99	...	1 055	1 635	3 168	6 008
100 -	...	...	146	325	...
Total	...	99 367	122 242	168 403	242 331
Both Sexes					
80 - 84	...	102 424	122 174	145 741	216 425
85 - 89	...	40 308	48 966	70 363	103 016
90 - 94	...	11 082	13 386	22 845	35 300
95 - 99	...	1 437	2 171	4 033	7 374
100 -	...	...	179	397	...
Total	...	155 251	186 876	243 379	362 115
Total population thousands	...	11 333	12 385	14 606	17 086
80 and over percent	...	1.37	1.51	1.67	2.12
100 and over per million	...	...	14.45	27.18	...

Annex Table 1. (cont.).

Austria

Sex and age	Population 1 January				
	1950	1960	1970	1980	1990
Male					
80 - 84	23 767	31 879	33 228	39 257	53 854
85 - 89	7 127	10 272	12 710	13 204	21 877
90 - 94	1 085	1 915	2 878	3 044	4 816
95 - 99	104	180	297	388	555
100 -	10	5	16	25	44
Total	32 093	44 251	49 129	55 918	81 146
Female					
80 - 84	34 249	54 249	70 877	92 585	119 642
85 - 89	11 301	18 501	28 001	38 029	58 244
90 - 94	2 090	3 794	6 772	9 782	16 132
95 - 99	229	410	816	1 322	2 456
100 -	7	20	47	83	188
Total	47 876	76 974	106 513	141 801	196 662
Both Sexes					
80 - 84	58 016	86 128	104 105	131 842	173 496
85 - 89	18 428	28 773	40 711	51 233	80 121
90 - 94	3 175	5 709	9 650	12 826	20 948
95 - 99	333	590	1 113	1 710	3 011
100 -	17	25	63	108	232
Total	79 969	121 225	155 642	197 719	277 808
Total population thousands	6 935	7 081	7 410	7 549	7 791
80 and over percent	1.15	1.71	2.10	2.62	3.57
100 and over per million	2.45	3.53	8.50	14.31	29.78

Annex Table 1. (cont.).

Belgium

Sex and age	Population 1 January				
	1950	1960	1970	1980	1990
Male					
80 - 84	34 919	47 815	49 474	55 825	67 008
85 - 89	10 649	16 595	19 884	20 801	27 698
90 - 94	1 827	2 806	4 447	5 324	7 418
95 - 99	175	310	570	755	1 074
100 -	...	...	...	43	93
Total	47 570	67 526	74 375	82 748	103 291
Female					
80 - 84	50 015	68 453	81 971	111 820	141 853
85 - 89	17 676	26 313	34 916	47 518	73 831
90 - 94	3 852	6 124	9 033	12 805	23 522
95 - 99	480	757	1 262	2 059	4 272
100 -	...	...	...	120	381
Total	72 023	101 647	127 182	174 322	243 859
Both Sexes					
80 - 84	84 934	116 268	131 445	167 645	208 861
85 - 89	28 325	42 908	54 800	68 319	101 529
90 - 94	5 679	8 930	13 480	18 129	30 940
95 - 99	655	1 067	1 832	2 814	5 346
100 -	...	...	...	163	474
Total	119 593	169 173	201 557	257 070	347 150
Total population thousands	8 639	9 153	9 655	9 842	9 845
80 and over percent	1.38	1.85	2.09	2.61	3.53
100 and over per million	...	...	...	16.56	48.15

Annex Table 1. (cont.).

Canada

Sex and age	Population 1 January				
	1950	1960	1970	1980	1990
Male					
80 - 84	45 918	67 669	87 168	90 234	124 990
85 - 89	17 385	25 569	38 687	43 294	54 954
90 - 94	4 217	6 494	10 294	15 400	16 408
95 - 99	645	983	1 608	3 039	3 640
Total	68 165	100 715	137 757	151 967	199 992
Female					
80 - 84	52 504	78 343	116 336	153 444	215 629
85 - 89	22 475	33 179	55 459	82 068	115 265
90 - 94	6 397	9 970	17 062	31 799	46 205
95 - 99	1 155	1 878	3 179	7 041	12 366
Total	82 531	123 370	192 036	274 352	389 465
Both Sexes					
80 - 84	98 422	146 012	203 504	243 678	340 619
85 - 89	39 860	58 748	94 146	125 362	170 219
90 - 94	10 614	16 464	27 356	47 199	62 613
95 - 99	1 800	2 861	4 787	10 080	16 006
Total	150 696	224 085	329 793	426 319	589 457
Total population thousands	13 712	17 814	21 175	23 895	26 065
80 - 99* percent	1.10	1.26	1.56	1.78	2.26

Annex Table 1. (cont.).

Czechoslovakia

Sex and age	Population 1 January				
	1950	1960	1970	1980	1990
Male					
80 - 84	34 777	40 657	45 537	57 382	77 250
85 - 89	10 252	13 857	16 025	17 090	25 296
90 - 94	1 810	2 476	3 413	3 567	5 204
95 - 99	168	238	376	415	425
Total	47 007	57 228	65 351	78 454	108 175
Female					
80 - 84	48 158	64 734	87 179	126 430	160 131
85 - 89	16 439	22 773	32 881	44 225	66 761
90 - 94	3 330	4 515	7 459	10 286	16 810
95 - 99	396	511	937	1 326	1 952
Total	68 323	92 533	128 456	182 267	245 654
Both Sexes					
80 - 84	82 935	105 391	132 716	183 812	237 381
85 - 89	26 691	36 630	48 906	61 315	92 057
90 - 94	5 140	6 991	10 872	13 853	22 014
95 - 99	564	749	1 313	1 741	2 377
Total	115 330	149 761	193 807	260 721	353 829
Total population thousands	12 389	13 654	14 375	15 274	15 661
80 - 99* percent	.93	1.10	1.35	1.71	2.26

Annex Table 1. (cont.).

Denmark

Sex and age	Population 1 January				
	1950	1960	1970	1980	1990
Male					
80 - 84	15 777	23 288	27 030	32 384	38 892
85 - 89	5 621	8 136	10 992	14 050	16 982
90 - 94	1 293	1 715	2 750	3 961	5 044
95 - 99	138	217	316	641	919
100 -	3	9	15	40	82
Total	22 832	33 365	41 103	51 076	61 919
Female					
80 - 84	19 458	27 110	37 625	55 528	71 656
85 - 89	7 273	10 122	15 891	26 257	38 350
90 - 94	1 855	2 494	4 099	7 953	13 564
95 - 99	241	308	586	1 346	2 674
100 -	14	10	31	116	243
Total	28 841	40 044	58 232	91 200	126 487
Both Sexes					
80 - 84	35 235	50 398	64 655	87 912	110 548
85 - 89	12 894	18 258	26 883	40 307	55 332
90 - 94	3 148	4 209	6 849	11 914	18 608
95 - 99	379	525	902	1 987	3 593
100 -	17	19	46	156	325
Total	51 673	73 409	99 335	142 276	188 406
Total population thousands	4 270	4 581	4 910	5 120	5 140
80 and over percent	1.21	1.60	2.02	2.78	3.67
100 and over per million	3.98	4.15	9.37	30.47	63.23

Annex Table 1. (cont.).

England & Wales

Sex and age	Population 1 January				
	1950	1960	1970	1980	1990
Male					
80 - 84	164 924	208 008	216 268	241 599	361 895
85 - 89	51 094	71 382	84 511	92 929	138 223
90 - 94	9 246	13 530	20 881	24 254	32 778
95 - 99	935	1 359	2 672	3 617	5 363
100 -	38	72	134	257	469
Total	226 237	294 351	324 466	362 656	538 728
Female					
80 - 84	282 402	395 766	484 739	582 471	741 239
85 - 89	108 300	158 148	227 383	284 412	397 821
90 - 94	26 101	40 262	68 328	94 538	140 095
95 - 99	3 554	6 119	11 347	18 362	30 560
100 -	227	459	935	1 883	3 573
Total	420 584	600 754	792 732	981 666	1 313 288
Both Sexes					
80 - 84	447 326	603 774	701 007	824 070	1 103 134
85 - 89	159 394	229 530	311 894	377 341	536 044
90 - 94	35 347	53 792	89 209	118 792	172 873
95 - 99	4 489	7 478	14 019	21 979	35 923
100 -	265	531	1 069	2 140	4 042
Total	646 821	895 105	1 117 198	1 344 322	1 852 016
Total population thousands	43 830	45 862	48 615	49 556	50 950
80 and over percent	1.48	1.95	2.30	2.71	3.63
100 and over per million	6.05	11.58	21.99	43.18	79.33

Annex Table 1. (cont.).

Estonia

Sex and age	Population 1 January				
	1950	1960	1970	1980	1990
Male					
80 - 84	2 766	3 405	4 311	4 861	6 349
80 - 89	1 002	1 231	1 620	1 761	2 490
90 - 94	169	236	330	462	528
95 - 99	18	29	47	76	75
100 -	...	...	...	...	2
Total	3 955	4 901	6 308	7 160	9 444
Female					
80 - 84	6 769	9 485	12 911	15 671	18 781
80 - 89	2 948	3 855	5 277	6 899	8 982
90 - 94	520	837	1 425	2 144	2 702
95 - 99	74	149	216	373	438
100 -	...	...	...	...	40
Total	10 311	14 326	19 829	25 087	30 943
Both Sexes					
80 - 84	9 535	12 890	17 222	20 532	25 130
80 - 89	3 950	5 086	6 897	8 660	11 472
90 - 94	689	1 073	1 755	2 606	3 230
95 - 99	92	178	263	449	513
100 -	...	...	...	...	42
Total	14 266	19 227	26 137	32 247	40 387
Total population thousands	1 097	1 206	1 352	1 472	1 572
80 and over percent	1.30	1.59	1.93	2.19	2.57
100 and over per million	...	...	...	...	26.72

Annex Table 1. (cont.).

Finland

Sex and age	Population 1 January				
	1950	1960	1970	1980	1990
Male					
80 - 84	6 336	9 359	11 256	16 398	26 003
85 - 89	2 279	3 011	3 493	5 363	9 379
90 - 94	391	486	744	1 206	2 294
95 - 99	28	66	74	127	274
100 -	2	2	9	5	22
Total	9 036	12 924	15 576	23 099	37 972
Female					
80 - 84	12 810	19 218	24 612	39 693	62 563
85 - 89	5 441	7 005	8 838	14 790	28 054
90 - 94	1 106	1 254	1 907	3 754	8 281
95 - 99	139	184	209	576	1 292
100 -	2	9	12	37	119
Total	19 498	27 670	35 578	58 850	100 309
Both Sexes					
80 - 84	19 146	28 577	35 868	56 091	88 566
85 - 89	7 720	10 016	12 331	20 153	37 433
90 - 94	1 497	1 740	2 651	4 960	10 575
95 - 99	167	250	283	703	1 566
100 -	4	11	21	42	141
Total	28 534	40 594	51 154	81 949	138 281
Total population thousands	3 986	4 429	4 615	4 772	4 986
80 and over percent	0.72	0.92	1.11	1.72	2.77
100 and over per million	1.00	2.48	4.55	8.80	28.28

Annex Table 1. (cont.).

France

Sex and age	Population 1 January				
	1950	1960	1970	1980	1990
Male					
80 - 84	164 330	212 648	227 031	290 692	410 434
85 - 89	51 780	72 601	89 221	102 841	179 069
90 - 94	8 814	13 344	21 686	27 960	43 786
95 - 99	863	1 322	2 740	4 295	5 926
100 -	47	67	155	264	466
Total	225 834	299 982	340 833	426 052	639 681
Female					
80 - 84	290 216	405 023	503 826	635 624	799 731
85 - 89	111 136	160 456	232 548	311 004	453 492
90 - 94	24 074	38 144	66 872	101 556	156 648
95 - 99	2 759	5 296	10 140	18 324	31 523
100 -	151	304	707	1 622	3 387
Total	428 336	609 223	814 093	1 068 130	1 444 781
Both Sexes					
80 - 84	454 546	617 671	730 857	926 316	1 210 165
85 - 89	162 916	233 057	321 769	413 845	632 561
90 - 94	32 888	51 488	88 558	129 516	200 434
95 - 99	3 622	6 618	12 880	22 619	37 449
100 -	198	371	862	1 886	3 853
Total	654 170	909 205	1 154 926	1 494 182	2 084 462
Total population thousands	41 736	45 542	50 545	53 743	56 735
80 and over percent	1.57	2.00	2.28	2.78	3.67
100 and over per million	4.74	8.15	17.05	35.09	67.91

Annex Table 1. (cont.).

Germany East

Sex and age	Population 1 January				
	1950	1960	1970	1980	1990
Male					
80 - 84	71 300	92 751	91 916	93 697	103 759
85 - 89	18 650	28 545	32 551	31 670	40 418
90 - 94	2 404	4 458	7 248	7 465	7 889
95 - 99	151	317	666	946	862
Total	92 505	126 071	132 381	133 778	152 928
Female					
80 - 84	99 875	136 142	170 791	211 916	250 098
85 - 89	30 356	43 445	60 330	81 782	107 081
90 - 94	5 025	8 379	13 840	18 906	27 471
95 - 99	342	761	1 409	2 262	3 456
Total	135 598	188 727	246 370	314 866	388 106
Both Sexes					
80 - 84	171 175	228 893	262 707	305 613	353 857
85 - 89	49 006	71 990	92 881	113 452	147 499
90 - 94	7 429	12 837	21 088	26 371	35 360
95 - 99	493	1 078	2 075	3 208	4 318
Total	228 103	314 798	378 751	448 644	541 034
Total population thousands	18 059	17 241	17 070	16 741	16 247
80 - 99* percent	1.26	1.83	2.22	2.68	3.33

Annex Table 1. (cont.).

Germany West

Sex and age	Population 1 January				
	1950	1960	1970	1980	1990
Male					
80 - 84	193 254	253 233	262 366	307 775	446 282
85 - 89	53 063	78 732	101 159	106 042	181 074
90 - 94	6 908	12 959	23 783	26 777	39 703
95 - 99	...	1 112	2 565	3 697	5 583
100 -	...	34	90	183	408
Total	253 225	346 070	389 963	444 474	673 050
Female					
80 - 84	249 947	352 862	496 589	729 065	1 047 783
85 - 89	77 400	112 777	184 979	298 608	497 125
90 - 94	11 881	22 478	44 174	73 949	147 529
95 - 99	...	2 366	5 193	9 877	26 617
100 -	...	85	228	539	2 120
Total	339 228	490 568	731 163	1 112 038	1 721 174
Both Sexes					
80 - 84	443 201	606 095	758 955	1 036 840	1 494 065
85 - 89	130 463	191 509	286 138	404 650	678 199
90 - 94	18 789	35 437	67 957	100 726	187 232
95 - 99	...	3 478	7 758	13 574	32 200
100 -	...	119	318	722	2 528
Total	592 453	836 638	1 121 126	1 556 512	2 394 224
Total population thousands	50 786	53 373	60 775	61 449	63 232
80 and over percent	1.17	1.57	1.84	2.53	3.79
100 and over per million	...	2.23	5.23	11.75	39.98

Annex Table 1. (cont.).

Hungary

Sex and age	Population 1 January				
	1950	1960	1970	1980	1990
Male					
80 - 84	25 526	32 487	38 653	49 744	57 685
85 - 89	7 893	9 714	13 838	15 415	20 063
90 - 94	1 318	1 932	2 622	3 378	4 441
95 - 99	146	192	231	399	466
Total	34 883	44 325	55 344	68 936	82 655
Female					
80 - 84	32 088	46 166	66 740	94 375	114 744
85 - 89	11 327	14 398	24 986	35 199	47 714
90 - 94	2 088	2 997	5 000	8 214	12 714
95 - 99	225	352	566	1 065	1 805
Total	45 728	63 913	97 292	138 853	176 977
Both Sexes					
80 - 84	57 614	78 653	105 393	144 119	172 429
85 - 89	19 220	24 112	38 824	50 614	67 777
90 - 94	3 406	4 929	7 622	11 592	17 155
95 - 99	371	544	797	1 464	2 271
Total	80 611	108 238	152 636	207 789	259 632
Total population thousands	9 334	9 999	10 322	10 704	10 365
80 - 99* percent	0.86	1.08	1.48	1.94	2.50

Annex Table 1. (cont.).

Iceland

Sex and age	Population 1 January				
	1950	1960	1970	1980	1990
Male					
80 - 84	...	657	835	1 223	1 402
85 - 89	...	245	295	596	754
90 - 94	...	75	98	163	252
95 - 99	...	16	18	25	51
100 -	...	...	2	...	2
Total	...	993	1 248	2 007	2 461
Female					
80 - 84	...	900	1 090	1 733	2 024
85 - 89	...	443	459	935	1 208
90 - 94	...	155	151	272	479
95 - 99	...	32	30	56	134
100 -	...	3	2	6	15
Total	...	1 533	1 732	3 002	3 860
Both Sexes					
80 - 84	...	1 557	1 925	2 956	3 426
85 - 89	...	688	754	1 531	1 962
90 - 94	...	230	249	435	731
95 - 99	...	48	48	81	185
100 -	...	...	4	...	17
Total	...	2 526	2 980	5 009	6 321
Total population thousands	...	176	205	227	255
80 and over percent	...	1.44	1.45	2.21	2.48
100 and over per million	...	...	19.51	...	66.67

Annex Table 1. (cont.).

Ireland

Sex and age	Population 1 January				
	1950	1960	1970	1980	1990
Male					
80 - 84	14 573	17 871	16 115	15 722	18 000
85 - 89	4 330	6 524	6 702	6 313	7 673
90 - 94	965	1 390	1 694	1 718	1 749
95 - 99	157	174	247	257	207
100 -	12	7	6	11	6
Total	20 037	25 966	24 764	24 021	27 635
Female					
80 - 84	16 163	21 090	21 631	25 330	28 342
85 - 89	5 622	8 591	10 066	11 453	15 120
90 - 94	1 479	2 239	3 178	3 542	5 113
95 - 99	283	356	554	644	944
100 -	19	24	25	54	81
Total	23 566	32 300	35 454	41 023	49 600
Both Sexes					
80 - 84	30 736	38 961	37 746	41 052	46 342
85 - 89	9 952	15 115	16 768	17 766	22 793
90 - 94	2 444	3 629	4 872	5 260	6 862
95 - 99	440	530	801	901	1 151
100 -	31	31	31	65	87
Total	43 603	58 266	60 218	65 044	77 235
Total population thousands	2 969	2 834	2 940	3 384	3 509
80 and over percent	1.47	2.06	2.05	1.92	2.20
100 and over per million	10.44	10.94	10.54	19.21	24.79

Annex Table 1. (cont.).

Italy

Sex and age	Population 1 January				
	1950	1960	1970	1980	1990
Male					
80 - 84	177 962	224 471	234 730	261 480	378 868
85 - 89	61 882	84 873	93 071	102 140	149 119
90 - 94	10 731	19 039	21 834	27 783	37 381
95 - 99	833	2 162	2 337	4 245	5 396
100 -	22	64	119	233	451
Total	251 430	330 609	352 091	395 881	571 215
Female					
80 - 84	222 118	292 134	384 307	514 413	700 052
85 - 89	84 501	119 426	154 911	226 243	344 651
90 - 94	17 967	30 618	38 468	64 103	109 295
95 - 99	1 839	4 359	5 143	10 007	18 704
100 -	82	201	366	645	1 596
Total	326 507	446 738	583 195	815 411	1 174 298
Both Sexes					
80 - 84	400 080	516 605	619 037	775 893	1 078 920
85 - 89	146 383	204 299	247 982	328 383	493 770
90 - 94	28 698	49 657	60 302	91 886	146 676
95 - 99	2 672	6 521	7 480	14 252	24 100
100 -	104	265	485	878	2 047
Total	577 937	777 347	935 286	1 211 292	1 745 513
Total population thousands	47 321	49 361	53 445	56 354	57 590
80 and over percent	1.22	1.57	1.75	2.15	3.03
100 and over per million	2.20	5.37	9.07	15.58	35.54

Annex Table 1. (cont.).

Japan

Sex and age	Population 1 January				
	1950	1960	1970	1980	1990
Male					
80 - 84	93 873	164 655	233 934	401 590	650 315
85 - 89	22 488	44 392	68 817	129 656	268 508
90 - 94	3 831	7 112	13 242	27 342	67 071
95 - 99	399	538	1 352	2 942	8 941
100 -	...	32	82	171	666
Total	120 591	216 729	317 427	561 701	995 501
Female					
80 - 84	175 674	301 953	399 819	648 769	1 098 745
85 - 89	50 028	98 438	155 357	252 137	535 616
90 - 94	10 040	20 116	38 540	69 193	165 128
95 - 99	1 096	2 050	4 579	9 742	25 937
100 -	61	123	263	747	2 460
Total	236 899	422 680	598 558	980 588	1 827 886
Both Sexes					
80 - 84	269 547	466 608	633 753	1 050 359	1 749 060
85 - 89	72 516	142 830	224 174	381 793	804 124
90 - 94	13 871	27 228	51 782	96 535	232 199
95 - 99	1 495	2 588	5 931	12 684	34 878
100 -	...	155	345	918	3 126
Total	357 490	639 409	915 985	1 542 289	2 823 387
Total population thousands	82 900	93 200	103 755	116 348	123 326
80 and over percent	0.43	0.69	0.88	1.33	2.29
100 and over per million	...	1.66	3.33	7.89	25.35

Annex Table 1. (cont.).

Latvia

Sex and age	Population 1 January				
	1950	1960	1970	1980	1990
Male					
80 - 84	5 098	7 555	8 550	8 674	12 554
85 - 89	1 943	2 984	3 894	3 945	5 061
90 - 94	362	513	944	1 078	1 009
95 - 99	48	101	188	257	249
Total	7 451	11 153	13 576	13 954	18 873
Female					
80 - 84	11 378	16 667	22 281	26 623	32 089
85 - 89	5 199	7 231	9 695	12 209	15 812
90 - 94	1 190	1 817	2 863	3 911	4 444
95 - 99	244	425	558	775	907
Total	18 011	26 140	35 397	43 518	53 252
Both Sexes					
80 - 84	16 476	24 222	30 831	35 297	44 643
85 - 89	7 142	10 215	13 589	16 154	20 873
90 - 94	1 552	2 330	3 807	4 989	5 453
95 - 99	292	526	746	1 032	1 156
Total	25 462	37 293	48 973	57 472	72 125
Total population thousands	1 884	2 104	2 352	2 509	2 673
80 - 99* percent	1.35	1.77	2.08	2.29	2.70

Annex Table 1. (cont.).

Luxembourg

Sex and age	Population 1 January				
	1950	1960	1970	1980	1990
Male					
80 - 84	1 136	1 428	1 519	1 748	2 184
85 - 89	347	452	565	579	857
90 - 94	51	64	135	149	214
95 - 99	1	4	20	20	20
Total	1 535	1 948	2 239	2 496	3 275
Female					
80 - 84	1 391	1 934	2 350	3 513	4 950
85 - 89	487	644	919	1 386	2 322
90 - 94	119	140	227	332	677
95 - 99	6	17	26	42	114
Total	2 003	2 735	3 522	5 273	8 063
Both Sexes					
80 - 84	2 527	3 362	3 869	5 261	7 134
85 - 89	834	1 096	1 484	1 965	3 179
90 - 94	170	204	362	481	891
95 - 99	7	21	46	62	134
Total	3 538	4 683	5 761	7 769	11 338
Total population thousands	304	314	340	364	379
80 - 99* percent	1.16	1.49	1.69	2.13	2.99

Annex Table 1. (cont.).

Netherlands

Sex and age	Population 1 January				
	1950	1960	1970	1980	1990
Male					
80 - 84	...	49 400	62 486	69 774	82 144
85 - 89	...	17 366	25 391	31 528	36 490
90 - 94	...	3 682	6 750	9 594	11 206
95 - 99	...	405	879	1 512	2 248
100 -	...	21	60	123	...
Total	...	70 874	95 566	112 531	132 088
Female					
80 - 84	...	57 170	81 628	120 944	167 917
85 - 89	...	21 329	34 568	56 437	89 708
90 - 94	...	5 205	9 384	16 962	31 105
95 - 99	...	721	1 491	2 820	6 328
100 -	...	41	99	269	...
Total	...	84 466	127 170	197 432	295 058
Both Sexes					
80 - 84	...	106 570	144 114	190 718	250 061
85 - 89	...	38 695	59 959	87 965	126 198
90 - 94	...	8 887	16 134	26 556	42 311
95 - 99	...	1 126	2 370	4 332	8 576
100 -	...	62	159	392	...
Total	...	155 340	222 736	309 963	427 146
Total population thousands	...	11 480	12 950	14 087	14 885
80 and over percent	...	1.35	1.72	2.20	2.87
100 and over per million	...	5.40	12.28	27.83	...

Annex Table 1. (cont.).

New Zealand

Sex and age	Population 1 January				
	1950	1960	1970	1980	1990
Male					
80 - 84	6 638	10 163	10 453	10 527	16 041
85 - 89	2 113	3 602	4 618	4 202	6 265
90 - 94	501	832	1 192	1 375	1 508
95 - 99	68	95	163	242	235
100 -	7	7	11	14	19
Total	9 327	14 699	16 437	16 360	24 068
Female					
80 - 84	8 224	13 695	17 444	20 039	28 474
85 - 89	2 963	5 221	8 399	10 568	13 479
90 - 94	784	1 452	2 488	3 848	4 692
95 - 99	133	200	378	805	1 202
100 -	7	9	39	67	177
Total	12 111	20 577	28 748	35 327	48 024
Both Sexes					
80 - 84	14 862	23 858	27 897	30 566	44 515
85 - 89	5 076	8 823	13 017	14 770	19 744
90 - 94	1 285	2 284	3 680	5 223	6 200
95 - 99	201	295	541	1 047	1 437
100 -	14	16	50	81	196
Total	21 438	35 276	45 185	51 687	72 092
Total population thousands	1 795	2 219	2 595	2 878	3 063
80 and over percent	1.19	1.59	1.74	1.80	2.35
100 and over per million	7.80	7.21	19.27	28.14	63.99

Annex Table 1. (cont.).

Norway

Sex and age	Population 1 January				
	1950	1960	1970	1980	1990
Male					
80 - 84	14 369	19 492	21 503	27 697	32 526
85 - 89	6 299	7 869	8 762	11 652	14 507
90 - 94	1 689	1 997	2 726	3 176	4 518
95 - 99	243	293	389	490	767
100 -	17	20	21	46	74
Total	22 617	29 671	33 401	43 061	52 392
Female					
80 - 84	20 114	25 602	31 455	45 683	58 488
85 - 89	9 374	10 974	14 111	21 096	31 856
90 - 94	2 741	3 276	4 413	6 243	11 102
95 - 99	498	560	724	1 165	2 215
100 -	31	53	48	108	226
Total	32 758	40 465	50 751	74 295	103 887
Both Sexes					
80 - 84	34 483	45 094	52 958	73 380	91 014
85 - 89	15 673	18 843	22 873	32 748	46 363
90 - 94	4 430	5 273	7 139	9 419	15 620
95 - 99	741	853	1 113	1 655	2 982
100 -	48	73	69	154	300
Total	55 375	70 136	84 152	117 356	156 279
Total population thousands	3 265	3 586	3 865	4 080	4 234
80 and over percent	1.70	1.96	2.18	2.88	3.69
100 and over per million	14.70	20.36	17.85	37.75	70.85

Annex Table 1. (cont.).

Poland

Sex and age	Population 1 January				
	1950	1960	1970	1980	1990
Male					
80 - 84	...	...	70 744	105 646	159 807
85 - 89	...	...	23 314	33 535	54 096
90 - 94	...	...	5 138	7 781	11 056
95 - 99	...	...	804	1 104	1 665
Total	...	...	100 000	148 066	226 624
Female					
80 - 84	...	...	149 996	230 296	330 205
85 - 89	...	...	55 960	86 362	136 859
90 - 94	...	...	13 839	23 257	34 581
95 - 99	...	...	2 100	3 481	5 407
Total	...	...	221 895	343 396	507 052
Both Sexes					
80 - 84	...	...	220 740	335 942	490 012
85 - 89	...	...	79 274	119 897	190 955
90 - 94	...	...	18 977	31 038	45 637
95 - 99	...	...	2 904	4 585	7 072
Total	...	...	321 895	491 462	733 676
Total population thousands	...	...	32 642	35 418	38 020
80 - 99* percent	...	...	0.99	1.39	1.93

Annex Table 1. (cont.).

Portugal

Sex and age	Population 1 January				
	1950	1960	1970	1980	1990
Male					
80 - 84	18 382	24 575	30 664	37 640	57 100
85 - 89	6 158	7 541	9 942	13 582	19 541
90 - 94	1 463	1 431	2 079	2 990	4 454
95 - 99	319	166	221	361	608
100 -	29	19	14	15	40
Total	26 351	33 732	42 920	54 588	81 743
Female					
80 - 84	37 148	48 754	61 325	74 261	104 800
85 - 89	15 902	19 326	24 696	32 738	44 564
90 - 94	4 934	4 826	6 582	9 003	13 615
95 - 99	1 199	848	1 115	1 418	2 597
100 -	195	89	92	112	229
Total	59 378	73 843	93 810	117 532	165 805
Both Sexes					
80 - 84	55 530	73 329	91 989	111 901	161 900
85 - 89	22 060	26 867	34 638	46 320	64 105
90 - 94	6 397	6 257	8 661	11 993	18 069
95 - 99	1 518	1 014	1 336	1 779	3 205
100 -	224	108	106	127	269
Total	85 729	107 575	136 730	172 120	247 548
Total population thousands	8 405	8 921	9 070	9 865	10 496
80 and over percent	1.02	1.21	1.51	1.74	2.36
100 and over per million	26.65	12.11	11.69	12.87	25.63

Annex Table 1. (cont.).

Scotland

Sex and age	Population 1 January				
	1950	1960	1970	1980	1990
Male					
80 - 84	17 769	22 070	20 385	21 936	32 105
85 - 89	5 092	7 164	8 164	8 111	11 555
90 - 94	961	1 312	1 914	2 083	2 429
95 - 99	85	112	206	291	374
Total	23 907	30 658	30 669	32 421	46 463
Female					
80 - 84	28 692	36 669	44 199	55 682	69 831
85 - 89	10 781	13 856	19 253	25 882	35 817
90 - 94	2 544	3 314	5 419	8 018	11 794
95 - 99	294	442	814	1 436	2 403
Total	42 311	54 281	69 685	91 018	119 845
Both Sexes					
80 - 84	46 461	58 739	64 584	77 618	101 936
85 - 89	15 873	21 020	27 417	33 993	47 372
90 - 94	3 505	4 626	7 333	10 101	14 223
95 - 99	379	554	1 020	1 727	2 777
Total	66 218	84 939	100 354	123 439	166 308
Total population thousands	5 126	5 254	5 210	5 160	4 970
80 - 99* percent	1.29	1.62	1.93	2.39	3.35

Annex Table 1. (cont.).

Singapore_Chinese

Sex and age	Population 1 January				
	1950	1960	1970	1980	1990
Male					
80 - 84	...	...	...	3 108	5 733
85 - 89	...	...	...	870	2 048
90 - 94	...	...	...	182	454
95 - 99	...	...	...	23	79
100 -	...	...	...	...	4
Total	...	...	...	4 183	8 318
Female					
80 - 84	...	...	...	5 767	9 303
85 - 89	...	...	...	2 444	4 209
90 - 94	...	...	...	730	1 258
95 - 99	...	...	...	147	305
100 -	...	...	...	16	41
Total	...	...	...	9 104	15 116
Both Sexes					
80 - 84	...	...	...	8 875	15 036
85 - 89	...	...	...	3 314	6 257
90 - 94	...	...	...	912	1 712
95 - 99	...	...	...	170	384
100 -	...	...	...	...	45
Total	...	...	...	13 287	23 434
Total population thousands	...	...	...	2 472	2 705
80 and over percent	...	...	...	0.54	0.87
100 and over per million	...	...	...	...	16.64

Annex Table 1. (cont.).

Spain

Sex and age	Population 1 January				
	1950	1960	1970	1980	1990
Male					
80 - 84	66 046	86 982	119 066	155 812	218 131
85 - 89	23 061	29 114	42 279	60 853	86 241
90 - 94	5 191	6 720	10 038	15 444	23 852
95 - 99	855	1 173	1 392	2 360	4 702
100 -	53	73	110	172	117
Total	95 206	124 062	172 885	234 641	333 043
Female					
80 - 84	116 593	157 929	212 601	278 535	382 928
85 - 89	49 399	63 599	88 271	130 021	176 404
90 - 94	15 249	18 244	26 576	38 426	56 692
95 - 99	3 419	3 914	5 117	6 887	11 741
100 -	385	359	487	707	276
Total	185 045	244 045	333 052	454 576	628 041
Both Sexes					
80 - 84	182 639	244 911	331 667	434 347	601 059
85 - 89	72 460	92 713	130 550	190 874	262 645
90 - 94	20 440	24 964	36 614	53 870	80 544
95 - 99	4 274	5 087	6 509	9 247	16 443
100 -	438	432	597	879	393
Total	280 251	368 107	505 937	689 217	961 084
Total population thousands	27 868	80 128	33 600	37 306	38 650
80 and over percent	1.01	0.46	1.51	1.85	2.49
100 and over per million	15.72	5.39	17.77	23.56	10.17

Annex Table 1. (cont.).

Sweden

Sex and age	Population 1 January				
	1950	1960	1970	1980	1990
Male					
80 - 84	30 405	42 143	49 726	60 412	80 744
85 - 89	12 717	14 976	19 579	24 515	33 598
90 - 94	2 837	3 189	5 068	6 847	8 966
95 - 99	302	432	630	1 017	1 429
100 -	13	23	32	94	114
Total	46 274	60 763	75 035	92 885	124 851
Female					
80 - 84	38 360	51 751	70 165	97 435	134 387
85 - 89	17 339	19 723	29 192	46 656	70 985
90 - 94	4 225	4 918	8 061	14 569	23 824
95 - 99	567	755	1 203	2 649	4 625
100 -	32	50	79	215	465
Total	60 523	77 197	108 700	161 524	234 286
Both Sexes					
80 - 84	68 765	93 894	119 891	157 847	215 131
85 - 89	30 056	34 699	48 771	71 171	104 583
90 - 94	7 062	8 107	13 129	21 416	32 790
95 - 99	869	1 187	1 833	3 666	6 054
100 -	45	73	111	309	579
Total	106 797	137 960	183 735	254 409	359 137
Total population thousands	7 014	7 480	8 005	8 302	8 526
80 and over percent	1.52	1.84	2.30	3.06	4.21
100 and over per million	6.42	9.76	13.87	37.22	67.91

Annex Table 1. (cont.).

Switzerland

Sex and age	Population 1 January				
	1950	1960	1970	1980	1990
Male					
80 - 84	14 424	21 833	25 525	34 902	49 842
85 - 89	4 470	6 998	10 073	13 457	21 363
90 - 94	731	1 248	2 245	3 391	5 396
95 - 99	65	135	232	483	820
100 -	2	8	9	33	68
Total	19 692	30 222	38 084	52 266	77 489
Female					
80 - 84	22 766	34 968	44 850	68 103	95 049
85 - 89	8 187	12 376	18 999	30 231	51 250
90 - 94	1 606	2 766	4 889	8 710	16 937
95 - 99	171	354	597	1 507	2 980
100 -	8	21	40	90	270
Total	32 738	50 485	69 375	108 641	166 486
Both Sexes					
80 - 84	37 190	56 801	70 375	103 005	144 891
85 - 89	12 657	19 374	29 072	43 688	72 613
90 - 94	2 337	4 014	7 134	12 101	22 333
95 - 99	236	489	829	1 990	3 800
100 -	10	29	49	123	338
Total	52 430	80 707	107 459	160 907	243 975
Total population thousands	4 694	5 351	6 165	6 368	6 680
80 and over percent	1.12	1.51	1.74	2.53	3.65
100 and over per million	2.13	5.42	7.95	19.32	50.60

Annex Table 2 DECENNIAL LIFE TABLES BY COUNTRY.

The 1980-1990 (or latest) life table is given in this Table for each of 30 countries. A full set of 108 decennial life tables since 1950 is available on request from the Secretariat, Aging Research Center, Winsløwparken 17, Odense Universitet, DK-5000 Odense C, Denmark, and contains the following:

Australia	England & Wales	Hungary	Luxembourg	Scotland
1970-1980	1950-1960	1950-1960	1953-1960	1950-1960
1980-1986	1960-1970	1960-1970	1960-1970	1960-1970
	1970-1980	1970-1980	1970-1980	1970-1980
Austria	1980-1990	1980-1990	1980-1989	1980-1990
1950-1960				
1960-1970	Estonia	Iceland	Netherlands	Singapore
1970-1980	1950-1960	1961-1970	1960-1970	1982-1990
1980-1990	1960-1970	1970-1980	1970-1980	
	1970-1980	1980-1989	1980-1990	Spain
Belgium	1980-1990			1950-1960
1950-1960		Ireland	New Zealand	1960-1970
1960-1970	Finland	1950-1960	1950-1960	1970-1980
1970-1980	1950-1960	1960-1970	1960-1970	1980-1986
1980-1990	1960-1970	1970-1980	1970-1980	
	1970-1980	1980-1989	1980-1990	Sweden
Canada	1980-1990			1950-1960
1950-1960		Italy	Norway	1960-1970
1960-1970	France	1952-1960	1950-1960	1970-1980
1970-1980	1950-1960	1960-1970	1960-1970	1980-1990
1980-1988	1960-1970	1970-1980	1970-1980	
	1970-1980	1980-1989	1980-1990	Switzerland
Chile	1980-1990			1950-1960
1980-1989		Japan	Poland	1960-1970
	Germany, East	1950-1960	1971-1980	1970-1980
Czechoslovakia	1954-1960	1960-1970	1980-1990	1980-1990
1950-1960	1960-1970	1970-1980		
1960-1970	1970-1980	1980-1990	Portugal	
1970-1980	1980-1990		1950-1960	
1980-1990		Latvia	1960-1970	
	Germany, West	1950-1960	1970-1980	
Denmark	1956-1960	1960-1970	1980-1990	
1950-1960	1964-1970	1970-1980		
1960-1970	1970-1980	1980-1990		
1970-1980	1980-1990			
1980-1990				

Annex Table 2 (cont.). Australia   1980 - 1986

Male

x	N_x	D_x	q_x	l_x	d_x	e_x
80	81225	7970	0.0981	1.0000	0.0981	6.4148
81	70332	7048	0.1002	0.9019	0.0904	6.0583
82	59940	6772	0.1130	0.8115	0.0917	5.6773
83	50391	6270	0.1244	0.7198	0.0896	5.3367
84	41626	5594	0.1344	0.6303	0.0847	5.0241
85	33564	4794	0.1428	0.5456	0.0779	4.7265
86	27318	4247	0.1555	0.4676	0.0727	4.4307
87	22413	3819	0.1704	0.3949	0.0673	4.1543
88	18290	3190	0.1744	0.3276	0.0571	3.9049
89	14817	2966	0.2002	0.2705	0.0541	3.6242
90	11673	2486	0.2130	0.2163	0.0461	3.4061
91	9039	2032	0.2248	0.1703	0.0383	3.1925
92	6871	1730	0.2518	0.1320	0.0332	2.9733
93	4971	1316	0.2647	0.0988	0.0261	2.8055
94	3523	988	0.2804	0.0726	0.0204	2.6356
95	2412	717	0.2973	0.0523	0.0155	2.4680
96	1620	523	0.3228	0.0367	0.0119	2.3005
97	1053	348	0.3305	0.0249	0.0082	2.1589
98	665	243	0.3654	0.0166	0.0061	1.9777
99	383	166	0.4334	0.0106	0.0046	1.8286
100	204	83	0.4069	0.0060	0.0024	1.8449
101	119	43	0.3613	0.0036	0.0013	1.7675
102	75	41	0.5467	0.0023	0.0012	1.4846
103	35	14	0.4000	0.0010	0.0004	1.6720
104	20	7	0.3500	0.0006	0.0002	1.4533
105	15	9	0.6000	0.0004	0.0002	0.9667
106	6	5	0.8333	0.0002	0.0001	0.6667
107	2	2	1.0000	0.0000	0.0000	0.5000

Female

x	N_x	D_x	q_x	l_x	d_x	e_x
80	136601	7879	0.0577	1.0000	0.0577	8.2767
81	125736	7989	0.0635	0.9423	0.0599	7.7528
82	114089	8302	0.0728	0.8824	0.0642	7.2448
83	102674	8343	0.0813	0.8182	0.0665	6.7742
84	90576	8182	0.0903	0.7517	0.0679	6.3291
85	77927	7841	0.1006	0.6838	0.0688	5.9079
86	67432	7669	0.1137	0.6150	0.0699	5.5130
87	57883	7116	0.1229	0.5451	0.0670	5.1562
88	49365	6518	0.1320	0.4781	0.0631	4.8089
89	41347	6276	0.1518	0.4149	0.0630	4.4644
90	33896	5416	0.1598	0.3520	0.0562	4.1738
91	27408	4807	0.1754	0.2957	0.0519	3.8724
92	21498	4153	0.1932	0.2439	0.0471	3.5897
93	16375	3517	0.2148	0.1968	0.0423	3.3295
94	12053	2750	0.2282	0.1545	0.0352	3.1035
95	8654	2166	0.2503	0.1192	0.0298	2.8731
96	5995	1603	0.2674	0.0894	0.0239	2.6653
97	4061	1215	0.2992	0.0655	0.0196	2.4556
98	2640	820	0.3106	0.0459	0.0143	2.2905
99	1662	614	0.3694	0.0316	0.0117	2.0972
100	968	354	0.3657	0.0200	0.0073	2.0329
101	582	231	0.3969	0.0127	0.0050	1.9167
102	347	138	0.3977	0.0076	0.0030	1.8491
103	203	89	0.4384	0.0046	0.0020	1.7398
104	115	48	0.4174	0.0026	0.0011	1.7078
105	70	30	0.4286	0.0015	0.0006	1.5730
106	38	15	0.3947	0.0009	0.0003	1.3778
107	22	14	0.6364	0.0005	0.0003	0.9502
108	7	6	0.8571	0.0002	0.0002	0.7381
109	3	2	0.6667	0.0000	0.0000	1.1667

Annex Table 2 (cont.).   Austria   1980 - 1990

	Male								Female					
x	N_x	D_x	q_x	l_x	d_x	e_x		x	N_x	D_x	q_x	l_x	d_x	e_x
80	136237	14666	0.1077	1.0000	0.1077	5.8594		80	280002	20873	0.0745	1.0000	0.0745	6.9880
81	118727	14003	0.1179	0.8923	0.1052	5.5060		81	253529	21280	0.0839	0.9255	0.0777	6.5106
82	101762	12894	0.1267	0.7871	0.0997	5.1753		82	226835	21240	0.0936	0.8478	0.0794	6.0613
83	85936	11957	0.1391	0.6874	0.0956	4.8537		83	199690	21089	0.1056	0.7684	0.0811	5.6358
84	71010	10757	0.1515	0.5917	0.0896	4.5573		84	172825	20188	0.1168	0.6872	0.0803	5.2423
85	57604	9445	0.1640	0.5021	0.0823	4.2817		85	148400	19272	0.1299	0.6070	0.0788	4.8695
86	45765	8083	0.1766	0.4198	0.0741	4.0234		86	124336	18174	0.1462	0.5281	0.0772	4.5216
87	35753	6803	0.1903	0.3456	0.0658	3.7791		87	101932	16401	0.1609	0.4509	0.0726	4.2101
88	27234	5469	0.2008	0.2799	0.0562	3.5497		88	81563	14445	0.1771	0.3784	0.0670	3.9215
89	20446	4542	0.2221	0.2237	0.0497	3.3160		89	63475	12287	0.1936	0.3114	0.0603	3.6579
90	15082	3590	0.2380	0.1740	0.0414	3.1203		90	48600	10199	0.2099	0.2511	0.0527	3.4159
91	10955	2738	0.2499	0.1326	0.0331	2.9388		91	36464	8255	0.2264	0.1984	0.0449	3.1903
92	7790	2099	0.2694	0.0994	0.0268	2.7514		92	26768	6528	0.2439	0.1535	0.0374	2.9776
93	5361	1493	0.2785	0.0726	0.0202	2.5818		93	19156	5038	0.2630	0.1161	0.0305	2.7767
94	3671	1194	0.3253	0.0524	0.0170	2.3854		94	13291	3855	0.2900	0.0855	0.0248	2.5892
95	2362	769	0.3256	0.0354	0.0115	2.2942		95	8934	2770	0.3101	0.0607	0.0188	2.4427
96	1550	560	0.3613	0.0239	0.0086	2.1604		96	5703	1849	0.3242	0.0419	0.0136	2.3158
97	952	363	0.3813	0.0152	0.0058	2.0996		97	3628	1235	0.3404	0.0283	0.0096	2.1869
98	563	206	0.3659	0.0094	0.0034	2.0854		98	2245	816	0.3635	0.0187	0.0068	2.0575
99	331	111	0.3353	0.0060	0.0020	2.0002		99	1360	524	0.3853	0.0119	0.0046	1.9468
100	203	86	0.4236	0.0040	0.0017	1.7572		100	793	313	0.3947	0.0073	0.0029	1.8537
101	109	49	0.4495	0.0023	0.0010	1.6813		101	440	173	0.3932	0.0044	0.0017	1.7364
102	57	24	0.4211	0.0013	0.0005	1.6460		102	238	111	0.4664	0.0027	0.0013	1.5375
103	27	13	0.4815	0.0007	0.0004	1.4794		103	119	57	0.4790	0.0014	0.0007	1.4443
104	15	7	0.4667	0.0004	0.0002	1.3889		104	57	30	0.5263	0.0007	0.0004	1.3124
105	8	4	0.5000	0.0002	0.0001	1.1667		105	25	14	0.5600	0.0004	0.0002	1.2150
106	3	2	0.6667	0.0001	0.0001	0.8333		106	10	5	0.5000	0.0002	0.0001	1.1250
107	1	1	1.0000	0.0000	0.0000	0.5000		107	4	3	0.7500	0.0001	0.0001	0.7500
108	1	0	0.0000	0.0000	0.0000	1.5000		108	1	1	1.0000	0.0000	0.0000	0.5000
109	1	1	1.0000	0.0000	0.0000	0.5000								

Annex Table 2 (cont.). Belgium 1980 - 1990

Male

x	N_x	D_x	q_x	l_x	d_x	e_x
80	173201	18662	0.1077	1.0000	0.1077	5.9185
81	152077	17889	0.1176	0.8923	0.1050	5.5728
82	131611	16680	0.1267	0.7873	0.0998	5.2490
83	112669	15563	0.1381	0.6875	0.0950	4.9383
84	95421	14171	0.1485	0.5925	0.0880	4.6496
85	79352	12784	0.1611	0.5045	0.0813	4.3733
86	64870	11203	0.1727	0.4233	0.0731	4.1172
87	52081	9734	0.1869	0.3502	0.0654	3.8723
88	41065	8136	0.1981	0.2847	0.0564	3.6474
89	31895	6741	0.2113	0.2283	0.0483	3.4251
90	24347	5610	0.2304	0.1801	0.0415	3.2090
91	18117	4522	0.2496	0.1386	0.0346	3.0201
92	13133	3390	0.2581	0.1040	0.0268	2.8583
93	9423	2668	0.2831	0.0771	0.0218	2.6789
94	6422	1868	0.2909	0.0553	0.0161	2.5395
95	4378	1417	0.3237	0.0392	0.0127	2.3760
96	2861	953	0.3331	0.0265	0.0088	2.2738
97	1853	649	0.3502	0.0177	0.0062	2.1597
98	1156	397	0.3434	0.0115	0.0039	2.0544
99	735	284	0.3864	0.0075	0.0029	1.8675
100	422	183	0.4336	0.0046	0.0020	1.7286
101	217	97	0.4470	0.0026	0.0012	1.6692
102	115	50	0.4348	0.0015	0.0006	1.6144
103	62	27	0.4355	0.0008	0.0004	1.4716
104	32	17	0.5313	0.0005	0.0002	1.2212
105	13	9	0.6923	0.0002	0.0002	1.0385
106	4	2	0.5000	0.0001	0.0000	1.2500
107	2	1	0.5000	0.0000	0.0000	1.0000
108	1	1	1.0000	0.0000	0.0000	0.5000

Female

x	N_x	D_x	q_x	l_x	d_x	e_x
80	328892	22549	0.0686	1.0000	0.0686	7.4766
81	300744	22896	0.0761	0.9314	0.0709	6.9901
82	271315	23171	0.0854	0.8605	0.0735	6.5249
83	241990	23160	0.0957	0.7870	0.0753	6.0875
84	212957	22746	0.1068	0.7117	0.0760	5.6789
85	184211	21855	0.1186	0.6357	0.0754	5.2982
86	156292	20610	0.1319	0.5603	0.0739	4.9441
87	130537	18747	0.1436	0.4864	0.0699	4.6191
88	106547	16746	0.1572	0.4165	0.0655	4.3099
89	84851	14766	0.1740	0.3511	0.0611	4.0204
90	66384	12694	0.1912	0.2900	0.0554	3.7620
91	50613	10192	0.2014	0.2345	0.0472	3.5333
92	38132	8507	0.2231	0.1873	0.0418	3.2981
93	27775	6500	0.2340	0.1455	0.0341	3.1016
94	19880	5177	0.2604	0.1115	0.0290	2.8965
95	13587	3656	0.2691	0.0824	0.0222	2.7403
96	9130	2712	0.2970	0.0603	0.0179	2.5650
97	5976	1855	0.3104	0.0424	0.0131	2.4376
98	3759	1213	0.3227	0.0292	0.0094	2.3098
99	2336	792	0.3390	0.0198	0.0067	2.1721
100	1419	495	0.3488	0.0131	0.0046	2.0298
101	812	310	0.3818	0.0085	0.0033	1.8493
102	469	193	0.4115	0.0053	0.0022	1.6826
103	245	114	0.4653	0.0031	0.0014	1.5095
104	117	58	0.4957	0.0017	0.0008	1.3880
105	51	24	0.4706	0.0008	0.0004	1.2610
106	24	17	0.7083	0.0004	0.0003	0.9375
107	6	4	0.6667	0.0001	0.0001	1.0000
108	2	1	0.5000	0.0000	0.0000	1.0000
109	1	1	1.0000	0.0000	0.0000	0.5000

Annex Table 2 (cont).   Canada   1980 - 1988

Male

x	N_x	D_x	q_x	l_x	d_x	e_x
80	233923	20682	0.0884	1.0000	0.0884	6.8867
81	205782	19581	0.0952	0.9116	0.0867	6.5061
82	178928	18344	0.1025	0.8248	0.0846	6.1377
83	154458	17206	0.1114	0.7403	0.0825	5.7817
84	132354	16081	0.1215	0.6578	0.0799	5.4438
85	112218	14629	0.1304	0.5779	0.0753	5.1276
86	94352	13381	0.1418	0.5026	0.0713	4.8213
87	78657	12015	0.1528	0.4313	0.0659	4.5354
88	65009	10756	0.1655	0.3654	0.0605	4.2629
89	53314	9440	0.1771	0.3049	0.0540	4.0089
90	43530	8368	0.1922	0.2510	0.0482	3.7639
91	34993	7272	0.2078	0.2027	0.0421	3.5407
92	27577	6063	0.2199	0.1606	0.0353	3.3384
93	21356	5023	0.2352	0.1253	0.0295	3.1383
94	16212	4100	0.2529	0.0958	0.0242	2.9496
95	12023	3311	0.2754	0.0716	0.0197	2.7789
96	8581	2432	0.2834	0.0519	0.0147	2.6449
97	6058	1804	0.2978	0.0372	0.0111	2.4933
98	4125	1291	0.3130	0.0261	0.0082	2.3386
99	2696	924	0.3427	0.0179	0.0061	2.1761
100	...	...	...	0.0118	...	2.0501

Female

x	N_x	D_x	q_x	l_x	d_x	e_x
80	361323	18911	0.0523	1.0000	0.0523	8.9620
81	329179	18986	0.0577	0.9477	0.0547	8.4294
82	298144	19330	0.0648	0.8930	0.0579	7.9147
83	268142	19094	0.0712	0.8351	0.0595	7.4288
84	240051	19122	0.0797	0.7756	0.0618	6.9600
85	213286	18602	0.0872	0.7139	0.0623	6.5191
86	187718	18464	0.0984	0.6516	0.0641	6.0942
87	163158	17608	0.1079	0.5875	0.0634	5.7045
88	139792	16385	0.1172	0.5241	0.0614	5.3341
89	118976	15492	0.1302	0.4627	0.0602	4.9759
90	99825	14313	0.1434	0.4024	0.0577	4.6460
91	82389	12978	0.1575	0.3447	0.0543	4.3400
92	66585	11512	0.1729	0.2904	0.0502	4.0579
93	52508	9790	0.1864	0.2402	0.0448	3.8017
94	40883	8281	0.2026	0.1954	0.0396	3.5583
95	31056	6823	0.2197	0.1558	0.0342	3.3352
96	23018	5399	0.2346	0.1216	0.0285	3.1334
97	16565	4165	0.2514	0.0931	0.0234	2.9404
98	11574	3079	0.2660	0.0697	0.0185	2.7601
99	7754	2307	0.2975	0.0511	0.0152	2.5792
100	...	...	...	0.0359	...	2.4599

Annex Table 2 (cont.).   Chile   1980 - 1989

Male

x	N_x	D_x	q_x	l_x	d_x	e_x
80	61370	6295	0.1026	1.0000	0.1026	6.3205
81	53252	5891	0.1106	0.8974	0.0993	5.9858
82	45753	5533	0.1209	0.7981	0.0965	5.6681
83	39071	5016	0.1284	0.7016	0.0901	5.3791
84	33217	4618	0.1390	0.6116	0.0850	5.0978
85	27659	3979	0.1439	0.5265	0.0757	4.8402
86	22845	3549	0.1554	0.4508	0.0700	4.5695
87	18398	3069	0.1668	0.3808	0.0635	4.3179
88	14405	2610	0.1812	0.3172	0.0575	4.0823
89	11262	2200	0.1953	0.2598	0.0507	3.8750
90	8769	1793	0.2045	0.2090	0.0427	3.6944
91	6716	1443	0.2149	0.1663	0.0357	3.5154
92	5008	1161	0.2318	0.1306	0.0303	3.3406
93	3638	838	0.2303	0.1003	0.0231	3.1979
94	2660	717	0.2695	0.0772	0.0208	3.0053
95	1854	549	0.2961	0.0564	0.0167	2.9298
96	1259	348	0.2764	0.0397	0.0110	2.9520
97	1044	222	0.2126	0.0287	0.0061	2.8887
98	729	165	0.2263	0.0226	0.0051	2.5338
99	501	198	0.3952	0.0175	0.0069	2.1288
100	...	...	0.2036	0.0106	0.0022	2.1931

Female

x	N_x	D_x	q_x	l_x	d_x	e_x
80	96618	6854	0.0709	1.0000	0.0709	7.6445
81	86102	6821	0.0792	0.9291	0.0736	7.1900
82	76178	6723	0.0883	0.8555	0.0755	6.7656
83	67174	6416	0.0955	0.7800	0.0745	6.3720
84	58786	6104	0.1038	0.7055	0.0733	5.9921
85	50663	5885	0.1162	0.6322	0.0734	5.6285
86	43038	5302	0.1232	0.5588	0.0688	5.3025
87	35740	4759	0.1332	0.4899	0.0652	4.9772
88	29078	4184	0.1439	0.4247	0.0611	4.6650
89	23788	3800	0.1597	0.3636	0.0581	4.3650
90	19185	3315	0.1728	0.3055	0.0528	4.0998
91	15130	2820	0.1864	0.2527	0.0471	3.8517
92	11634	2382	0.2047	0.2056	0.0421	3.6196
93	8729	1878	0.2151	0.1635	0.0352	3.4227
94	6528	1545	0.2367	0.1283	0.0304	3.2239
95	4792	1128	0.2354	0.0980	0.0231	3.0684
96	3520	912	0.2591	0.0749	0.0194	2.8592
97	2493	662	0.2655	0.0555	0.0147	2.6842
98	1545	449	0.2906	0.0408	0.0118	2.4738
99	907	314	0.3462	0.0289	0.0100	2.2825
100	...	...	0.2811	0.0189	0.0053	2.2263

Annex Table 2 (cont.).   Czechoslovakia   1980 - 1990

Male

x	N_x	D_x	q_x	l_x	d_x	e_x
80	206077	27657	0.1342	1.0000	0.1342	5.0905
81	173557	24930	0.1436	0.8658	0.1244	4.8020
82	143768	22062	0.1535	0.7414	0.1138	4.5237
83	117793	19646	0.1668	0.6277	0.1047	4.2530
84	94928	17075	0.1799	0.5230	0.0941	4.0043
85	75525	14576	0.1930	0.4289	0.0828	3.7728
86	58940	12232	0.2075	0.3461	0.0718	3.5556
87	44818	9876	0.2204	0.2743	0.0604	3.3557
88	33506	7745	0.2312	0.2139	0.0494	3.1629
89	24608	5999	0.2438	0.1644	0.0401	2.9635
90	17540	4635	0.2643	0.1243	0.0329	2.7576
91	12160	3405	0.2800	0.0915	0.0256	2.5685
92	8427	2595	0.3079	0.0659	0.0203	2.3730
93	5599	1894	0.3383	0.0456	0.0154	2.2064
94	3548	1263	0.3560	0.0302	0.0107	2.0787
95	2228	842	0.3779	0.0194	0.0073	1.9513
96	1335	546	0.4090	0.0121	0.0049	1.8330
97	828	336	0.4058	0.0071	0.0029	1.7555
98	492	234	0.4756	0.0042	0.0020	1.6129
99	266	112	0.4211	0.0022	0.0009	1.6223
100	...	...	...	0.0013	...	1.4385

Female

x	N_x	D_x	q_x	l_x	d_x	e_x
80	395768	37975	0.0960	1.0000	0.0960	6.1326
81	349594	36866	0.1055	0.9040	0.0953	5.7305
82	305068	35789	0.1173	0.8087	0.0949	5.3471
83	262815	33842	0.1288	0.7138	0.0919	4.9913
84	222973	31786	0.1426	0.6219	0.0887	4.6551
85	186362	29435	0.1579	0.5333	0.0842	4.3459
86	151878	25659	0.1689	0.4490	0.0759	4.0673
87	121287	22450	0.1851	0.3732	0.0691	3.7925
88	94357	18924	0.2006	0.3041	0.0610	3.5403
89	71757	15441	0.2152	0.2431	0.0523	3.3031
90	53062	12461	0.2348	0.1908	0.0448	3.0716
91	38436	9864	0.2566	0.1460	0.0375	2.8609
92	27057	7449	0.2753	0.1085	0.0299	2.6759
93	18618	5498	0.2953	0.0786	0.0232	2.5025
94	12389	3911	0.3157	0.0554	0.0175	2.3417
95	7944	2710	0.3411	0.0379	0.0129	2.1913
96	4897	1735	0.3543	0.0250	0.0089	2.0671
97	3068	1169	0.3810	0.0161	0.0061	1.9269
98	1858	769	0.4139	0.0100	0.0041	1.8053
99	1061	438	0.4128	0.0059	0.0024	1.7270
100	...	...	...	0.0034	...	1.5897

Annex Table 2 (cont.). Denmark 1980 - 1990

Male

x	N_x	D_x	q_x	l_x	d_x	e_x
80	95974	9579	0.0998	1.0000	0.0998	6.3588
81	84169	8999	0.1069	0.9002	0.0962	6.0084
82	73849	8487	0.1149	0.8039	0.0924	5.6678
83	64312	8002	0.1244	0.7116	0.0885	5.3388
84	55581	7362	0.1325	0.6230	0.0825	5.0265
85	47529	6780	0.1426	0.5405	0.0771	4.7176
86	40172	6288	0.1565	0.4634	0.0725	4.4193
87	33313	5542	0.1664	0.3909	0.0650	4.1466
88	26990	4891	0.1812	0.3258	0.0590	3.8744
89	21710	4308	0.1984	0.2668	0.0529	3.6212
90	17017	3552	0.2087	0.2139	0.0446	3.3938
91	13252	3033	0.2289	0.1692	0.0387	3.1572
92	9976	2547	0.2553	0.1305	0.0333	2.9459
93	7258	1942	0.2676	0.0972	0.0260	2.7844
94	5135	1421	0.2767	0.0712	0.0197	2.6190
95	3600	1146	0.3183	0.0515	0.0164	2.4297
96	2388	768	0.3216	0.0351	0.0113	2.3309
97	1540	529	0.3435	0.0238	0.0082	2.1989
98	965	337	0.3492	0.0156	0.0055	2.0878
99	606	221	0.3647	0.0102	0.0037	1.9398
100	373	157	0.4209	0.0065	0.0027	1.7663
101	194	75	0.3866	0.0037	0.0014	1.6867
102	113	56	0.4956	0.0023	0.0011	1.4346
103	50	24	0.4800	0.0012	0.0006	1.3528
104	25	16	0.6400	0.0006	0.0004	1.1400
105	9	6	0.6667	0.0002	0.0001	1.2778
106	3	1	0.3333	0.0001	0.0000	1.8333
107	1	0	0.0000	0.0000	0.0000	1.5000
108	1	1	1.0000	0.0000	0.0000	0.5000

Female

x	N_x	D_x	q_x	l_x	d_x	e_x
80	160082	9849	0.0615	1.0000	0.0615	7.9995
81	146387	9867	0.0674	0.9385	0.0633	7.4911
82	133147	9979	0.0749	0.8752	0.0656	6.9964
83	120145	10260	0.0854	0.8096	0.0691	6.5227
84	107131	10097	0.0942	0.7405	0.0698	6.0851
85	94354	9994	0.1059	0.6707	0.0710	5.6662
86	81708	9436	0.1155	0.5997	0.0693	5.2783
87	69820	8981	0.1286	0.5304	0.0682	4.9021
88	58353	8286	0.1420	0.4622	0.0656	4.5520
89	47891	7558	0.1578	0.3965	0.0626	4.2226
90	38722	6752	0.1744	0.3340	0.0582	3.9201
91	30422	5854	0.1924	0.2757	0.0531	3.6425
92	23329	4941	0.2118	0.2227	0.0472	3.3912
93	17485	4031	0.2305	0.1755	0.0405	3.1681
94	12600	3037	0.2410	0.1351	0.0326	2.9675
95	9008	2393	0.2657	0.1025	0.0272	2.7512
96	6170	1819	0.2948	0.0753	0.0222	2.5656
97	4083	1250	0.3061	0.0531	0.0163	2.4291
98	2661	838	0.3149	0.0368	0.0116	2.2803
99	1697	576	0.3394	0.0252	0.0086	2.0986
100	1022	395	0.3865	0.0167	0.0064	1.9201
101	568	226	0.3979	0.0102	0.0041	1.8147
102	334	143	0.4281	0.0062	0.0026	1.6834
103	185	76	0.4108	0.0035	0.0014	1.5694
104	101	54	0.5347	0.0021	0.0011	1.3151
105	41	22	0.5366	0.0010	0.0005	1.2516
106	17	11	0.6471	0.0004	0.0003	1.1218
107	7	3	0.4286	0.0002	0.0001	1.2619
108	3	2	0.6667	0.0001	0.0001	0.8333
109	1	1	1.0000	0.0000	0.0000	0.5000

Annex Table 2 (cont.). England & Wales   1980 - 1990

Male

x	N_x	D_x	q_x	l_x	d_x	e_x
80	889298	95870	0.1078	1.0000	0.1078	5.9674
81	766401	88898	0.1160	0.8922	0.1035	5.6280
82	649484	81992	0.1262	0.7887	0.0996	5.3008
83	544003	74338	0.1366	0.6891	0.0942	4.9945
84	449131	66285	0.1476	0.5950	0.0878	4.7059
85	366671	58498	0.1595	0.5072	0.0809	4.4341
86	294506	50858	0.1727	0.4262	0.0736	4.1808
87	233328	42718	0.1831	0.3526	0.0646	3.9491
88	182529	35856	0.1964	0.2881	0.0566	3.7221
89	140983	29574	0.2098	0.2315	0.0486	3.5098
90	107164	23869	0.2227	0.1829	0.0407	3.3088
91	80842	19172	0.2372	0.1422	0.0337	3.1137
92	59766	15280	0.2557	0.1085	0.0277	2.9262
93	43109	11688	0.2711	0.0807	0.0219	2.7596
94	30233	8852	0.2928	0.0588	0.0172	2.6001
95	20600	6293	0.3055	0.0416	0.0127	2.4696
96	13695	4493	0.3281	0.0289	0.0095	2.3359
97	8824	2994	0.3393	0.0194	0.0066	2.2323
98	5598	2010	0.3591	0.0128	0.0046	2.1219
99	3433	1260	0.3670	0.0082	0.0030	2.0305
100	2073	836	0.4033	0.0052	0.0021	1.9179
101	1174	486	0.4140	0.0031	0.0013	1.8762
102	641	263	0.4103	0.0018	0.0007	1.8483
103	355	155	0.4366	0.0011	0.0005	1.7864
104	190	79	0.4158	0.0006	0.0003	1.7834
105	104	45	0.4327	0.0004	0.0002	1.6968
106	53	25	0.4717	0.0002	0.0001	1.6096
107	22	8	0.3636	0.0001	0.0000	1.6004
108	12	7	0.5833	0.0001	0.0000	1.2292
109	4	3	0.7500	0.0000	0.0000	1.2500

Female

x	N_x	D_x	q_x	l_x	d_x	e_x
80	1694492	110658	0.0653	1.0000	0.0653	7.8542
81	1555548	112244	0.0722	0.9347	0.0674	7.3680
82	1408157	113229	0.0804	0.8673	0.0697	6.9021
83	1261502	112442	0.0891	0.7975	0.0711	6.4619
84	1118355	110288	0.0986	0.7264	0.0716	6.0453
85	978650	106382	0.1087	0.6548	0.0712	5.6520
86	844013	102065	0.1209	0.5836	0.0706	5.2804
87	716736	94636	0.1320	0.5130	0.0677	4.9380
88	600083	86402	0.1440	0.4453	0.0641	4.6131
89	495009	78954	0.1595	0.3812	0.0608	4.3049
90	400728	69597	0.1737	0.3204	0.0556	4.0270
91	318759	59607	0.1870	0.2647	0.0495	3.7683
92	248933	51146	0.2055	0.2152	0.0442	3.5200
93	189776	42107	0.2219	0.1710	0.0379	3.3010
94	141003	33604	0.2383	0.1331	0.0317	3.0996
95	102371	26007	0.2540	0.1014	0.0257	2.9130
96	72557	19983	0.2754	0.0756	0.0208	2.7348
97	49932	14435	0.2891	0.0548	0.0158	2.5843
98	33505	10131	0.3024	0.0389	0.0118	2.4319
99	21821	7089	0.3249	0.0272	0.0088	2.2692
100	14105	4989	0.3537	0.0183	0.0065	2.1205
101	8548	3190	0.3732	0.0119	0.0044	2.0074
102	4978	1944	0.3905	0.0074	0.0029	1.9049
103	2818	1123	0.3985	0.0045	0.0018	1.8050
104	1583	685	0.4327	0.0027	0.0012	1.6696
105	837	393	0.4695	0.0015	0.0007	1.5618
106	415	190	0.4578	0.0008	0.0004	1.5017
107	213	101	0.4742	0.0004	0.0002	1.3475
108	99	67	0.6768	0.0002	0.0002	1.1118
109	28	16	0.5714	0.0001	0.0000	1.3929

Annex Table 2 (cont). Estonia 1980 - 1990

Male

x	N_x	D_x	q_x	l_x	d_x	e_x
80	16845	1961	0.1164	1.0000	0.1164	5.5793
81	14543	1837	0.1263	0.8836	0.1116	5.2485
82	12449	1755	0.1410	0.7720	0.1088	4.9350
83	10380	1523	0.1467	0.6631	0.0973	4.6628
84	8571	1414	0.1650	0.5658	0.0934	4.3787
85	6937	1220	0.1759	0.4725	0.0831	4.1450
86	5508	1000	0.1816	0.3894	0.0707	3.9228
87	4298	893	0.2078	0.3187	0.0662	3.6821
88	3278	673	0.2053	0.2525	0.0518	3.5166
89	2545	579	0.2275	0.2006	0.0456	3.2959
90	1919	475	0.2475	0.1550	0.0384	3.1194
91	1419	361	0.2544	0.1166	0.0297	2.9810
92	1046	287	0.2744	0.870	0.0239	2.8275
93	754	220	0.2918	0.0631	0.0184	2.7076
94	529	156	0.2949	0.0447	0.0132	2.6172
95	362	98	0.2707	0.0315	0.0085	2.5026
96	262	91	0.3473	0.0230	0.0080	2.2460
97	175	59	0.3371	0.0150	0.0051	2.1752
98	117	44	0.3761	0.0099	0.0037	2.0272
99	73	27	0.3699	0.0062	0.0023	1.9478
100	0	0	...	0.0039	...	1.7976

Female

x	N_x	D_x	q_x	l_x	d_x	e_x
80	46481	3921	0.0844	1.0000	0.0844	6.7090
81	42116	4044	0.0960	0.9156	0.0879	6.2810
82	37613	3820	0.1016	0.8277	0.0841	5.8950
83	33096	3763	0.1137	0.7437	0.0846	5.5049
84	28576	3681	0.1288	0.6591	0.0849	5.1470
85	24284	3389	0.1396	0.5742	0.0801	4.8341
86	20324	3099	0.1525	0.4941	0.0753	4.5370
87	16750	2735	0.1633	0.4187	0.0684	4.2633
88	13645	2380	0.1744	0.3504	0.0611	3.9977
89	10961	2059	0.1878	0.2892	0.0543	3.7367
90	8663	1793	0.2070	0.2349	0.0486	3.4854
91	6721	1500	0.2232	0.1863	0.0416	3.2645
92	5083	1211	0.2382	0.1447	0.0345	3.0588
93	3778	992	0.2626	0.1102	0.0289	2.8590
94	2719	773	0.2843	0.0813	0.0231	2.6990
95	1893	553	0.2921	0.0582	0.0170	2.5725
96	1307	421	0.3221	0.0412	0.0133	2.4278
97	876	290	0.3311	0.0279	0.0092	2.3439
98	582	194	0.3333	0.0187	0.0062	2.2564
99	387	126	0.3256	0.0125	0.0041	2.1346
100	0	0	...	0.0084	...	1.9237

Annex Table 2 (cont). Finland 1980 - 1990

Male

x	N_x	D_x	q_x	l_x	d_x	e_x
80	61620	6643	0.1078	1.0000	0.1078	6.0046
81	52719	6149	0.1166	0.8922	0.1041	5.6697
82	44572	5529	0.1240	0.7881	0.0978	5.3523
83	37024	4953	0.1338	0.6904	0.0924	5.0395
84	30439	4318	0.1419	0.5980	0.0848	4.7406
85	24921	3843	0.1542	0.5132	0.0791	4.4416
86	20024	3410	0.1703	0.4340	0.0739	4.1602
87	15687	2808	0.1790	0.3601	0.0645	3.9115
88	12238	2438	0.1992	0.2957	0.0589	3.6553
89	9266	1949	0.2103	0.2368	0.0498	3.4402
90	6877	1573	0.2287	0.1870	0.0428	3.2234
91	4913	1164	0.2369	0.1442	0.0342	3.0311
92	3524	911	0.2585	0.1100	0.0284	2.8169
93	2497	698	0.2795	0.0816	0.0228	2.6247
94	1691	515	0.3046	0.0588	0.0179	2.4491
95	1088	364	0.3346	0.0409	0.0137	2.3026
96	686	223	0.3251	0.0272	0.0088	2.2089
97	430	148	0.3442	0.0184	0.0063	2.0320
98	264	110	0.4167	0.0120	0.0050	1.8360
99	138	56	0.4058	0.0070	0.0029	1.7903
100	74	29	0.3919	0.0042	0.0016	1.6715
101	36	17	0.4722	0.0025	0.0012	1.4265
102	15	7	0.4667	0.0013	0.0006	1.2556
103	6	4	0.6667	0.0007	0.0005	0.9167
104	2	1	0.5000	0.0002	0.0001	0.7500

Female

x	N_x	D_x	q_x	l_x	d_x	e_x
80	136936	9685	0.0707	1.0000	0.0707	7.4178
81	122109	9501	0.0778	0.9293	0.0723	6.9443
82	108116	9514	0.0880	0.8570	0.0754	6.4881
83	93812	9190	0.0980	0.7816	0.0766	6.0658
84	80381	8685	0.1080	0.7050	0.0762	5.6703
85	68232	8170	0.1197	0.6288	0.0753	5.2966
86	56670	7383	0.1303	0.5535	0.0721	4.9491
87	46474	6663	0.1434	0.4814	0.0690	4.6155
88	37337	5929	0.1588	0.4124	0.0655	4.3043
89	29321	5047	0.1721	0.3469	0.0597	4.0225
90	22632	4247	0.1877	0.2872	0.0539	3.7549
91	16988	3536	0.2081	0.2333	0.0486	3.5068
92	12361	2736	0.2213	0.1847	0.0409	3.2971
93	8947	2163	0.2418	0.1438	0.0348	3.0922
94	6330	1673	0.2643	0.1091	0.0288	2.9187
95	4253	1169	0.2749	0.0802	0.0221	2.7877
96	2836	807	0.2846	0.0582	0.0166	2.6548
97	1902	579	0.3044	0.0416	0.0127	2.5119
98	1235	404	0.3271	0.0290	0.0095	2.3923
99	758	253	0.3338	0.0195	0.0065	2.3123
100	463	164	0.3542	0.0130	0.0046	2.2202
101	276	106	0.3841	0.0084	0.0032	2.1638
102	165	55	0.3333	0.0052	0.0017	2.2012
103	93	33	0.3548	0.0034	0.0012	2.0518
104	57	25	0.4386	0.0022	0.0010	1.9053
105	30	13	0.4333	0.0012	0.0005	2.0032
106	12	5	0.4167	0.0007	0.0003	2.1528
107	6	2	0.3333	0.0004	0.0001	2.3333
108	4	2	0.5000	0.0003	0.0001	2.2500
109	1	0	0.0000	0.0001	0.0000	3.0000

Annex Table 2 (cont.).   France   1980 - 1990

Male

x	N_x	D_x	q_x	l_x	d_x	e_x
80	995230	91804	0.0922	1.0000	0.0922	6.3995
81	881312	89851	0.1020	0.9078	0.0925	5.9990
82	765612	85397	0.1115	0.8152	0.0909	5.6233
83	658054	80593	0.1225	0.7243	0.0887	5.2665
84	555441	74013	0.1333	0.6356	0.0847	4.9317
85	457131	66600	0.1457	0.5509	0.0803	4.6130
86	370794	58785	0.1585	0.4706	0.0746	4.3144
87	295487	51140	0.1731	0.3960	0.0685	4.0331
88	228954	42810	0.1870	0.3275	0.0612	3.7725
89	175126	35613	0.2034	0.2662	0.0541	3.5252
90	131605	28955	0.2200	0.2121	0.0467	3.2974
91	97252	23310	0.2397	0.1654	0.0397	3.0865
92	70360	17768	0.2525	0.1258	0.0318	2.9019
93	49869	13779	0.2763	0.0940	0.0260	2.7133
94	34323	10130	0.2951	0.0680	0.0201	2.5583
95	23545	7256	0.3082	0.0480	0.0148	2.4202
96	15717	5228	0.3326	0.0332	0.0110	2.2756
97	10101	3462	0.3427	0.0221	0.0076	2.1605
98	6487	2251	0.3470	0.0146	0.0051	2.0265
99	4048	1562	0.3859	0.0095	0.0037	1.8376
100	2426	1113	0.4588	0.0058	0.0027	1.6780
101	1246	568	0.4559	0.0032	0.0014	1.6767
102	630	284	0.4508	0.0017	0.0008	1.6624
103	333	160	0.4805	0.0009	0.0005	1.6165
104	168	72	0.4286	0.0005	0.0002	1.6491
105	93	43	0.4624	0.0003	0.0001	1.5110
106	46	21	0.4565	0.0002	0.0001	1.3804
107	25	16	0.6400	0.0001	0.0001	1.1200
108	9	5	0.5556	0.0000	0.0000	1.2222
109	4	2	0.5000	0.0000	0.0000	1.1250

Female

x	N_x	D_x	q_x	l_x	d_x	e_x
80	1796647	100649	0.0560	1.0000	0.0560	8.1287
81	1663861	106215	0.0638	0.9440	0.0603	7.5814
82	1520181	110013	0.0724	0.8837	0.0640	7.0643
83	1380128	112992	0.0819	0.8198	0.0671	6.5764
84	1237190	113618	0.0918	0.7527	0.0691	6.1183
85	1089075	112327	0.1031	0.6835	0.0705	5.6854
86	945953	108927	0.1152	0.6130	0.0706	5.2828
87	808722	104027	0.1286	0.5424	0.0698	4.9052
88	673725	96635	0.1434	0.4727	0.0678	4.5555
89	550296	87377	0.1588	0.4049	0.0643	4.2347
90	442702	77416	0.1749	0.3406	0.0596	3.9396
91	350216	67018	0.1914	0.2810	0.0538	3.6685
92	271762	57002	0.2097	0.2272	0.0477	3.4184
93	204650	46369	0.2266	0.1796	0.0407	3.1930
94	150125	37187	0.2477	0.1389	0.0344	2.9819
95	107477	28371	0.2640	0.1045	0.0276	2.7991
96	74824	21440	0.2865	0.0769	0.0220	2.6236
97	50148	15149	0.3021	0.0549	0.0166	2.4765
98	33167	10711	0.3229	0.0383	0.0124	2.3320
99	21317	7067	0.3315	0.0259	0.0086	2.2058
100	13425	5089	0.3791	0.0173	0.0066	2.0518
101	7800	2988	0.3831	0.0108	0.0041	1.9992
102	4415	1702	0.3855	0.0066	0.0026	1.9301
103	2549	1089	0.4272	0.0041	0.0017	1.8273
104	1335	575	0.4307	0.0023	0.0010	1.8173
105	695	299	0.4302	0.0013	0.0006	1.8139
106	360	142	0.3944	0.0008	0.0003	1.8059
107	190	89	0.4684	0.0005	0.0002	1.6566
108	88	47	0.5341	0.0002	0.0001	1.6757
109	34	20	0.5882	0.0001	0.0001	2.0235

Annex Table 2 (cont.). Germany, East 1980 - 1990

Male

x	N_x	D_x	q_x	l_x	d_x	e_x
80	299988	38044	0.1268	1.0000	0.1268	5.1481
81	261293	36288	0.1389	0.8732	0.1213	4.8232
82	223937	33686	0.1504	0.7519	0.1131	4.5204
83	187390	30791	0.1643	0.6388	0.1050	4.2322
84	154038	27426	0.1780	0.5338	0.0950	3.9661
85	123552	23880	0.1933	0.4388	0.0848	3.7169
86	96928	19965	0.2060	0.3540	0.0729	3.4876
87	75021	16775	0.2236	0.2811	0.0628	3.2626
88	56314	13520	0.2401	0.2182	0.0524	3.0583
89	41740	10814	0.2591	0.1658	0.0430	2.8665
90	30354	8360	0.2754	0.1229	0.0338	2.6940
91	21633	6330	0.2926	0.0890	0.0261	2.5280
92	15240	4800	0.3150	0.0630	0.0198	2.3669
93	10422	3565	0.3421	0.0431	0.0148	2.2252
94	6808	2397	0.3521	0.0284	0.0100	2.1221
95	4398	1639	0.3727	0.0184	0.0069	2.0036
96	2751	1056	0.3839	0.0115	0.0044	1.8968
97	1718	721	0.4197	0.0071	0.0030	1.7670
98	981	405	0.4128	0.0041	0.0017	1.6833
99	596	286	0.4799	0.0024	0.0012	1.5154
100	...	...	...	0.0013		1.4521

Female

x	N_x	D_x	q_x	l_x	d_x	e_x
80	622533	57663	0.0926	1.0000	0.0926	6.1620
81	556341	57444	0.1033	0.9074	0.0937	5.7400
82	491113	56187	0.1144	0.8137	0.0931	5.3434
83	426649	54187	0.1270	0.7206	0.0915	4.9691
84	364373	52036	0.1428	0.6291	0.0898	4.6192
85	306243	47548	0.1553	0.5392	0.0837	4.3055
86	252548	43738	0.1732	0.4555	0.0789	4.0050
87	203628	38379	0.1885	0.3766	0.0710	3.7391
88	159437	32804	0.2057	0.3056	0.0629	3.4914
89	122417	27090	0.2213	0.2428	0.0537	3.2663
90	92113	21840	0.2371	0.1890	0.0448	3.0525
91	67571	17385	0.2573	0.1442	0.0371	2.8457
92	48321	13473	0.2788	0.1071	0.0299	2.6583
93	33410	10142	0.3036	0.0772	0.0234	2.4928
94	22139	7008	0.3165	0.0538	0.0170	2.3614
95	14337	4911	0.3425	0.0368	0.0126	2.2235
96	8979	3172	0.3533	0.0242	0.0085	2.1215
97	5520	2008	0.3638	0.0156	0.0057	2.0072
98	3358	1279	0.3809	0.0099	0.0038	1.8690
99	1977	848	0.4289	0.0062	0.0026	1.7112
100	...	...	...	0.0035		1.6209

Annex Table 2 (cont.).   Germany, West   1980 - 1990

Male

x	N_x	D_x	q_x	l_x	d_x	e_x
80	1129893	120437	0.1066	1.0000	0.1066	5.9243
81	983828	115122	0.1170	0.8934	0.1045	5.5715
82	841628	106561	0.1266	0.7889	0.0999	5.2436
83	705740	96707	0.1370	0.6890	0.0944	4.9312
84	583887	86662	0.1484	0.5946	0.0882	4.6349
85	472420	75707	0.1603	0.5063	0.0811	4.3555
86	374991	65148	0.1737	0.4252	0.0739	4.0913
87	293960	55090	0.1874	0.3513	0.0658	3.8464
88	225593	45251	0.2006	0.2855	0.0573	3.6182
89	170274	36289	0.2131	0.2282	0.0486	3.4006
90	126813	29543	0.2330	0.1796	0.0418	3.1863
91	92758	22959	0.2475	0.1377	0.0341	3.0021
92	66990	17735	0.2647	0.1036	0.0274	2.8251
93	47513	13662	0.2875	0.0762	0.0219	2.6624
94	32508	9753	0.3000	0.0543	0.0163	2.5351
95	22038	7032	0.3191	0.0380	0.0121	2.4073
96	14512	4800	0.3308	0.0259	0.0086	2.3011
97	9364	3087	0.3297	0.0173	0.0057	2.1912
98	5980	2041	0.3413	0.0116	0.0040	2.0230
99	3713	1508	0.4061	0.0076	0.0031	1.8121
100	2075	932	0.4492	0.0045	0.0020	1.7095
101	1055	456	0.4322	0.0025	0.0011	1.6957
102	562	263	0.4680	0.0014	0.0007	1.6060
103	277	131	0.4729	0.0008	0.0004	1.5789
104	143	65	0.4545	0.0004	0.0002	1.5469
105	66	32	0.4848	0.0002	0.0001	1.4193
106	31	14	0.4516	0.0001	0.0001	1.2846
107	13	9	0.6923	0.0001	0.0000	0.9308
108	5	3	0.6000	0.0000	0.0000	0.9000
109	2	2	1.0000	0.0000	0.0000	0.5000

Female

x	N_x	D_x	q_x	l_x	d_x	e_x
80	2333437	161458	0.0692	1.0000	0.0692	7.3779
81	2102093	164569	0.0783	0.9308	0.0729	6.8892
82	1870182	162822	0.0871	0.8579	0.0747	6.4319
83	1642681	160324	0.0976	0.7832	0.0764	5.9976
84	1424056	155082	0.1089	0.7068	0.0770	5.5922
85	1218175	147488	0.1211	0.6298	0.0763	5.2145
86	1023043	136434	0.1334	0.5536	0.0738	4.8639
87	846876	124734	0.1473	0.4797	0.0707	4.5354
88	682640	110712	0.1622	0.4091	0.0663	4.2325
89	539881	95520	0.1769	0.3427	0.0606	3.9550
90	417296	80989	0.1941	0.2821	0.0548	3.6977
91	316302	66391	0.2099	0.2273	0.0477	3.4677
92	233685	52926	0.2265	0.1796	0.0407	3.2561
93	168484	41091	0.2439	0.1389	0.0339	3.0631
94	117862	30710	0.2606	0.1051	0.0274	2.8899
95	80859	22248	0.2751	0.0777	0.0214	2.7320
96	53105	15372	0.2895	0.0563	0.0163	2.5792
97	34045	10375	0.3047	0.0400	0.0122	2.4263
98	21266	6816	0.3205	0.0278	0.0089	2.2706
99	12851	4654	0.3622	0.0189	0.0068	2.1058
100	7317	2771	0.3787	0.0121	0.0046	2.0175
101	3977	1570	0.3948	0.0075	0.0030	1.9425
102	2064	832	0.4031	0.0045	0.0018	1.8833
103	1046	434	0.4149	0.0027	0.0011	1.8176
104	517	217	0.4197	0.0016	0.0007	1.7519
105	246	107	0.4350	0.0009	0.0004	1.6574
106	113	50	0.4425	0.0005	0.0002	1.5484
107	53	18	0.3396	0.0003	0.0001	1.3805
108	30	20	0.6667	0.0002	0.0001	0.8333
109	8	8	1.0000	0.0001	0.0001	0.5000

Annex Table 2 (cont.).   Hungary   1980 - 1990

Male

x	N_x	D_x	q_x	l_x	d_x	e_x
80	156702	20295	0.1295	1.0000	0.1295	5.1558
81	134291	18956	0.1412	0.8705	0.1229	4.8485
82	113404	17355	0.1530	0.7476	0.1144	4.5632
83	94731	15589	0.1646	0.6332	0.1042	4.2974
84	77566	13891	0.1791	0.5290	0.0947	4.0454
85	62834	12048	0.1917	0.4343	0.0833	3.8189
86	49710	9946	0.2001	0.3510	0.0702	3.6062
87	38931	8474	0.2177	0.2808	0.0611	3.3832
88	29582	6742	0.2279	0.2197	0.0501	3.1854
89	22007	5462	0.2482	0.1696	0.0421	2.9780
90	15775	4209	0.2668	0.1275	0.0340	2.7961
91	11224	3307	0.2946	0.0935	0.0275	2.6317
92	7675	2318	0.3020	0.0659	0.0199	2.5221
93	5222	1605	0.3074	0.0460	0.0141	2.3971
94	3519	1226	0.3484	0.0319	0.0111	2.2389
95	2228	787	0.3532	0.0208	0.0073	2.1686
96	1415	496	0.3505	0.0134	0.0047	2.0799
97	888	360	0.4054	0.0087	0.0035	1.9325
98	519	198	0.3815	0.0052	0.0020	1.9093
99	315	124	0.3937	0.0032	0.0013	1.7786
100	...	...	...	0.0019	...	1.6086

Female

x	N_x	D_x	q_x	l_x	d_x	e_x
80	280496	26648	0.0950	1.0000	0.0950	6.1865
81	248279	26130	0.1052	0.9050	0.0952	5.7835
82	217339	25309	0.1164	0.8098	0.0943	5.4049
83	188284	24095	0.1280	0.7155	0.0916	5.0514
84	160898	22897	0.1423	0.6239	0.0888	4.7193
85	135555	20708	0.1528	0.5351	0.0817	4.4194
86	112735	18807	0.1668	0.4534	0.0756	4.1261
87	91575	16782	0.1833	0.3777	0.0692	3.8521
88	72098	14411	0.1999	0.3085	0.0617	3.6042
89	55580	11854	0.2133	0.2468	0.0526	3.3797
90	41305	9624	0.2330	0.1942	0.0452	3.1604
91	30385	7558	0.2487	0.1490	0.0371	2.9686
92	21939	5812	0.2649	0.1119	0.0296	2.7859
93	15349	4414	0.2876	0.0823	0.0237	2.6098
94	10376	3126	0.3013	0.0586	0.0177	2.4614
95	6866	2277	0.3316	0.0409	0.0136	2.3071
96	4373	1442	0.3298	0.0274	0.0090	2.2037
97	2741	993	0.3623	0.0183	0.0066	2.0419
98	1628	619	0.3802	0.0117	0.0044	1.9178
99	952	389	0.4086	0.0072	0.0030	1.7876
100	...	...	...	0.0043	...	1.6773

Annex Table 2 (cont). Iceland 1980 – 1989

Male

x	N_x	D_x	q_x	l_x	d_x	e_x
80	3040	223	0.0734	1.0000	0.0734	7.2137
81	2744	239	0.0871	0.9266	0.0807	6.7451
82	2500	231	0.0924	0.8459	0.0782	6.3410
83	2242	225	0.1004	0.7678	0.0771	5.9356
84	2002	223	0.1114	0.6907	0.0769	5.5420
85	1723	202	0.1172	0.6138	0.0720	5.1740
86	1482	214	0.1444	0.5418	0.0782	4.7947
87	1252	176	0.1406	0.4636	0.0652	4.5196
88	1062	188	0.1770	0.3984	0.0705	4.1770
89	867	148	0.1707	0.3279	0.0560	3.9680
90	684	136	0.1988	0.2719	0.0541	3.6818
91	538	109	0.2026	0.2179	0.0441	3.4715
92	414	100	0.2415	0.1737	0.0420	3.2264
93	294	64	0.2177	0.1318	0.0287	3.0947
94	220	61	0.2773	0.1031	0.0286	2.8168
95	149	40	0.2685	0.0745	0.0200	2.7056
96	103	34	0.3301	0.0545	0.0180	2.5150
97	62	18	0.2903	0.0365	0.0106	2.5079
98	36	11	0.3056	0.0259	0.0079	2.3292
99	25	7	0.2800	0.0180	0.0050	2.1341
100	17	10	0.5882	0.0130	0.0076	1.7696
101	6	1	0.1667	0.0053	0.0009	2.5833
102	5	1	0.2000	0.0044	0.0009	2.0000
103	4	1	0.2500	0.0036	0.0009	1.3750
104	3	2	0.6667	0.0027	0.0018	0.6667

Female

x	N_x	D_x	q_x	l_x	d_x	e_x
80	4045	198	0.0489	1.0000	0.0489	8.7039
81	3766	230	0.0611	0.9511	0.0581	8.1261
82	3498	234	0.0669	0.8930	0.0597	7.6222
83	3204	244	0.0762	0.8332	0.0635	7.1328
84	2939	247	0.0840	0.7698	0.0647	6.6795
85	2624	248	0.0945	0.7051	0.0666	6.2465
86	2319	254	0.1095	0.6384	0.0699	5.8463
87	2021	223	0.1103	0.5685	0.0627	5.5039
88	1768	213	0.1205	0.5058	0.0609	5.1246
89	1510	217	0.1437	0.4449	0.0639	4.7580
90	1261	186	0.1475	0.3809	0.0562	4.4726
91	1033	162	0.1568	0.3247	0.0509	4.1600
92	822	140	0.1703	0.2738	0.0466	3.8407
93	639	152	0.2379	0.2272	0.0540	3.5265
94	452	95	0.2102	0.1731	0.0364	3.4711
95	324	72	0.2222	0.1367	0.0304	3.2618
96	246	67	0.2724	0.1064	0.0290	3.0509
97	162	38	0.2346	0.0774	0.0182	3.0057
98	100	23	0.2300	0.0592	0.0136	2.7735
99	73	16	0.2192	0.0456	0.0100	2.4526
100	49	20	0.4082	0.0356	0.0145	2.0007
101	28	9	0.3214	0.0211	0.0068	2.0357
102	19	7	0.3684	0.0143	0.0053	1.7632
103	10	6	0.6000	0.0090	0.0054	1.5000
104	4	1	0.2500	0.0036	0.0009	2.0000
105	2	0	0.0000	0.0027	0.0000	1.5000
106	2	2	1.0000	0.0027	0.0027	0.5000
107	1	0	0.0000	0.0000	0.0000	1.5000
108	1	1	1.0000	0.0000	0.0000	0.5000

Annex Table 2 (cont).   Ireland   1980 - 1989

Male

x	N_x	D_x	q_x	l_x	d_x	e_x
80	43180	5008	0.1160	1.0000	0.1160	5.6737
81	37915	4293	0.1132	0.8840	0.1001	5.3525
82	33359	4444	0.1332	0.7839	0.1044	4.9720
83	28099	4014	0.1429	0.6795	0.0971	4.6594
84	23685	3885	0.1640	0.5824	0.0955	4.3526
85	19619	3153	0.1607	0.4869	0.0782	4.1085
86	15747	2998	0.1904	0.4086	0.0778	3.7994
87	12427	2563	0.2062	0.3308	0.0682	3.5753
88	9751	2093	0.2146	0.2626	0.0564	3.3744
89	7603	1739	0.2287	0.2062	0.0472	3.1600
90	5850	1443	0.2467	0.1591	0.0392	2.9489
91	4347	1071	0.2464	0.1198	0.0295	2.7507
92	3317	989	0.2982	0.0903	0.0269	2.4865
93	2332	739	0.3169	0.0634	0.0201	2.3304
94	1601	527	0.3292	0.0433	0.0143	2.1795
95	1096	390	0.3558	0.0290	0.0103	2.0037
96	710	265	0.3732	0.0187	0.0070	1.8343
97	450	191	0.4244	0.0117	0.0050	1.6289
98	269	142	0.5279	0.0067	0.0036	1.4614
99	130	67	0.5154	0.0032	0.0016	1.5364
100	63	27	0.4286	0.0015	0.0007	1.6386
101	39	17	0.4359	0.0009	0.0004	1.4926
102	22	14	0.6364	0.0005	0.0003	1.2596
103	9	4	0.4444	0.0002	0.0001	1.5889
104	5	2	0.4000	0.0001	0.0000	1.4600
105	5	3	0.6000	0.0001	0.0000	1.1000
106	2	1	0.5000	0.0000	0.0000	1.0000
107	1	1	1.0000	0.0000	0.0000	0.5000

Female

x	N_x	D_x	q_x	l_x	d_x	e_x
80	63393	5248	0.0828	1.0000	0.0828	7.1239
81	58269	4576	0.0785	0.9172	0.0720	6.7217
82	53328	5173	0.0970	0.8452	0.0820	6.2519
83	47047	4822	0.1025	0.7632	0.0782	5.8698
84	41290	4932	0.1194	0.6850	0.0818	5.4831
85	35842	4420	0.1233	0.6032	0.0744	5.1590
86	30912	4460	0.1443	0.5288	0.0763	4.8144
87	25754	3862	0.1500	0.4525	0.0679	4.5418
88	20928	3379	0.1615	0.3846	0.0621	4.2549
89	16705	2801	0.1677	0.3225	0.0541	3.9778
90	13160	2594	0.1971	0.2684	0.0529	3.6785
91	10276	2010	0.1956	0.2155	0.0422	3.4588
92	8102	1920	0.2370	0.1734	0.0411	3.1783
93	6016	1399	0.2325	0.1323	0.0308	3.0101
94	4449	1178	0.2648	0.1015	0.0269	2.7707
95	3163	877	0.2773	0.0746	0.0207	2.5884
96	2199	656	0.2983	0.0539	0.0161	2.3896
97	1489	494	0.3318	0.0379	0.0126	2.1930
98	950	357	0.3758	0.0253	0.0095	2.0335
99	565	213	0.3770	0.0158	0.0060	1.9567
100	339	137	0.4041	0.0098	0.0040	1.8382
101	188	83	0.4415	0.0059	0.0026	1.7458
102	102	44	0.4314	0.0033	0.0014	1.7306
103	55	20	0.3636	0.0019	0.0007	1.6641
104	36	17	0.4722	0.0012	0.0006	1.3294
105	21	12	0.5714	0.0006	0.0004	1.0714
106	9	7	0.7778	0.0003	0.0002	0.8333
107	2	1	0.5000	0.0001	0.0000	1.0000
108	1	1	1.0000	0.0000	0.0000	0.5000

Annex Table 2 (cont.).   Italy   1980 - 1989

	Male								Female					
x	N_x	D_x	q_x	l_x	d_x	e_x	x	N_x	D_x	q_x	l_x	d_x	e_x
80	795169	80239	0.1009	1.0000	0.1009	6.1736	80	1370059	91554	0.0668	1.0000	0.0668	7.5183
81	690636	75151	0.1088	0.8991	0.0978	5.8104	81	1241875	92694	0.0746	0.9332	0.0697	7.0208
82	593727	70537	0.1188	0.8013	0.0952	5.4588	82	1114424	93097	0.0835	0.8635	0.0721	6.5468
83	503644	64955	0.1290	0.7061	0.0911	5.1273	83	989773	92687	0.0936	0.7914	0.0741	6.0980
84	421049	58790	0.1396	0.6150	0.0859	4.8124	84	868310	91034	0.1048	0.7173	0.0752	5.6764
85	345531	52171	0.1510	0.5291	0.0799	4.5123	85	747601	87422	0.1169	0.6421	0.0751	5.2826
86	282385	46323	0.1640	0.4492	0.0737	4.2258	86	637210	82226	0.1290	0.5670	0.0732	4.9160
87	226469	40125	0.1772	0.3755	0.0665	3.9570	87	531225	76078	0.1432	0.4938	0.0707	4.5702
88	179314	34736	0.1937	0.3090	0.0599	3.7014	88	435160	68717	0.1579	0.4231	0.0668	4.2506
89	138658	28772	0.2075	0.2491	0.0517	3.4705	89	349024	61015	0.1748	0.3563	0.0623	3.9539
90	105572	23649	0.2240	0.1974	0.0442	3.2483	90	273324	52276	0.1913	0.2940	0.0562	3.6856
91	79452	19292	0.2428	0.1532	0.0372	3.0417	91	209929	43600	0.2077	0.2378	0.0494	3.4390
92	58024	15144	0.2610	0.1160	0.0303	2.8567	92	156942	35323	0.2251	0.1884	0.0424	3.2094
93	41679	11622	0.2788	0.0857	0.0239	2.6890	93	114796	28204	0.2457	0.1460	0.0359	2.9963
94	29362	8717	0.2969	0.0618	0.0184	2.5354	94	81529	21383	0.2623	0.1101	0.0289	2.8093
95	20219	6356	0.3144	0.0435	0.0137	2.3949	95	56537	16075	0.2843	0.0812	0.0231	2.6303
96	13526	4429	0.3274	0.0298	0.0098	2.2636	96	38028	11444	0.3009	0.0581	0.0175	2.4767
97	8801	3103	0.3526	0.0200	0.0071	2.1223	97	24839	7987	0.3216	0.0406	0.0131	2.3276
98	5509	2022	0.3670	0.0130	0.0048	2.0058	98	15702	5178	0.3298	0.0276	0.0091	2.1939
99	3379	1341	0.3969	0.0082	0.0033	1.8789	99	9821	3627	0.3693	0.0185	0.0068	2.0273
100	1937	828	0.4275	0.0050	0.0021	1.7863	100	5678	2166	0.3815	0.0117	0.0044	1.9216
101	1055	448	0.4246	0.0028	0.0012	1.7466	101	3172	1291	0.4070	0.0072	0.0029	1.7983
102	548	243	0.4434	0.0016	0.0007	1.6667	102	1705	744	0.4364	0.0043	0.0019	1.6894
103	282	143	0.5071	0.0009	0.0005	1.5962	103	895	404	0.4514	0.0024	0.0011	1.6102
104	123	59	0.4797	0.0004	0.0002	1.7239	104	447	205	0.4586	0.0013	0.0006	1.5238
105	59	20	0.3390	0.0002	0.0001	1.8522	105	215	110	0.5116	0.0007	0.0004	1.3910
106	34	16	0.4706	0.0001	0.0001	1.5456	106	98	56	0.5714	0.0003	0.0002	1.3244
107	15	6	0.4000	0.0001	0.0000	1.4750	107	36	15	0.4167	0.0001	0.0001	1.4236
108	8	3	0.3750	0.0000	0.0000	1.1250	108	18	11	0.6111	0.0001	0.0001	1.0833
109	3	3	1.0000	0.0000	0.0000	0.5000	109	6	3	0.5000	0.0000	0.0000	1.0000

Annex Table 2 (cont.). Japan 1980 - 1990

Male

x	N_x	D_x	q_x	l_x	d_x	e_x
80	1488902	129059	0.0867	1.0000	0.0867	6.6587
81	1297356	124697	0.0961	0.9133	0.0878	6.2432
82	1118653	118437	0.1059	0.8255	0.0874	5.8539
83	944822	109827	0.1158	0.7381	0.0854	5.4878
84	801055	101416	0.1266	0.6527	0.0826	5.1408
85	665127	92095	0.1385	0.5701	0.0789	4.8135
86	540835	81528	0.1507	0.4911	0.0740	4.5067
87	428401	71832	0.1677	0.4171	0.0699	4.2179
88	329268	58712	0.1783	0.3472	0.0619	3.9669
89	247987	48086	0.1939	0.2853	0.0553	3.7192
90	183667	38599	0.2102	0.2299	0.0483	3.4936
91	133629	30014	0.2246	0.1816	0.0408	3.2901
92	94682	22923	0.2421	0.1408	0.0341	3.0983
93	65001	16576	0.2550	0.1067	0.0272	2.9283
94	43645	11898	0.2726	0.0795	0.0217	2.7596
95	28379	8297	0.2924	0.0578	0.0169	2.6064
96	18018	5524	0.3066	0.0409	0.0125	2.4766
97	11186	3633	0.3248	0.0284	0.0092	2.3506
98	6755	2253	0.3335	0.0192	0.0064	2.2407
99	3987	1440	0.3612	0.0128	0.0046	2.1118
100	2223	822	0.3698	0.0082	0.0030	2.0231
101	1210	484	0.4000	0.0051	0.0021	1.9168
102	625	244	0.3904	0.0031	0.0012	1.8613
103	333	148	0.4444	0.0019	0.0008	1.7330
104	155	63	0.4065	0.0010	0.0004	1.7195
105	84	40	0.4762	0.0006	0.0003	1.5545
106	38	17	0.4474	0.0003	0.0001	1.5132
107	16	6	0.3750	0.0002	0.0001	1.3333
108	9	6	0.6667	0.0001	0.0001	0.8333
109	2	2	1.0000	0.0000	0.0000	0.5000

Female

x	N_x	D_x	q_x	l_x	d_x	e_x
80	2279129	126441	0.0555	1.0000	0.0555	8.2085
81	2036619	128381	0.0630	0.9445	0.0595	7.6612
82	1812149	129726	0.0716	0.8850	0.0634	7.1430
83	1588477	127449	0.0802	0.8216	0.0659	6.6552
84	1390925	126474	0.0909	0.7557	0.0687	6.1922
85	1196430	121484	0.1015	0.6870	0.0698	5.7615
86	1011111	114666	0.1134	0.6172	0.0700	5.3561
87	833773	105224	0.1262	0.5472	0.0691	4.9773
88	672933	94422	0.1403	0.4782	0.0671	4.6239
89	527470	81957	0.1554	0.4111	0.0639	4.2970
90	407028	69510	0.1708	0.3472	0.0593	3.9955
91	310400	58898	0.1897	0.2879	0.0546	3.7154
92	229520	47014	0.2048	0.2333	0.0478	3.4684
93	164793	36839	0.2235	0.1855	0.0415	3.2331
94	115337	28269	0.2451	0.1440	0.0353	3.0200
95	78227	20575	0.2630	0.1087	0.0286	2.8382
96	51922	14539	0.2800	0.0801	0.0224	2.6726
97	33750	10112	0.2996	0.0577	0.0173	2.5176
98	21355	6865	0.3215	0.0404	0.0130	2.3807
99	13107	4380	0.3342	0.0274	0.0092	2.2717
100	7877	2729	0.3465	0.0183	0.0063	2.1609
101	4538	1666	0.3671	0.0119	0.0044	2.0414
102	2539	984	0.3876	0.0076	0.0029	1.9355
103	1377	576	0.4183	0.0046	0.0019	1.8438
104	694	284	0.4092	0.0027	0.0011	1.8102
105	360	153	0.4250	0.0016	0.0007	1.7177
106	176	78	0.4432	0.0009	0.0004	1.6178
107	81	43	0.5309	0.0005	0.0003	1.5075
108	33	7	0.2121	0.0002	0.0001	1.6476
109	23	14	0.6087	0.0002	0.0001	0.9565

Annex Table 2 (cont). Latvia   1980 - 1990

Male

x	N_x	D_x	q_x	l_x	d_x	e_x
80	33152	3846	0.1160	1.0000	0.1160	5.7449
81	28651	3558	0.1242	0.8840	0.1098	5.4333
82	24449	3239	0.1325	0.7742	0.1026	5.1328
83	20235	2895	0.1431	0.6716	0.0961	4.8402
84	16613	2598	0.1564	0.5756	0.0900	4.5649
85	13406	2311	0.1724	0.4855	0.0837	4.3184
86	10638	1959	0.1842	0.4018	0.0740	4.1137
87	8441	1575	0.1866	0.3278	0.0612	3.9294
88	6698	1322	0.1974	0.2667	0.0526	3.7161
89	5306	1182	0.2228	0.2140	0.0477	3.5069
90	4103	944	0.2301	0.1664	0.0383	3.3688
91	3187	765	0.2400	0.1281	0.0307	3.2261
92	2439	587	0.2407	0.0973	0.0234	3.0871
93	1883	500	0.2655	0.0739	0.0196	2.9071
94	1378	389	0.2823	0.0543	0.0153	2.7773
95	984	298	0.3028	0.0390	0.0118	2.6731
96	679	185	0.2725	0.0272	0.0074	2.6171
97	496	167	0.3367	0.0198	0.0067	2.4099
98	340	110	0.3235	0.0131	0.0042	2.3793
99	237	70	0.2954	0.0089	0.0026	2.2782
100	...	...	...	0.0062	...	2.0235

Female

x	N_x	D_x	q_x	l_x	d_x	e_x
80	79215	6579	0.0831	1.0000	0.0831	6.8141
81	71712	6594	0.0920	0.9169	0.0843	6.3859
82	64228	6497	0.1012	0.8326	0.0842	5.9820
83	56580	6371	0.1126	0.7484	0.0843	5.5989
84	48954	6030	0.1232	0.6641	0.0818	5.2459
85	41933	5644	0.1346	0.5823	0.0784	4.9126
86	35213	5167	0.1467	0.5040	0.0739	4.5989
87	29270	4772	0.1630	0.4300	0.0701	4.3038
88	23661	4294	0.1815	0.3599	0.0653	4.0447
89	19068	3604	0.1890	0.2946	0.0557	3.8307
90	15097	3083	0.2042	0.2389	0.0488	3.6069
91	11957	2622	0.2193	0.1901	0.0417	3.4042
92	9111	2126	0.2333	0.1484	0.0346	3.2199
93	6963	1767	0.2538	0.1138	0.0289	3.0478
94	5154	1335	0.2590	0.0849	0.0220	2.9142
95	3747	1042	0.2781	0.0629	0.0175	2.7581
96	2691	789	0.2932	0.0454	0.0133	2.6280
97	1897	552	0.2910	0.0321	0.0093	2.5107
98	1298	420	0.3236	0.0228	0.0074	2.3359
99	879	288	0.3276	0.0154	0.0050	2.2141
100	...	...	...	0.0104	...	2.0494

Annex Table 2 (cont.).   Luxembourg   1980 - 1989

Male

x	N_x	D_x	q_x	l_x	d_x	e_x
80	5116	600	0.1173	1.0000	0.1173	5.6473
81	4446	564	0.1269	0.8827	0.1120	5.3312
82	3787	514	0.1357	0.7707	0.1046	5.0331
83	3169	458	0.1445	0.6661	0.0963	4.7450
84	2642	411	0.1556	0.5699	0.0886	4.4621
85	2178	365	0.1676	0.4812	0.0806	4.1920
86	1766	313	0.1772	0.4006	0.0710	3.9353
87	1391	255	0.1833	0.3296	0.0604	3.6754
88	1078	241	0.2236	0.2692	0.0602	3.3882
89	796	178	0.2236	0.2090	0.0467	3.2198
90	605	140	0.2314	0.1622	0.0375	3.0031
91	442	106	0.2398	0.1247	0.0299	2.7567
92	323	94	0.2910	0.0948	0.0276	2.4687
93	227	63	0.2775	0.0672	0.0187	2.2768
94	154	53	0.3442	0.0486	0.0167	1.9593
95	93	49	0.5269	0.0318	0.0168	1.7251
96	42	15	0.3571	0.0151	0.0054	2.0894
97	29	10	0.3448	0.0097	0.0033	1.9725
98	18	7	0.3889	0.0063	0.0025	1.7475
99	13	6	0.4615	0.0039	0.0018	1.5413
100	...	...	...	0.0021	...	1.4339

Female

x	N_x	D_x	q_x	l_x	d_x	e_x
80	10047	750	0.0746	1.0000	0.0746	7.1346
81	9035	778	0.0861	0.9254	0.0797	6.6698
82	7920	716	0.0904	0.8457	0.0765	6.2511
83	6947	721	0.1038	0.7692	0.0798	5.8227
84	5956	667	0.1120	0.6894	0.0772	5.4391
85	5061	622	0.1229	0.6122	0.0752	5.0620
86	4190	606	0.1446	0.5369	0.0777	4.7012
87	3449	522	0.1513	0.4593	0.0695	4.4116
88	2763	469	0.1697	0.3898	0.0662	4.1092
89	2160	390	0.1806	0.3236	0.0584	3.8470
90	1647	369	0.2240	0.2652	0.0594	3.5845
91	1179	229	0.1942	0.2058	0.0400	3.4751
92	876	216	0.2466	0.1658	0.0409	3.1923
93	620	156	0.2516	0.1249	0.0314	3.0734
94	441	106	0.2404	0.0935	0.0225	2.9386
95	307	89	0.2899	0.0710	0.0206	2.7102
96	198	55	0.2778	0.0504	0.0140	2.6125
97	128	40	0.3125	0.0364	0.0114	2.4250
98	79	29	0.3671	0.0250	0.0092	2.3000
99	44	12	0.2727	0.0158	0.0043	2.3440
100	...	...	...	0.0115	...	2.0355

Annex Table 2 (cont.). Netherlands 1980 - 1990

Male

x	N_x	D_x	q_x	l_x	d_x	e_x
80	207072	20241	0.0977	1.0000	0.0977	6.3922
81	183518	19433	0.1059	0.9023	0.0955	6.0305
82	161188	18297	0.1135	0.8067	0.0916	5.6855
83	140401	17322	0.1234	0.7151	0.0882	5.3495
84	121504	16315	0.1343	0.6269	0.0842	5.0320
85	103599	15047	0.1452	0.5427	0.0788	4.7350
86	86860	13733	0.1581	0.4639	0.0733	4.4546
87	72260	12269	0.1698	0.3906	0.0663	4.1972
88	59035	10631	0.1801	0.3242	0.0584	3.9534
89	47789	9196	0.1924	0.2659	0.0512	3.7118
90	38068	7935	0.2084	0.2147	0.0448	3.4772
91	29698	6645	0.2238	0.1699	0.0380	3.2611
92	22768	5441	0.2390	0.1319	0.0315	3.0570
93	17056	4342	0.2546	0.1004	0.0256	2.8600
94	12353	3471	0.2810	0.0748	0.0210	2.6660
95	8677	2555	0.2945	0.0538	0.0158	2.5124
96	5983	1923	0.3214	0.0380	0.0122	2.3523
97	3886	1300	0.3345	0.0258	0.0086	2.2296
98	2473	897	0.3627	0.0171	0.0062	2.0991
99	1497	568	0.3794	0.0109	0.0041	2.0093
100	912	358	0.3925	0.0068	0.0027	1.9321
101	543	216	0.3978	0.0041	0.0016	1.8576
102	307	120	0.3909	0.0025	0.0010	1.7543
103	172	78	0.4535	0.0015	0.0007	1.5592
104	91	44	0.4835	0.0008	0.0004	1.4381
105	44	23	0.5227	0.0004	0.0002	1.3164
106	19	12	0.6316	0.0002	0.0001	1.2105
107	7	4	0.5714	0.0001	0.0000	1.4286
108	3	2	0.6667	0.0000	0.0000	1.6667
109	1	0	0.0000	0.0000	0.0000	3.0000

Female

x	N_x	D_x	q_x	l_x	d_x	e_x
80	367867	20887	0.0568	1.0000	0.0568	8.2246
81	336602	21517	0.0639	0.9432	0.0603	7.6896
82	305149	21972	0.0720	0.8829	0.0636	7.1806
83	274071	22248	0.0812	0.8194	0.0665	6.6990
84	243610	22074	0.0906	0.7528	0.0682	6.2466
85	213270	21467	0.1007	0.6846	0.0689	5.8192
86	184097	20803	0.1130	0.6157	0.0696	5.4146
87	156797	19678	0.1255	0.5461	0.0685	5.0407
88	130409	18023	0.1382	0.4776	0.0660	4.6923
89	106865	16407	0.1535	0.4116	0.0632	4.3646
90	85840	14315	0.1668	0.3484	0.0581	4.0656
91	67721	12582	0.1858	0.2903	0.0539	3.7792
92	52166	10558	0.2024	0.2364	0.0478	3.5274
93	39147	8518	0.2176	0.1885	0.0410	3.2957
94	28536	6728	0.2358	0.1475	0.0348	3.0731
95	20407	5173	0.2535	0.1127	0.0286	2.8670
96	14083	3880	0.2755	0.0842	0.0232	2.6707
97	9403	2903	0.3087	0.0610	0.0188	2.4962
98	6016	1910	0.3175	0.0421	0.0134	2.3877
99	3737	1238	0.3313	0.0288	0.0095	2.2658
100	2275	765	0.3363	0.0192	0.0065	2.1406
101	1396	531	0.3804	0.0128	0.0049	1.9718
102	784	311	0.3967	0.0079	0.0031	1.8754
103	423	184	0.4350	0.0048	0.0021	1.7797
104	221	89	0.4027	0.0027	0.0011	1.7648
105	124	56	0.4516	0.0016	0.0007	1.6176
106	62	28	0.4516	0.0009	0.0004	1.5380
107	33	18	0.5455	0.0005	0.0003	1.3929
108	12	6	0.5000	0.0002	0.0001	1.4643
109	7	1	0.1429	0.0001	0.0000	1.4286

Annex Table 2 (cont).   New Zealand   1980 - 1990

Male

x	N_x	D_x	q_x	l_x	d_x	e_x
80	38444	3978	0.1035	1.0000	0.1035	6.2162
81	33424	3658	0.1094	0.8965	0.0981	5.8760
82	28505	3363	0.1180	0.7984	0.0942	5.5366
83	23953	2977	0.1243	0.7042	0.0875	5.2103
84	20007	2683	0.1341	0.6167	0.0827	4.8789
85	16439	2491	0.1515	0.5340	0.0809	4.5570
86	13411	2162	0.1612	0.4531	0.0730	4.2816
87	10650	1956	0.1837	0.3800	0.0698	4.0084
88	8304	1603	0.1930	0.3102	0.0599	3.7977
89	6500	1254	0.1929	0.2503	0.0483	3.5866
90	4998	1096	0.2193	0.2020	0.0443	3.3244
91	3766	878	0.2331	0.1577	0.0368	3.1177
92	2875	714	0.2483	0.1210	0.0300	2.9135
93	2150	618	0.2874	0.0909	0.0261	2.7109
94	1530	437	0.2856	0.0648	0.0185	2.6028
95	1096	332	0.3029	0.0463	0.0140	2.4436
96	761	232	0.3049	0.0323	0.0098	2.2882
97	532	185	0.3477	0.0224	0.0078	2.0724
98	349	130	0.3725	0.0146	0.0054	1.9107
99	214	79	0.3692	0.0092	0.0034	1.7481
100	132	67	0.5076	0.0058	0.0029	1.4784
101	63	28	0.4444	0.0029	0.0013	1.4870
102	36	19	0.5278	0.0016	0.0008	1.2765
103	18	12	0.6667	0.0007	0.0005	1.1444
104	5	1	0.2000	0.0002	0.0000	1.4333
105	3	2	0.6667	0.0002	0.0001	0.6667

Female

x	N_x	D_x	q_x	l_x	d_x	e_x
80	61584	4006	0.0650	1.0000	0.0650	7.9206
81	55703	3863	0.0693	0.9350	0.0648	7.4369
82	49635	4000	0.0806	0.8701	0.0701	6.9538
83	44043	3918	0.0890	0.8000	0.0712	6.5195
84	38764	3852	0.0994	0.7288	0.0724	6.1073
85	33646	3659	0.1087	0.6564	0.0714	5.7260
86	29287	3385	0.1156	0.5850	0.0676	5.3636
87	25299	3271	0.1293	0.5174	0.0669	4.9992
88	21566	3085	0.1430	0.4505	0.0644	4.6673
89	17881	2775	0.1552	0.3861	0.0599	4.3630
90	14668	2577	0.1757	0.3261	0.0573	4.0726
91	11833	2159	0.1825	0.2688	0.0491	3.8341
92	9562	1943	0.2032	0.2198	0.0447	3.5781
93	7459	1604	0.2150	0.1751	0.0377	3.3631
94	5729	1342	0.2342	0.1375	0.0322	3.1475
95	4270	1069	0.2504	0.1053	0.0264	2.9574
96	3104	819	0.2639	0.0789	0.0208	2.7780
97	2213	693	0.3131	0.0581	0.0182	2.5945
98	1447	421	0.2909	0.0399	0.0116	2.5495
99	969	294	0.3034	0.0283	0.0086	2.3904
100	626	218	0.3482	0.0197	0.0069	2.2138
101	374	130	0.3476	0.0128	0.0045	2.1295
102	221	90	0.4072	0.0084	0.0034	1.9977
103	119	47	0.3950	0.0050	0.0020	2.0266
104	66	22	0.3333	0.0030	0.0010	2.0232
105	40	14	0.3500	0.0020	0.0007	1.7848
106	24	9	0.3750	0.0013	0.0005	1.4766
107	16	11	0.6875	0.0008	0.0006	1.0625
108	5	2	0.4000	0.0003	0.0001	1.3000
109	3	2	0.6667	0.0002	0.0001	0.8333

Annex Table 2 (cont).   Norway   1980 - 1990

	Male							Female						
x	N_x	D_x	q_x	l_x	d_x	e_x	x	N_x	D_x	q_x	l_x	d_x	e_x
80	80634	7591	0.0941	1.0000	0.0941	6.4621	80	131754	7773	0.0590	1.0000	0.0590	8.0421
81	71465	7280	0.1019	0.9059	0.0923	6.0817	81	120921	8040	0.0665	0.9410	0.0626	7.5149
82	63314	7130	0.1126	0.8136	0.0916	5.7148	82	110598	8339	0.0754	0.8784	0.0662	7.0146
83	55334	6650	0.1202	0.7220	0.0868	5.3766	83	99725	8344	0.0837	0.8122	0.0680	6.5458
84	47900	6454	0.1347	0.6352	0.0856	5.0427	84	88945	8345	0.0938	0.7442	0.0698	6.0978
85	41000	5729	0.1397	0.5496	0.0768	4.7501	85	78373	8169	0.1042	0.6744	0.0703	5.6774
86	34634	5385	0.1555	0.4728	0.0735	4.4405	86	67786	8006	0.1181	0.6041	0.0714	5.2799
87	28608	4820	0.1685	0.3993	0.0673	4.1659	87	57623	7502	0.1302	0.5328	0.0694	4.9200
88	23296	4246	0.1823	0.3320	0.0605	3.9088	88	48083	6751	0.1404	0.4634	0.0651	4.5816
89	18611	3670	0.1972	0.2715	0.0535	3.6685	89	39372	6348	0.1612	0.3983	0.0642	4.2483
90	14583	3066	0.2102	0.2180	0.0458	3.4468	90	31526	5616	0.1781	0.3341	0.0595	3.9688
91	11217	2552	0.2275	0.1721	0.0392	3.2313	91	24633	4667	0.1895	0.2746	0.0520	3.7206
92	8299	2039	0.2457	0.1330	0.0327	3.0357	92	18802	3840	0.2042	0.2226	0.0455	3.4735
93	6079	1562	0.2570	0.1003	0.0258	2.8617	93	14145	3167	0.2239	0.1771	0.0397	3.2366
94	4419	1209	0.2736	0.0745	0.0204	2.6783	94	10334	2516	0.2435	0.1375	0.0335	3.0261
95	3041	964	0.3170	0.0541	0.0172	2.4988	95	7386	1940	0.2627	0.1040	0.0273	2.8390
96	2005	607	0.3027	0.0370	0.0112	2.4264	96	5121	1454	0.2839	0.0767	0.0218	2.6722
97	1347	455	0.3378	0.0258	0.0087	2.2629	97	3438	1036	0.3013	0.0549	0.0165	2.5335
98	833	293	0.3517	0.0171	0.0060	2.1621	98	2264	716	0.3163	0.0384	0.0121	2.4106
99	517	194	0.3752	0.0111	0.0042	2.0640	99	1426	479	0.3359	0.0262	0.0088	2.2943
100	323	118	0.3653	0.0069	0.0025	2.0033	100	891	300	0.3367	0.0174	0.0059	2.2018
101	189	76	0.4021	0.0044	0.0018	1.8686	101	557	193	0.3465	0.0116	0.0040	2.0657
102	109	48	0.4404	0.0026	0.0012	1.7891	102	334	120	0.3593	0.0076	0.0027	1.8959
103	55	28	0.5091	0.0015	0.0007	1.8035	103	199	86	0.4322	0.0048	0.0021	1.6786
104	26	12	0.4615	0.0007	0.0003	2.1553	104	113	46	0.4071	0.0027	0.0011	1.5756
105	12	4	0.3333	0.0004	0.0001	2.5741	105	61	29	0.4754	0.0016	0.0008	1.3141
106	8	0	0.0000	0.0003	0.0000	2.6111	106	31	20	0.6452	0.0009	0.0006	1.0520
107	9	4	0.4444	0.0003	0.0001	1.6111	107	9	6	0.6667	0.0003	0.0002	1.0556
108	4	2	0.5000	0.0001	0.0001	1.5000	108	3	1	0.3333	0.0001	0.0000	1.1667
109	2	1	0.5000	0.0001	0.0000	1.5000	109	2	2	1.0000	0.0001	0.0001	0.5000

Annex Table 2 (cont.). Poland 1980 – 1990

	Male							Female						
x	N_x	D_x	q_x	l_x	d_x	e_x	x	N_x	D_x	q_x	l_x	d_x	e_x
80	408537	49434	0.1210	1.0000	0.1210	5.4865	80	777573	66225	0.0852	1.0000	0.0852	6.5663
81	346001	45216	0.1307	0.8790	0.1149	5.1730	81	689349	64895	0.0941	0.9148	0.0861	6.1310
82	289292	40667	0.1406	0.7641	0.1074	4.8755	82	603537	63539	0.1053	0.8287	0.0872	5.7162
83	237656	36240	0.1525	0.6567	0.1001	4.5911	83	520589	60216	0.1157	0.7415	0.0858	5.3300
84	192655	31833	0.1652	0.5566	0.0920	4.3272	84	441666	57746	0.1307	0.6557	0.0857	4.9618
85	153924	27277	0.1772	0.4646	0.0823	4.0848	85	368081	53121	0.1443	0.5700	0.0823	4.6329
86	120322	23027	0.1914	0.3823	0.0732	3.8569	86	299237	47503	0.1587	0.4877	0.0774	4.3299
87	92820	19082	0.2056	0.3091	0.0635	3.6514	87	241043	42405	0.1759	0.4103	0.0722	4.0526
88	70029	15441	0.2205	0.2456	0.0541	3.4669	88	189772	36120	0.1903	0.3381	0.0644	3.8111
89	52439	12323	0.2350	0.1914	0.0450	3.3061	89	147443	30247	0.2051	0.2738	0.0562	3.5894
90	38352	9335	0.2434	0.1464	0.0356	3.1681	90	111872	24700	0.2208	0.2176	0.0480	3.3867
91	28067	7276	0.2592	0.1108	0.0287	3.0265	91	84273	19838	0.2354	0.1696	0.0399	3.2047
92	20130	5392	0.2679	0.0821	0.0220	2.9107	92	61650	15509	0.2516	0.1296	0.0326	3.0374
93	14221	4037	0.2839	0.0601	0.0171	2.7926	93	44374	11863	0.2673	0.0970	0.0259	2.8903
94	9816	2852	0.2905	0.0430	0.0125	2.7014	94	31222	8732	0.2797	0.0711	0.0199	2.7625
95	6721	2034	0.3026	0.0305	0.0092	2.6030	95	21613	6418	0.2970	0.0512	0.0152	2.6409
96	4534	1446	0.3189	0.0213	0.0068	2.5156	96	14557	4524	0.3108	0.0360	0.0112	2.5452
97	2954	953	0.3226	0.0145	0.0047	2.4595	97	9697	3108	0.3205	0.0248	0.0080	2.4674
98	1933	596	0.3083	0.0098	0.0030	2.3927	98	6369	2047	0.3214	0.0169	0.0054	2.3954
99	1271	385	0.3029	0.0068	0.0021	2.2364	99	4123	1185	0.2874	0.0114	0.0033	2.2931
100	...	...	...	0.0047	...	1.9909	100	...	...	...	0.0082	...	2.0163

Annex Table 2 (cont.).   Portugal   1980 - 1990

Male

x	N_x	D_x	q_x	l_x	d_x	e_x
80	137489	14817	0.1078	1.0000	0.1078	5.7680
81	117399	13894	0.1183	0.8922	0.1056	5.4043
82	99547	12747	0.1281	0.7866	0.1007	5.0627
83	83174	11839	0.1423	0.6859	0.0976	4.7327
84	68072	10522	0.1546	0.5883	0.0909	4.4352
85	55335	9373	0.1694	0.4973	0.0842	4.1547
86	44386	8145	0.1835	0.4131	0.0758	3.9000
87	35018	6880	0.1965	0.3373	0.0663	3.6641
88	27165	5822	0.2143	0.2710	0.0581	3.4377
89	20582	4694	0.2281	0.2129	0.0486	3.2391
90	15262	3753	0.2459	0.1644	0.0404	3.0483
91	11092	2808	0.2532	0.1240	0.0314	2.8793
92	8015	2203	0.2749	0.0926	0.0254	2.6859
93	5573	1659	0.2977	0.0671	0.0200	2.5144
94	3752	1169	0.3116	0.0471	0.0147	2.3682
95	2477	822	0.3319	0.0325	0.0108	2.2137
96	1578	596	0.3777	0.0217	0.0082	2.0649
97	926	351	0.3790	0.0135	0.0051	2.0146
98	546	214	0.3919	0.0084	0.0033	1.9392
99	329	135	0.4103	0.0051	0.0021	1.8669
100	184	78	0.4239	0.0030	0.0013	1.8181
101	101	43	0.4257	0.0017	0.0007	1.7880
102	51	23	0.4510	0.0010	0.0004	1.7429
103	24	10	0.4167	0.0005	0.0002	1.7639
104	12	6	0.5000	0.0003	0.0002	1.6667
105	6	2	0.3333	0.0002	0.0001	1.8333
106	4	1	0.2500	0.0001	0.0000	1.5000
107	3	2	0.6667	0.0001	0.0001	0.8333
108	1	1	1.0000	0.0000	0.0000	0.5000

Female

x	N_x	D_x	q_x	l_x	d_x	e_x
80	237654	18567	0.0781	1.0000	0.0781	6.9335
81	211572	18411	0.0870	0.9219	0.0802	6.4787
82	187738	18191	0.0969	0.8417	0.0816	6.0486
83	163357	17928	0.1097	0.7601	0.0834	5.6439
84	139928	16978	0.1213	0.6767	0.0821	5.2780
85	118435	16019	0.1353	0.5946	0.0804	4.9378
86	99621	14786	0.1484	0.5142	0.0763	4.6319
87	82047	13062	0.1592	0.4378	0.0697	4.3521
88	66996	11450	0.1709	0.3681	0.0629	4.0815
89	53985	10124	0.1875	0.3052	0.0572	3.8197
90	42502	8661	0.2038	0.2480	0.0505	3.5860
91	32618	7098	0.2176	0.1974	0.0430	3.3758
92	24576	5756	0.2342	0.1545	0.0362	3.1756
93	18115	4465	0.2465	0.1183	0.0292	2.9940
94	13124	3419	0.2605	0.0891	0.0232	2.8098
95	9218	2655	0.2880	0.0659	0.0190	2.6235
96	6223	1854	0.2979	0.0469	0.0140	2.4825
97	4094	1316	0.3214	0.0330	0.0106	2.3238
98	2616	910	0.3479	0.0224	0.0078	2.1878
99	1590	559	0.3516	0.0146	0.0051	2.0881
100	973	355	0.3649	0.0095	0.0034	1.9492
101	579	259	0.4473	0.0060	0.0027	1.7817
102	297	124	0.4175	0.0033	0.0014	1.8191
103	161	61	0.3789	0.0019	0.0007	1.7645
104	93	47	0.5054	0.0012	0.0006	1.5359
105	42	19	0.4524	0.0006	0.0003	1.5943
106	23	10	0.4348	0.0003	0.0001	1.4983
107	11	6	0.5455	0.0002	0.0001	1.2662
108	7	4	0.5714	0.0001	0.0000	1.1857
109	5	3	0.6000	0.0000	0.0000	1.1000

Annex Table 2 (cont.).   Scotland   1980 - 1990

Male

x	N_x	D_x	q_x	l_x	d_x	e_x
80	81019	9453	0.1167	1.0000	0.1167	5.6335
81	69212	8690	0.1256	0.8833	0.1109	5.3116
82	58044	7905	0.1362	0.7724	0.1052	5.0025
83	48182	7116	0.1477	0.6672	0.0985	4.7123
84	39475	6262	0.1586	0.5687	0.0902	4.4423
85	31868	5450	0.1710	0.4785	0.0818	4.1855
86	25386	4612	0.1817	0.3966	0.0721	3.9458
87	19937	3894	0.1953	0.3246	0.0634	3.7109
88	15423	3258	0.2112	0.2612	0.0552	3.4902
89	11677	2611	0.2236	0.2060	0.0461	3.2910
90	8846	2123	0.2400	0.1599	0.0384	3.0948
91	6605	1696	0.2568	0.1216	0.0312	2.9143
92	4841	1303	0.2692	0.0903	0.0243	2.7483
93	3486	1011	0.2900	0.0660	0.0191	2.5764
94	2443	732	0.2996	0.0469	0.0140	2.4246
95	1683	579	0.3440	0.0328	0.0113	2.2479
96	1076	371	0.3448	0.0215	0.0074	2.1646
97	691	243	0.3517	0.0141	0.0050	2.0406
98	444	177	0.3986	0.0091	0.0036	1.8763
99	252	101	0.4008	0.0055	0.0022	1.7886
100	...	...	...	0.0033	...	1.6505

Female

x	N_x	D_x	q_x	l_x	d_x	e_x
80	163918	12112	0.0739	1.0000	0.0739	7.4217
81	149083	11933	0.0800	0.9261	0.0741	6.9740
82	134134	12103	0.0902	0.8520	0.0769	6.5372
83	119368	11760	0.0985	0.7751	0.0764	6.1360
84	104838	11261	0.1074	0.6987	0.0751	5.7520
85	90911	10645	0.1171	0.6237	0.0730	5.3840
86	77703	10092	0.1299	0.5507	0.0715	5.0317
87	65586	9306	0.1419	0.4791	0.0680	4.7081
88	54462	8548	0.1570	0.4112	0.0645	4.4039
89	44162	7504	0.1699	0.3466	0.0589	4.1307
90	35404	6624	0.1871	0.2877	0.0538	3.8740
91	27765	5607	0.2019	0.2339	0.0472	3.6505
92	21359	4579	0.2144	0.1867	0.0400	3.4477
93	16094	3795	0.2358	0.1466	0.0346	3.2521
94	11806	2973	0.2518	0.1121	0.0282	3.1013
95	8499	2223	0.2616	0.0838	0.0219	2.9769
96	6015	1619	0.2692	0.0619	0.0167	2.8542
97	4202	1197	0.2849	0.0452	0.0129	2.7213
98	2846	827	0.2906	0.0324	0.0094	2.6061
99	1896	537	0.2832	0.0230	0.0065	2.4687
100	...	...	...	0.0165	...	2.2467

Annex Table 2 (cont.).   Singapore Chinese   1982 - 1990

Male

x	N_x	D_x	q_x	l_x	d_x	e_x
80	10468	974	0.0930	1.0000	0.0930	6.7904
81	8873	900	0.1014	0.9070	0.0920	6.4358
82	7395	825	0.1116	0.8150	0.0909	6.1058
83	6013	697	0.1159	0.7240	0.0839	5.8097
84	4894	624	0.1275	0.6401	0.0816	5.5059
85	3921	516	0.1316	0.5585	0.0735	5.2375
86	3101	447	0.1441	0.4850	0.0699	4.9554
87	2379	370	0.1555	0.4151	0.0646	4.7058
88	1756	275	0.1566	0.3505	0.0549	4.4804
89	1305	224	0.1716	0.2956	0.0507	4.2195
90	976	170	0.1742	0.2449	0.0427	3.9902
91	737	147	0.1995	0.2022	0.0403	3.7263
92	518	119	0.2297	0.1619	0.0372	3.5302
93	347	65	0.1873	0.1247	0.0234	3.4339
94	245	59	0.2408	0.1013	0.0244	3.1102
95	166	37	0.2229	0.0769	0.0171	2.9382
96	113	30	0.2655	0.0598	0.0159	2.6375
97	67	19	0.2836	0.0439	0.0125	2.4101
98	40	11	0.2750	0.0315	0.0087	2.1662
99	23	11	0.4783	0.0228	0.0109	1.7981
100	11	6	0.5455	0.0119	0.0065	1.9881
101	5	2	0.4000	0.0054	0.0022	...
102	3	0	0.0000	0.0032	0.0000	...
103	2	0	0.0000	0.0032	0.0000	...
104	2	0	0.0000	0.0032	0.0000	...
105	1	0	0.0000	0.0032	0.0000	...
106	1	0	0.0000	0.0032	0.0000	...
107	0	0	...	0.0032	...	...

Female

x	N_x	D_x	q_x	l_x	d_x	e_x
80	16430	1122	0.0683	1.0000	0.0683	8.0209
81	14452	1118	0.0774	0.9317	0.0721	7.5721
82	12582	1033	0.0821	0.8596	0.0706	7.1651
83	10828	990	0.0914	0.7891	0.0721	6.7612
84	9250	888	0.0960	0.7169	0.0688	6.3913
85	7865	834	0.1060	0.6481	0.0687	6.0169
86	6544	743	0.1135	0.5794	0.0658	5.6713
87	5395	692	0.1283	0.5136	0.0659	5.3337
88	4371	558	0.1277	0.4477	0.0572	5.0449
89	3541	513	0.1449	0.3906	0.0566	4.7100
90	2829	487	0.1721	0.3340	0.0575	4.4232
91	2195	389	0.1772	0.2765	0.0490	4.2391
92	1677	296	0.1765	0.2275	0.0402	4.0444
93	1278	246	0.1925	0.1873	0.0361	3.8041
94	968	201	0.2076	0.1513	0.0314	3.5917
95	727	165	0.2270	0.1199	0.0272	3.4020
96	523	134	0.2562	0.0927	0.0237	3.2540
97	345	79	0.2290	0.0689	0.0158	3.2026
98	235	51	0.2170	0.0531	0.0115	3.0053
99	162	46	0.2840	0.0416	0.0118	2.6997
100	107	31	0.2897	0.0298	0.0086	2.5720
101	70	27	0.3857	0.0212	0.0082	...
102	38	14	0.3684	0.0130	0.0048	...
103	20	8	0.4000	0.0082	0.0033	...
104	9	2	0.2222	0.0049	0.0011	...
105	4	0	0.0000	0.0038	0.0000	...
106	2	0	0.0000	0.0038	0.0000	...
107	2	0	0.0000	0.0038	0.0000	...
108	2	0	0.0000	0.0038	0.0000	...
109	...	...	1.0000	0.0038	0.0038	...

Annex Table 2 (cont.). Spain 1980 - 1986

Male

x	N_x	D_x	q_x	l_x	d_x	e_x
80	320203	29638	0.0926	1.0000	0.0926	6.5785
81	276977	27706	0.1000	0.9074	0.0908	6.1985
82	236591	26090	0.1103	0.8167	0.0901	5.8319
83	198930	23346	0.1174	0.7266	0.0853	5.4928
84	167201	21964	0.1314	0.6413	0.0842	5.1566
85	137854	19739	0.1432	0.5571	0.0798	4.8608
86	112317	17079	0.1521	0.4773	0.0726	4.5896
87	90791	15036	0.1656	0.4047	0.0670	4.3230
88	72608	12809	0.1764	0.3377	0.0596	4.0818
89	57102	10764	0.1885	0.2781	0.0524	3.8490
90	44468	9199	0.2069	0.2257	0.0467	3.6269
91	33665	6829	0.2029	0.1790	0.0363	3.4425
92	25452	5700	0.2240	0.1427	0.0320	3.1913
93	18273	4277	0.2341	0.1107	0.0259	2.9679
94	12743	3076	0.2414	0.0848	0.0205	2.7221
95	8704	2413	0.2772	0.0643	0.0178	2.4292
96	5646	1604	0.2841	0.0465	0.0132	2.1691
97	3588	1102	0.3071	0.0333	0.0102	1.8315
98	2270	675	0.2974	0.0231	0.0069	1.4217
99	1538	579	0.3765	0.0162	0.0061	0.8118

Female

x	N_x	D_x	q_x	l_x	d_x	e_x
80	528158	34878	0.0660	1.0000	0.0660	7.6333
81	471032	34427	0.0731	0.9340	0.0683	7.1376
82	415770	34479	0.0829	0.8657	0.0718	6.6610
83	361551	33644	0.0931	0.7939	0.0739	6.2181
84	313069	32862	0.1050	0.7200	0.0756	5.8048
85	267176	31032	0.1161	0.6445	0.0749	5.4270
86	225786	28425	0.1259	0.5696	0.0717	5.0744
87	188851	26263	0.1391	0.4979	0.0692	4.7333
88	157092	23993	0.1527	0.4287	0.0655	4.4171
89	127965	21190	0.1656	0.3632	0.0601	4.1232
90	103298	18823	0.1822	0.3030	0.0552	3.8422
91	80915	15098	0.1866	0.2478	0.0462	3.5870
92	62635	12817	0.2046	0.2016	0.0412	3.2951
93	46433	10283	0.2215	0.1603	0.0355	3.0142
94	33289	8041	0.2416	0.1248	0.0302	2.7294
95	23193	6167	0.2659	0.0947	0.0252	2.4394
96	15614	4488	0.2874	0.0695	0.0200	2.1419
97	10152	3146	0.3099	0.0495	0.0153	1.8042
98	6613	2165	0.3274	0.0342	0.0112	1.3898
99	4373	1549	0.3542	0.0230	0.0081	0.8229

Annex Table 2 (cont.).   Sweden   1980 - 1990

		Male								Female					
x	N_x	D_x	q_x	l_x	d_x	e_x		x	N_x	D_x	q_x	l_x	d_x	e_x
80	193023	17780	0.0921	1.0000	0.0921	6.3884		80	295468	17127	0.0580	1.0000	0.0580	8.0747
81	169454	17276	0.1020	0.9079	0.0926	5.9858		81	270006	17654	0.0654	0.9420	0.0616	7.5408
82	148048	16587	0.1120	0.8153	0.0913	5.6086		82	244513	17837	0.0729	0.8804	0.0642	7.0333
83	127452	15651	0.1228	0.7240	0.0889	5.2532		83	219330	17859	0.0814	0.8162	0.0665	6.5475
84	108777	14712	0.1352	0.6351	0.0859	4.9186		84	194656	18189	0.0934	0.7498	0.0701	6.0835
85	91448	13309	0.1455	0.5492	0.0799	4.6096		85	170561	18215	0.1068	0.6797	0.0726	5.6590
86	75634	11890	0.1572	0.4693	0.0738	4.3096		86	146440	17018	0.1162	0.6071	0.0706	5.2759
87	62028	10830	0.1746	0.3955	0.0691	4.0202		87	124570	15894	0.1276	0.5366	0.0685	4.9038
88	49383	9321	0.1887	0.3264	0.0616	3.7649		88	103719	14992	0.1445	0.4681	0.0677	4.5479
89	38810	7947	0.2048	0.2648	0.0542	3.5245		89	84776	13484	0.1591	0.4004	0.0637	4.2319
90	29823	6522	0.2187	0.2106	0.0461	3.3033		90	67817	11799	0.1740	0.3367	0.0586	3.9377
91	22575	5439	0.2409	0.1645	0.0396	3.0879		91	53421	10271	0.1923	0.2782	0.0535	3.6618
92	16604	4212	0.2537	0.1249	0.0317	2.9093		92	41084	8632	0.2101	0.2247	0.0472	3.4144
93	12111	3329	0.2749	0.0932	0.0256	2.7282		93	30908	7067	0.2286	0.1775	0.0406	3.1896
94	8459	2440	0.2885	0.0676	0.0195	2.5729		94	22660	5470	0.2414	0.1369	0.0330	2.9869
95	5890	1829	0.3105	0.0481	0.0149	2.4132		95	16281	4288	0.2634	0.1038	0.0274	2.7782
96	3977	1271	0.3196	0.0332	0.0106	2.2748		96	11459	3378	0.2948	0.0765	0.0226	2.5928
97	2617	933	0.3565	0.0226	0.0080	2.1085		97	7618	2306	0.3027	0.0539	0.0163	2.4676
98	1610	588	0.3652	0.0145	0.0053	1.9996		98	5031	1604	0.3188	0.0376	0.0120	2.3218
99	980	390	0.3980	0.0092	0.0037	1.8624		99	3174	1057	0.3330	0.0256	0.0085	2.1745
100	553	228	0.4123	0.0055	0.0023	1.7629		100	1995	736	0.3689	0.0171	0.0063	2.0106
101	327	146	0.4465	0.0033	0.0015	1.6489		101	1193	467	0.3915	0.0108	0.0042	1.8936
102	171	78	0.4561	0.0018	0.0008	1.5757		102	671	272	0.4054	0.0066	0.0027	1.7901
103	86	41	0.4767	0.0010	0.0005	1.4779		103	361	154	0.4266	0.0039	0.0017	1.6695
104	41	21	0.5122	0.0005	0.0003	1.3689		104	190	81	0.4263	0.0022	0.0010	1.5396
105	16	6	0.3750	0.0003	0.0001	1.2813		105	109	61	0.5596	0.0013	0.0007	1.3122
106	8	6	0.7500	0.0002	0.0001	0.7500		106	43	18	0.4186	0.0006	0.0002	1.3444
107	1	1	1.0000	0.0000	0.0000	0.5000		107	21	14	0.6667	0.0003	0.0002	1.7901
								108	7	5	0.7143	0.0001	0.0001	0.8571
								109	4	2	0.5000	0.0000	0.0000	0.7500

Annex Table 2 (cont.). Switzerland 1980 - 1990

Male

x	N_x	D_x	q_x	l_x	d_x	e_x
80	117644	10558	0.0897	1.0000	0.0897	6.5047
81	104158	10280	0.0987	0.9103	0.0898	6.0967
82	90317	9746	0.1079	0.8204	0.0885	5.7096
83	77705	9258	0.1191	0.7319	0.0872	5.3397
84	65865	8389	0.1274	0.6447	0.0821	4.9943
85	55056	7873	0.1430	0.5626	0.0804	4.6503
86	45127	6962	0.1543	0.4821	0.0744	4.3429
87	36578	6242	0.1706	0.4077	0.0696	4.0439
88	28917	5412	0.1872	0.3382	0.0633	3.7730
89	22352	4523	0.2024	0.2749	0.0556	3.5267
90	16919	3857	0.2280	0.2193	0.0500	3.2945
91	12409	2897	0.2335	0.1693	0.0395	3.1197
92	9130	2362	0.2587	0.1298	0.0336	2.9175
93	6493	1745	0.2688	0.0962	0.0258	2.7612
94	4570	1334	0.2919	0.0703	0.0205	2.5923
95	3081	950	0.3083	0.0498	0.0154	2.4548
96	2020	662	0.3277	0.0344	0.0113	2.3262
97	1282	425	0.3315	0.0232	0.0077	2.2165
98	821	292	0.3557	0.0155	0.0055	2.0677
99	495	189	0.3818	0.0100	0.0038	1.9330
100	294	128	0.4354	0.0062	0.0027	1.8181
101	154	57	0.3701	0.0035	0.0013	1.8344
102	89	40	0.4494	0.0022	0.0010	1.6186
103	45	20	0.4444	0.0012	0.0005	1.5317
104	21	9	0.4286	0.0007	0.0003	1.3571
105	8	6	0.7500	0.0004	0.0003	1.0000
106	2	0	0.0000	0.0001	0.0000	1.5000
107	2	2	1.0000	0.0001	0.0001	0.5000

Female

x	N_x	D_x	q_x	l_x	d_x	e_x
80	207392	11424	0.0551	1.0000	0.0551	8.1370
81	191247	12083	0.0632	0.9449	0.0597	7.5822
82	173325	12546	0.0724	0.8852	0.0641	7.0599
83	155338	12648	0.0814	0.8211	0.0669	6.5717
84	137668	12743	0.0926	0.7543	0.0698	6.1099
85	119565	12036	0.1007	0.6845	0.0689	5.6822
86	102779	11802	0.1148	0.6156	0.0707	5.2622
87	86929	11160	0.1284	0.5449	0.0700	4.8800
88	71537	10097	0.1411	0.4749	0.0670	4.5251
89	57948	9186	0.1585	0.4079	0.0647	4.1866
90	45633	8072	0.1769	0.3432	0.0607	3.8811
91	35194	6848	0.1946	0.2825	0.0550	3.6077
92	26510	5602	0.2113	0.2275	0.0481	3.3585
93	19529	4563	0.2337	0.1795	0.0419	3.1244
94	13881	3485	0.2511	0.1375	0.0345	2.9246
95	9777	2662	0.2723	0.1030	0.0280	2.7374
96	6649	1900	0.2858	0.0750	0.0214	2.5745
97	4434	1312	0.2959	0.0535	0.0158	2.4045
98	2896	973	0.3360	0.0377	0.0127	2.2048
99	1778	663	0.3729	0.0250	0.0093	2.0674
100	1031	417	0.4045	0.0157	0.0063	1.9994
101	557	207	0.3716	0.0093	0.0035	2.0177
102	310	123	0.3968	0.0059	0.0023	1.9153
103	177	75	0.4237	0.0035	0.0015	1.8463
104	89	38	0.4270	0.0020	0.0009	1.8362
105	42	18	0.4286	0.0012	0.0005	1.8318
106	22	8	0.3636	0.0007	0.0002	1.8306
107	11	5	0.4545	0.0004	0.0002	1.5909
108	3	0	0.0000	0.0002	0.0000	1.5000
109	2	2	1.0000	0.0002	0.0002	0.5000

Annex Table 3. Decennial life tables for aggregates.
Thirteen countries with good data   1950 - 1960

Male

x	N_x	D_x	q_x	l_x	d_x	e_x
80	2965900	367026	0.1237	1.0000	0.1237	5.2507
81	2528425	338916	0.1340	0.8763	0.1175	4.9216
82	2121444	312381	0.1472	0.7588	0.1117	4.6060
83	1743838	278514	0.1597	0.6471	0.1033	4.3150
84	1407009	244287	0.1736	0.5437	0.0944	4.0402
85	1112149	209589	0.1885	0.4493	0.0847	3.7839
86	863268	176555	0.2045	0.3646	0.0746	3.5465
87	658566	145356	0.2207	0.2901	0.0640	3.3298
88	489548	115799	0.2365	0.2260	0.0535	3.1313
89	358303	90528	0.2527	0.1726	0.0436	2.9465
90	256389	69014	0.2692	0.1290	0.0347	2.7736
91	176662	50647	0.2867	0.0943	0.0270	2.6111
92	118481	36194	0.3055	0.0672	0.0205	2.4595
93	77126	24967	0.3237	0.0467	0.0151	2.3215
94	48544	16484	0.3396	0.0316	0.0107	2.1933
95	29577	10764	0.3639	0.0209	0.0076	2.0640
96	17813	6690	0.3756	0.0133	0.0050	1.9588
97	10472	4170	0.3982	0.0083	0.0033	1.8362
98	5900	2483	0.4208	0.0050	0.0021	1.7204
99	3232	1514	0.4684	0.0029	0.0014	1.6072
100	1643	820	0.4991	0.0015	0.0008	1.5829
101	771	336	0.4358	0.0008	0.0003	1.6619
102	402	190	0.4726	0.0004	0.0002	1.5594
103	190	93	0.4895	0.0002	0.0001	1.5088
104	93	45	0.4839	0.0001	0.0001	1.4760
105	45	24	0.5333	0.0001	0.0000	1.3909
106	22	12	0.5455	0.0000	0.0000	1.4091
107	9	2	0.2222	0.0000	0.0000	1.5000
108	7	5	0.7143	0.0000	0.0000	0.7857
109	2	2	1.0000	0.0000	0.0000	0.5000

Female

x	N_x	D_x	q_x	l_x	d_x	e_x
80	4447961	444621	0.1000	1.0000	0.1000	6.0387
81	3860398	422119	0.1093	0.9000	0.0984	5.6539
82	3305262	399631	0.1209	0.8016	0.0969	5.2866
83	2785155	370763	0.1331	0.7047	0.0938	4.9449
84	2308214	337103	0.1460	0.6109	0.0892	4.6275
85	1882329	298640	0.1587	0.5217	0.0828	4.3334
86	1511727	263087	0.1740	0.4389	0.0764	4.0563
87	1193460	224277	0.1879	0.3625	0.0681	3.8056
88	924399	187065	0.2024	0.2944	0.0596	3.5705
89	707441	154574	0.2185	0.2348	0.0513	3.3495
90	528866	123993	0.2345	0.1835	0.0430	3.1462
91	382272	95104	0.2488	0.1405	0.0350	2.9566
92	270210	72869	0.2697	0.1055	0.0285	2.7702
93	185691	53004	0.2854	0.0771	0.0220	2.6085
94	124104	37669	0.3035	0.0551	0.0167	2.4508
95	80372	26001	0.3235	0.0384	0.0124	2.3009
96	51108	17552	0.3434	0.0259	0.0089	2.1621
97	31456	11539	0.3668	0.0170	0.0062	2.0315
98	18648	7208	0.3865	0.0108	0.0042	1.9188
99	10674	4383	0.4106	0.0066	0.0027	1.8128
100	5933	2632	0.4436	0.0039	0.0017	1.7275
101	3072	1343	0.4372	0.0022	0.0009	1.7062
102	1592	711	0.4466	0.0012	0.0005	1.6430
103	793	383	0.4830	0.0007	0.0003	1.5655
104	376	174	0.4628	0.0003	0.0002	1.5609
105	173	82	0.4740	0.0002	0.0001	1.4747
106	79	34	0.4304	0.0001	0.0000	1.3529
107	47	30	0.6383	0.0001	0.0000	0.9973
108	16	10	0.6250	0.0000	0.0000	0.8750
109	5	5	1.0000	0.0000	0.0000	0.5000

Annex Table 3 (cont.).   Thirteen countries with good data 1960 - 1970

Male

x	N_x	D_x	q_x	l_x	d_x	e_x
80	3759342	444050	0.1181	1.0000	0.1181	5.4503
81	3274209	420568	0.1284	0.8819	0.1133	5.1133
82	2818161	396580	0.1407	0.7686	0.1082	4.7932
83	2394777	363967	0.1520	0.6604	0.1004	4.4963
84	2012364	333305	0.1656	0.5601	0.0928	4.2125
85	1658486	295946	0.1784	0.4673	0.0834	3.9495
86	1340245	260410	0.1943	0.3839	0.0746	3.6987
87	1057032	220782	0.2089	0.3093	0.0646	3.4701
88	816847	184204	0.2255	0.2447	0.0552	3.2543
89	611738	147466	0.2411	0.1895	0.0457	3.0563
90	449228	115765	0.2577	0.1438	0.0371	2.8682
91	320491	88903	0.2774	0.1068	0.0296	2.6904
92	221819	65777	0.2965	0.0772	0.0229	2.5312
93	148221	46494	0.3137	0.0543	0.0170	2.3874
94	96697	32241	0.3334	0.0373	0.0124	2.2501
95	61107	21531	0.3523	0.0248	0.0087	2.1255
96	37323	13826	0.3704	0.0161	0.0060	2.0098
97	22213	8615	0.3878	0.0101	0.0039	1.8982
98	12689	5164	0.4070	0.0062	0.0025	1.7840
99	7111	3209	0.4513	0.0037	0.0017	1.6651
100	3623	1663	0.4590	0.0020	0.0009	1.6232
101	1773	831	0.4687	0.0011	0.0005	1.5762
102	880	412	0.4682	0.0006	0.0003	1.5256
103	442	219	0.4955	0.0003	0.0002	1.4285
104	197	110	0.5584	0.0002	0.0001	1.3403
105	82	41	0.5000	0.0001	0.0000	1.4028
106	38	23	0.6053	0.0000	0.0000	1.3057
107	13	6	0.4615	0.0000	0.0000	1.5410
108	6	2	0.3333	0.0000	0.0000	1.4333
109	5	4	0.8000	0.0000	0.0000	0.9000

Female

x	N_x	D_x	q_x	l_x	d_x	e_x
80	6304878	568967	0.0902	1.0000	0.0902	6.3924
81	5583726	556607	0.0997	0.9098	0.0907	5.9769
82	4890807	541254	0.1107	0.8191	0.0906	5.5833
83	4232048	518193	0.1224	0.7284	0.0892	5.2159
84	3616606	487048	0.1347	0.6392	0.0861	4.8739
85	3038785	448216	0.1475	0.5531	0.0816	4.5546
86	2506183	406447	0.1622	0.4716	0.0765	4.2561
87	2023476	356698	0.1763	0.3951	0.0696	3.9832
88	1601013	305820	0.1910	0.3254	0.0622	3.7286
89	1233898	254990	0.2067	0.2633	0.0544	3.4910
90	934506	209033	0.2237	0.2089	0.0467	3.2701
91	689902	165144	0.2394	0.1621	0.0388	3.0682
92	498292	128599	0.2581	0.1233	0.0318	2.8764
93	348690	96427	0.2765	0.0915	0.0253	2.7031
94	237673	69908	0.2941	0.0662	0.0195	2.5452
95	158328	49479	0.3125	0.0467	0.0146	2.3974
96	102763	34355	0.3343	0.0321	0.0107	2.2599
97	64353	22524	0.3500	0.0214	0.0075	2.1438
98	38976	14535	0.3729	0.0139	0.0052	2.0289
99	23044	8830	0.3832	0.0087	0.0033	1.9381
100	13134	5476	0.4169	0.0054	0.0022	1.8315
101	7166	3000	0.4186	0.0031	0.0013	1.7837
102	3907	1661	0.4251	0.0018	0.0008	1.7080
103	2059	940	0.4565	0.0010	0.0005	1.6014
104	1032	486	0.4709	0.0006	0.0003	1.5267
105	513	254	0.4951	0.0003	0.0001	1.4406
106	237	118	0.4979	0.0002	0.0001	1.3630
107	105	62	0.5905	0.0001	0.0000	1.2187
108	38	21	0.5526	0.0000	0.0000	1.2549
109	16	12	0.7500	0.0000	0.0000	1.1875

Annex Table 3 (cont). Thirteen countries with good data   1970 - 1980

Male

x	N_x	D_x	q_x	l_x	d_x	e_x
80	4418380	491979	0.1113	1.0000	0.1113	5.7487
81	3815635	459662	0.1205	0.8887	0.1071	5.4063
82	3269932	428912	0.1312	0.7816	0.1025	5.0783
83	2770947	394111	0.1422	0.6791	0.0966	4.7695
84	2318115	357750	0.1543	0.5825	0.0899	4.4775
85	1922579	320678	0.1668	0.4926	0.0822	4.2033
86	1571413	283255	0.1803	0.4104	0.0740	3.9447
87	1259864	245305	0.1947	0.3365	0.0655	3.7021
88	992168	207167	0.2088	0.2709	0.0566	3.4764
89	768009	171982	0.2239	0.2144	0.0480	3.2618
90	581125	140464	0.2417	0.1664	0.0402	3.0588
91	428487	111059	0.2592	0.1262	0.0327	2.8744
92	307781	85263	0.2770	0.0935	0.0259	2.7051
93	216206	63857	0.2954	0.0676	0.0200	2.5500
94	147709	45967	0.3112	0.0476	0.0148	2.4093
95	98283	32514	0.3308	0.0328	0.0108	2.2719
96	62968	21803	0.3463	0.0219	0.0076	2.1479
97	39122	14218	0.3634	0.0143	0.0052	2.0207
98	23693	8963	0.3783	0.0091	0.0035	1.8890
99	13898	5946	0.4278	0.0057	0.0024	1.7341
100	7491	3397	0.4535	0.0032	0.0015	1.6569
101	3843	1764	0.4590	0.0018	0.0008	1.6168
102	1964	902	0.4593	0.0010	0.0004	1.5645
103	987	488	0.4944	0.0005	0.0003	1.4685
104	465	231	0.4968	0.0003	0.0001	1.4157
105	224	125	0.5580	0.0001	0.0001	1.3197
106	94	46	0.4894	0.0001	0.0000	1.3547
107	44	23	0.5227	0.0000	0.0000	1.1738
108	17	11	0.6471	0.0000	0.0000	0.9118
109	6	5	0.8333	0.0000	0.0000	0.6667

Female

x	N_x	D_x	q_x	l_x	d_x	e_x
80	8245250	640452	0.0777	1.0000	0.0777	6.9568
81	7376400	638925	0.0866	0.9223	0.0799	6.5006
82	6523358	629649	0.0965	0.8424	0.0813	6.0697
83	5694696	612901	0.1076	0.7611	0.0819	5.6647
84	4894762	584349	0.1194	0.6792	0.0811	5.2876
85	4159233	545433	0.1311	0.5981	0.0784	4.9366
86	3481684	503668	0.1447	0.5197	0.0752	4.6063
87	2862374	452517	0.1581	0.4445	0.0703	4.3007
88	2317794	400196	0.1727	0.3742	0.0646	4.0144
89	1842386	348428	0.1891	0.3096	0.0586	3.7479
90	1433385	293554	0.2048	0.2511	0.0514	3.5054
91	1088144	241059	0.2215	0.1996	0.0442	3.2794
92	806287	193647	0.2402	0.1554	0.0373	3.0703
93	584096	150205	0.2572	0.1181	0.0304	2.8828
94	413310	113852	0.2755	0.0877	0.0242	2.7077
95	283576	83355	0.2939	0.0636	0.0187	2.5470
96	188831	59262	0.3138	0.0449	0.0141	2.3992
97	121672	40150	0.3300	0.0308	0.0102	2.2679
98	76460	26537	0.3471	0.0206	0.0072	2.1386
99	46370	17286	0.3728	0.0135	0.0050	2.0095
100	27145	10720	0.3949	0.0084	0.0033	1.9067
101	15235	6219	0.4082	0.0051	0.0021	1.8249
102	8369	3544	0.4235	0.0030	0.0013	1.7387
103	4421	1929	0.4363	0.0017	0.0008	1.6486
104	2295	1074	0.4680	0.0010	0.0005	1.5377
105	1114	557	0.5000	0.0005	0.0003	1.4505
106	513	258	0.5029	0.0003	0.0001	1.4009
107	242	126	0.5207	0.0001	0.0001	1.3124
108	111	67	0.6036	0.0001	0.0000	1.1948
109	37	24	0.6486	0.0000	0.0000	1.2529

Annex Table 3 (cont.). Thirteen countries with good data 1980 - 1990

Male

x	N_x	D_x	q_x	l_x	d_x	e_x
80	6171300	602450	0.0976	1.0000	0.0976	6.2670
81	5386660	575263	0.1068	0.9024	0.0964	5.8909
82	4637269	539856	0.1164	0.8060	0.0938	5.5354
83	3935705	498531	0.1267	0.7122	0.0902	5.1989
84	3300704	453904	0.1375	0.6220	0.0855	4.8804
85	2718510	405671	0.1492	0.5364	0.0800	4.5788
86	2203932	357107	0.1620	0.4564	0.0739	4.2943
87	1755371	309010	0.1760	0.3824	0.0673	4.0279
88	1367630	258807	0.1892	0.3151	0.0596	3.7817
89	1048111	213666	0.2039	0.2555	0.0521	3.5476
90	790000	173994	0.2202	0.2034	0.0448	3.3280
91	586574	138558	0.2362	0.1586	0.0375	3.1268
92	426200	107969	0.2533	0.1211	0.0307	2.9391
93	302759	82024	0.2709	0.0905	0.0245	2.7667
94	209593	60627	0.2893	0.0659	0.0191	2.6090
95	142067	43595	0.3069	0.0469	0.0144	2.4673
96	93741	30306	0.3233	0.0325	0.0105	2.3383
97	60141	20295	0.3375	0.0220	0.0074	2.2165
98	37828	13209	0.3492	0.0146	0.0051	2.0908
99	23170	8784	0.3791	0.0095	0.0036	1.9444
100	13066	5486	0.4199	0.0059	0.0025	1.8263
101	7048	2979	0.4227	0.0034	0.0014	1.7862
102	3732	1606	0.4303	0.0020	0.0008	1.7278
103	1958	914	0.4668	0.0011	0.0005	1.6553
104	963	428	0.4444	0.0006	0.0003	1.6667
105	482	216	0.4481	0.0003	0.0001	1.6001
106	236	108	0.4576	0.0002	0.0001	1.4933
107	109	54	0.4954	0.0001	0.0000	1.3314
108	50	28	0.5600	0.0001	0.0000	1.1478
109	18	14	0.7778	0.0000	0.0000	0.9722

Female

x	N_x	D_x	q_x	l_x	d_x	e_x
80	11016260	686248	0.0623	1.0000	0.0623	7.8267
81	10006889	701865	0.0701	0.9377	0.0658	7.3134
82	8995877	708061	0.0787	0.8719	0.0686	6.8274
83	7996893	705263	0.0882	0.8033	0.0708	6.3679
84	7039045	694516	0.0987	0.7325	0.0723	5.9355
85	6100389	670136	0.1099	0.6602	0.0725	5.5305
86	5205902	634694	0.1219	0.5877	0.0716	5.1513
87	4364637	588790	0.1349	0.5160	0.0696	4.7971
88	3581333	533373	0.1489	0.4464	0.0665	4.4672
89	2880082	473395	0.1644	0.3799	0.0624	4.1614
90	2272608	409177	0.1800	0.3175	0.0572	3.8816
91	1763145	346114	0.1963	0.2603	0.0511	3.6242
92	1336032	285000	0.2133	0.2092	0.0446	3.3873
93	987352	228189	0.2311	0.1646	0.0380	3.1702
94	710422	177138	0.2493	0.1265	0.0316	2.9728
95	499268	133062	0.2665	0.0950	0.0253	2.7941
96	340859	97381	0.2857	0.0697	0.0199	2.6277
97	226248	68334	0.3020	0.0498	0.0150	2.4787
98	146702	46706	0.3184	0.0347	0.0111	2.3349
99	92505	31437	0.3398	0.0237	0.0080	2.1920
100	55761	20472	0.3671	0.0156	0.0057	2.0630
101	32349	12361	0.3821	0.0099	0.0038	1.9698
102	18150	7189	0.3961	0.0061	0.0024	1.8788
103	10035	4206	0.4191	0.0037	0.0015	1.7830
104	5295	2281	0.4308	0.0021	0.0009	1.7088
105	2723	1248	0.4583	0.0012	0.0006	1.6237
106	1325	595	0.4491	0.0007	0.0003	1.5744
107	645	305	0.4729	0.0004	0.0002	1.4502
108	297	166	0.5589	0.0002	0.0001	1.3026
109	115	69	0.6000	0.0001	0.0001	1.3196

Annex Table 3 (cont.). Low mortality countries 1950 - 1960

Male							Female						
x	N_x	D_x	q_x	l_x	d_x	e_x	x	N_x	D_x	q_x	l_x	d_x	e_x
80	1235701	156542	0.1267	1.0000	0.1267	5.1776	80	1987270	198286	0.0998	1.0000	0.0998	6.0139
81	1041923	143276	0.1375	0.8733	0.1201	4.8561	81	1720503	189014	0.1099	0.9002	0.0989	5.6251
82	867940	130390	0.1502	0.7532	0.1132	4.5506	82	1471964	177848	0.1208	0.8013	0.0968	5.2576
83	709024	115001	0.1622	0.6401	0.1038	4.2667	83	1239959	165657	0.1336	0.7045	0.0941	4.9115
84	570113	99791	0.1750	0.5363	0.0939	3.9960	84	1027012	149681	0.1457	0.6104	0.0890	4.5917
85	451670	86112	0.1907	0.4424	0.0843	3.7377	85	842287	133859	0.1589	0.5214	0.0829	4.2898
86	350837	72696	0.2072	0.3580	0.0742	3.5004	86	677967	118289	0.1745	0.4386	0.0765	4.0059
87	266620	59342	0.2226	0.2839	0.0632	3.2846	87	533819	101119	0.1894	0.3620	0.0686	3.7468
88	197638	47597	0.2408	0.2207	0.0531	3.0819	88	412060	84685	0.2055	0.2935	0.0603	3.5056
89	144432	37278	0.2581	0.1675	0.0432	2.9009	89	315625	70016	0.2218	0.2331	0.0517	3.2831
90	103480	28237	0.2729	0.1243	0.0339	2.7361	90	235901	56279	0.2386	0.1814	0.0433	3.0765
91	72701	21396	0.2943	0.0904	0.0266	2.5753	91	172347	44088	0.2558	0.1381	0.0353	2.8837
92	49340	15422	0.3126	0.0638	0.0199	2.4408	92	122524	34020	0.2777	0.1028	0.0285	2.7031
93	32488	10609	0.3266	0.0438	0.0143	2.3232	93	84324	24697	0.2929	0.0743	0.0217	2.5499
94	20818	7223	0.3470	0.0295	0.0102	2.2073	94	56508	17700	0.3132	0.0525	0.0164	2.3990
95	12919	4745	0.3673	0.0193	0.0071	2.1144	95	36492	12147	0.3329	0.0361	0.0120	2.2651
96	7886	2910	0.3690	0.0122	0.0045	2.0516	96	22999	8093	0.3519	0.0241	0.0085	2.1458
97	4805	1809	0.3765	0.0077	0.0029	1.9590	97	14160	5236	0.3698	0.0156	0.0058	2.0394
98	2858	1135	0.3971	0.0048	0.0019	1.8399	98	8464	3216	0.3800	0.0098	0.0037	1.9426
99	1674	690	0.4122	0.0029	0.0012	1.7226	99	4937	1888	0.3824	0.0061	0.0023	1.8267
100	950	479	0.5042	0.0017	0.0009	1.5799	100	2882	1354	0.4698	0.0038	0.0018	1.6482
101	445	198	0.4449	0.0008	0.0004	1.6782	101	1430	630	0.4406	0.0020	0.0009	1.6656
102	231	109	0.4719	0.0005	0.0002	1.6226	102	744	349	0.4691	0.0011	0.0005	1.5835
103	115	56	0.4870	0.0002	0.0001	1.6256	103	374	179	0.4786	0.0006	0.0003	1.5408
104	57	24	0.4211	0.0001	0.0001	1.6939	104	184	100	0.5435	0.0003	0.0002	1.4962
105	33	15	0.4545	0.0001	0.0000	1.5622	105	69	26	0.3768	0.0001	0.0001	1.6821
106	19	10	0.5263	0.0000	0.0000	1.4474	106	36	14	0.3889	0.0001	0.0000	1.3968
107	8	2	0.2500	0.0000	0.0000	1.5000	107	22	14	0.6364	0.0001	0.0000	0.9675
108	6	4	0.6667	0.0000	0.0000	0.8333	108	7	5	0.7143	0.0000	0.0000	0.7857
109	2	2	1.0000	0.0000	0.0000	0.5000	109	2	2	1.0000	0.0000	0.0000	0.5000

Annex Table 3 (cont.). Low mortality countries   1960 - 1970

Male

x	N_x	D_x	q_x	l_x	d_x	e_x
80	1669973	196318	0.1176	1.0000	0.1176	5.4865
81	1442864	184751	0.1280	0.8824	0.1130	5.1508
82	1229334	172220	0.1401	0.7695	0.1078	4.8338
83	1037171	156662	0.1510	0.6617	0.0999	4.5398
84	864939	141753	0.1639	0.5617	0.0921	4.2586
85	707674	125348	0.1771	0.4697	0.0832	3.9953
86	567815	109452	0.1928	0.3865	0.0745	3.7477
87	445740	91642	0.2056	0.3120	0.0641	3.5232
88	343753	76595	0.2228	0.2478	0.0552	3.3056
89	256021	60842	0.2376	0.1926	0.0458	3.1100
90	186957	47534	0.2543	0.1468	0.0373	2.9236
91	132656	36405	0.2744	0.1095	0.0301	2.7499
92	91415	26649	0.2915	0.0795	0.0232	2.6008
93	60793	18597	0.3059	0.0563	0.0172	2.4652
94	39821	13039	0.3274	0.0391	0.0128	2.3314
95	25157	8663	0.3444	0.0263	0.0090	2.2230
96	15289	5457	0.3569	0.0172	0.0061	2.1279
97	9157	3373	0.3684	0.0111	0.0041	2.0314
98	5377	2036	0.3786	0.0070	0.0026	1.9245
99	3147	1240	0.3940	0.0043	0.0017	1.7926
100	1772	828	0.4673	0.0026	0.0012	1.6331
101	846	383	0.4527	0.0014	0.0006	1.6269
102	433	192	0.4434	0.0008	0.0003	1.5590
103	226	105	0.4646	0.0004	0.0002	1.4028
104	103	60	0.5825	0.0002	0.0001	1.1861
105	41	25	0.6098	0.0001	0.0001	1.1436
106	19	12	0.6316	0.0000	0.0000	1.1491
107	7	3	0.4286	0.0000	0.0000	1.2619
108	3	2	0.6667	0.0000	0.0000	0.8333
109	2	2	1.0000	0.0000	0.0000	0.5000

Female

x	N_x	D_x	q_x	l_x	d_x	e_x
80	2785995	246419	0.0884	1.0000	0.0884	6.4670
81	2474713	242494	0.0980	0.9116	0.0893	6.0460
82	2171922	235591	0.1085	0.8222	0.0892	5.6485
83	1886417	226791	0.1202	0.7330	0.0881	5.2749
84	1617076	213923	0.1323	0.6449	0.0853	4.9274
85	1360663	197053	0.1448	0.5596	0.0810	4.6024
86	1124767	179395	0.1595	0.4786	0.0763	4.2971
87	910404	158356	0.1739	0.4022	0.0700	4.0176
88	721647	136323	0.1889	0.3323	0.0628	3.7583
89	554316	113663	0.2051	0.2695	0.0553	3.5172
90	418911	92973	0.2219	0.2142	0.0475	3.2955
91	308274	73525	0.2385	0.1667	0.0398	3.0929
92	221621	56810	0.2563	0.1269	0.0325	2.9050
93	154358	42364	0.2745	0.0944	0.0259	2.7340
94	104833	30438	0.2903	0.0685	0.0199	2.5791
95	69842	21592	0.3092	0.0486	0.0150	2.4297
96	45203	14944	0.3306	0.0336	0.0111	2.2933
97	28099	9743	0.3467	0.0225	0.0078	2.1789
98	16954	6157	0.3632	0.0147	0.0053	2.0700
99	10153	3664	0.3609	0.0094	0.0034	1.9653
100	6008	2601	0.4329	0.0060	0.0026	1.7927
101	3212	1349	0.4200	0.0034	0.0014	1.7795
102	1734	744	0.4291	0.0020	0.0008	1.7061
103	911	419	0.4599	0.0011	0.0005	1.6124
104	451	212	0.4701	0.0006	0.0003	1.5598
105	222	103	0.4640	0.0003	0.0001	1.4998
106	110	57	0.5182	0.0002	0.0001	1.3652
107	50	29	0.5800	0.0001	0.0000	1.2958
108	19	11	0.5789	0.0000	0.0000	1.3947
109	8	5	0.6250	0.0000	0.0000	1.6250

Annex Table 3 (cont).   Low mortality countries   1970 - 1980

Male

x	N_x	D_x	q_x	l_x	d_x	e_x
80	2174796	228658	0.1051	1.0000	0.1051	5.9479
81	1875990	214341	0.1143	0.8949	0.1022	5.5880
82	1601757	200031	0.1249	0.7926	0.0990	5.2444
83	1348884	183261	0.1359	0.6936	0.0942	4.9214
84	1121022	165285	0.1474	0.5994	0.0884	4.6165
85	922987	147965	0.1603	0.5110	0.0819	4.3285
86	748669	130496	0.1743	0.4291	0.0748	4.0594
87	596304	112179	0.1881	0.3543	0.0667	3.8108
88	467150	94276	0.2018	0.2877	0.0581	3.5779
89	359813	78241	0.2174	0.2296	0.0499	3.3561
90	270937	63386	0.2340	0.1797	0.0420	3.1497
91	198927	50057	0.2516	0.1376	0.0346	2.9590
92	142164	38082	0.2679	0.1030	0.0276	2.7858
93	100124	28843	0.2881	0.0754	0.0217	2.6221
94	68128	20470	0.3005	0.0537	0.0161	2.4808
95	45545	14734	0.3235	0.0376	0.0121	2.3316
96	29262	9935	0.3395	0.0254	0.0086	2.2075
97	18216	6500	0.3568	0.0168	0.0060	2.0852
98	11016	4069	0.3694	0.0108	0.0040	1.9647
99	6539	2608	0.3988	0.0068	0.0027	1.8226
100	3716	1661	0.4470	0.0041	0.0018	1.7000
101	1906	838	0.4397	0.0023	0.0010	1.6700
102	1002	462	0.4611	0.0013	0.0006	1.5880
103	499	238	0.4770	0.0007	0.0003	1.5188
104	256	129	0.5039	0.0004	0.0002	1.4477
105	124	64	0.5161	0.0002	0.0001	1.4104
106	56	25	0.4464	0.0001	0.0000	1.3815
107	26	15	0.5769	0.0000	0.0000	1.0923
108	10	7	0.7000	0.0000	0.0000	0.9000
109	3	2	0.6667	0.0000	0.0000	0.8333

Female

x	N_x	D_x	q_x	l_x	d_x	e_x
80	3693577	267716	0.0725	1.0000	0.0725	7.1957
81	3312834	269403	0.0813	0.9275	0.0754	6.7189
82	2933935	266011	0.0907	0.8521	0.0773	6.2694
83	2565068	260565	0.1016	0.7748	0.0787	5.8447
84	2210322	250202	0.1132	0.6961	0.0788	5.4490
85	1884628	235177	0.1248	0.6173	0.0770	5.0807
86	1583560	218085	0.1377	0.5403	0.0744	4.7338
87	1308725	199298	0.1523	0.4659	0.0709	4.4100
88	1064487	177032	0.1663	0.3949	0.0657	4.1124
89	852040	156287	0.1834	0.3293	0.0604	3.8330
90	665608	132210	0.1986	0.2689	0.0534	3.5817
91	506843	109401	0.2158	0.2155	0.0465	3.3456
92	376328	88474	0.2351	0.1690	0.0397	3.1289
93	273816	68674	0.2508	0.1292	0.0324	2.9369
94	194471	52693	0.2710	0.0968	0.0262	2.7527
95	133655	38610	0.2889	0.0706	0.0204	2.5899
96	89303	27602	0.3091	0.0502	0.0155	2.4389
97	57623	18750	0.3254	0.0347	0.0113	2.3063
98	36279	12419	0.3423	0.0234	0.0080	2.1775
99	21990	7981	0.3629	0.0154	0.0056	2.0506
100	13036	5092	0.3906	0.0098	0.0038	1.9340
101	7268	2888	0.3974	0.0060	0.0024	1.8531
102	4023	1681	0.4178	0.0036	0.0015	1.7453
103	2094	925	0.4417	0.0021	0.0009	1.6392
104	1057	488	0.4617	0.0012	0.0005	1.5406
105	511	255	0.4990	0.0006	0.0003	1.4331
106	238	124	0.5210	0.0003	0.0002	1.3627
107	110	56	0.5091	0.0002	0.0001	1.3010
108	53	34	0.6415	0.0001	0.0000	1.1316
109	14	10	0.7143	0.0000	0.0000	1.2619

Annex Table 3 (cont).   Low mortality countries   1980 - 1990

Male

x	N_x	D_x	q_x	l_x	d_x	e_x
80	3159083	284595	0.0901	1.0000	0.0901	6.5227
81	2774349	275940	0.0995	0.9099	0.0905	6.1190
82	2406096	262343	0.1090	0.8194	0.0893	5.7395
83	2059358	245621	0.1193	0.7301	0.0871	5.3807
84	1745188	227092	0.1301	0.6430	0.0837	5.0417
85	1451363	206007	0.1419	0.5593	0.0794	4.7211
86	1186261	183285	0.1545	0.4799	0.0742	4.4193
87	950174	161466	0.1699	0.4058	0.0690	4.1356
88	740722	135057	0.1823	0.3368	0.0614	3.8798
89	568484	112540	0.1980	0.2754	0.0545	3.6335
90	428492	91770	0.2142	0.2209	0.0473	3.4070
91	317654	73233	0.2305	0.1736	0.0400	3.1992
92	230106	56800	0.2468	0.1336	0.0330	3.0080
93	162600	42861	0.2636	0.1006	0.0265	2.8299
94	112128	31596	0.2818	0.0741	0.0209	2.6639
95	75760	22781	0.3007	0.0532	0.0160	2.5129
96	49772	15801	0.3175	0.0372	0.0118	2.3785
97	31770	10600	0.3336	0.0254	0.0085	2.2523
98	19914	6820	0.3425	0.0169	0.0058	2.1296
99	12176	4508	0.3702	0.0111	0.0041	1.9784
100	6704	2775	0.4139	0.0070	0.0029	1.8476
101	3619	1523	0.4208	0.0041	0.0017	1.7993
102	1909	806	0.4222	0.0024	0.0010	1.7435
103	1011	468	0.4629	0.0014	0.0006	1.6521
104	490	217	0.4429	0.0007	0.0003	1.6451
105	245	115	0.4694	0.0004	0.0002	1.5553
106	115	51	0.4435	0.0002	0.0001	1.4889
107	58	30	0.5172	0.0001	0.0001	1.2769
108	24	15	0.6250	0.0001	0.0000	1.1094
109	8	5	0.6250	0.0000	0.0000	1.1250

Female

x	N_x	D_x	q_x	l_x	d_x	e_x
80	5201334	292020	0.0561	1.0000	0.0561	8.1581
81	4731735	301577	0.0637	0.9439	0.0602	7.6136
82	4268163	308159	0.0722	0.8837	0.0638	7.0979
83	3809435	309531	0.0813	0.8199	0.0666	6.6113
84	3375118	309239	0.0916	0.7533	0.0690	6.1518
85	2939331	301402	0.1025	0.6843	0.0702	5.7219
86	2520630	288412	0.1144	0.6141	0.0703	5.3185
87	2121394	270278	0.1274	0.5438	0.0693	4.9411
88	1744550	247168	0.1417	0.4745	0.0672	4.5895
89	1403372	220572	0.1572	0.4073	0.0640	4.2646
90	1110028	191869	0.1729	0.3433	0.0593	3.9666
91	864703	164725	0.1905	0.2840	0.0541	3.6910
92	657343	136341	0.2074	0.2299	0.0477	3.4420
93	486193	109586	0.2254	0.1822	0.0411	3.2119
94	350407	85913	0.2452	0.1411	0.0346	3.0010
95	246314	64793	0.2631	0.1065	0.0280	2.8133
96	168630	47926	0.2842	0.0785	0.0223	2.6391
97	111902	33723	0.3014	0.0562	0.0169	2.4884
98	72749	23361	0.3211	0.0393	0.0126	2.3461
99	45894	15290	0.3332	0.0267	0.0089	2.2194
100	27405	10069	0.3674	0.0178	0.0065	2.0784
101	15936	6031	0.3785	0.0112	0.0043	1.9951
102	9000	3503	0.3892	0.0070	0.0027	1.9055
103	5064	2155	0.4256	0.0043	0.0018	1.8012
104	2634	1119	0.4248	0.0025	0.0010	1.7651
105	1370	611	0.4460	0.0014	0.0006	1.6995
106	677	289	0.4269	0.0008	0.0003	1.6650
107	333	166	0.4985	0.0004	0.0002	1.5328
108	145	65	0.4483	0.0002	0.0001	1.5594
109	72	42	0.5833	0.0001	0.0001	1.4201

Annex Table 3 (cont.). Medium mortality countries 1950 - 1960

Male

x	N_x	D_x	q_x	l_x	d_x	e_x
80	1730199	210484	0.1217	1.0000	0.1217	5.3023
81	1486502	195640	0.1316	0.8783	0.1156	4.9674
82	1253504	181991	0.1452	0.7627	0.1107	4.6445
83	1034814	163513	0.1580	0.6520	0.1030	4.3484
84	836896	144496	0.1727	0.5490	0.0948	4.0706
85	660479	123477	0.1870	0.4542	0.0849	3.8157
86	512431	103859	0.2027	0.3693	0.0748	3.5782
87	391946	86014	0.2195	0.2944	0.0646	3.3606
88	291910	68202	0.2336	0.2298	0.0537	3.1649
89	213871	53250	0.2490	0.1761	0.0439	2.9773
90	152909	40777	0.2667	0.1323	0.0353	2.7986
91	103961	29251	0.2814	0.0970	0.0273	2.6346
92	69141	20772	0.3004	0.0697	0.0209	2.4703
93	44638	14358	0.3217	0.0488	0.0157	2.3164
94	27726	9261	0.3340	0.0331	0.0110	2.1777
95	16658	6019	0.3613	0.0220	0.0080	2.0192
96	9927	3780	0.3808	0.0141	0.0054	1.8787
97	5667	2361	0.4166	0.0087	0.0036	1.7265
98	3042	1348	0.4431	0.0051	0.0023	1.6024
99	1558	824	0.5289	0.0028	0.0015	1.4796
100	693	341	0.4921	0.0013	0.0007	1.5792
101	326	138	0.4233	0.0007	0.0003	1.6248
102	171	81	0.4737	0.0004	0.0002	1.4504
103	75	37	0.4933	0.0002	0.0001	1.3057
104	36	21	0.5833	0.0001	0.0001	1.0903
105	12	9	0.7500	0.0000	0.0000	0.9167
106	3	2	0.6667	0.0000	0.0000	1.1667
107	1	0	0.0000	0.0000	0.0000	1.5000
108	1	1	1.0000	0.0000	0.0000	0.5000

Female

x	N_x	D_x	q_x	l_x	d_x	e_x
80	2460691	246335	0.1001	1.0000	0.1001	6.0595
81	2139895	233105	0.1089	0.8999	0.0980	5.6780
82	1833298	221783	0.1210	0.8019	0.0970	5.3110
83	1545196	205106	0.1327	0.7049	0.0936	4.9731
84	1281202	187422	0.1463	0.6113	0.0894	4.6577
85	1040042	164781	0.1584	0.5219	0.0827	4.3702
86	833760	144798	0.1737	0.4392	0.0763	4.0988
87	659641	123158	0.1867	0.3629	0.0678	3.8551
88	512339	102380	0.1998	0.2952	0.0590	3.6253
89	391816	84558	0.2158	0.2362	0.0510	3.4058
90	292965	67714	0.2311	0.1852	0.0428	3.2055
91	209925	51016	0.2430	0.1424	0.0346	3.0188
92	147686	38849	0.2631	0.1078	0.0284	2.8275
93	101367	28307	0.2793	0.0794	0.0222	2.6583
94	67596	19969	0.2954	0.0573	0.0169	2.4945
95	43880	13854	0.3157	0.0403	0.0127	2.3307
96	28109	9459	0.3365	0.0276	0.0093	2.1754
97	17296	6303	0.3644	0.0183	0.0067	2.0252
98	10184	3992	0.3920	0.0116	0.0046	1.8997
99	5737	2495	0.4349	0.0071	0.0031	1.8021
100	3051	1278	0.4189	0.0040	0.0017	1.8042
101	1642	713	0.4342	0.0023	0.0010	1.7442
102	848	362	0.4269	0.0013	0.0006	1.6992
103	419	204	0.4869	0.0008	0.0004	1.5924
104	192	74	0.3854	0.0004	0.0001	1.6289
105	104	56	0.5385	0.0002	0.0001	1.3368
106	43	20	0.4651	0.0001	0.0001	1.3130
107	25	16	0.6400	0.0001	0.0000	1.0200
108	9	5	0.5556	0.0000	0.0000	0.9444
109	3	3	1.0000	0.0000	0.0000	0.5000

Annex Table 3 (cont.). Medium mortality countries 1960 - 1970

Male

x	N_x	D_x	q_x	l_x	d_x	e_x
80	2089369	247732	0.1186	1.0000	0.1186	5.4240
81	1831345	235817	0.1288	0.8814	0.1135	5.0864
82	1588827	224360	0.1412	0.7679	0.1084	4.7642
83	1357606	207305	0.1527	0.6595	0.1007	4.4654
84	1147425	191552	0.1669	0.5588	0.0933	4.1800
85	950812	170598	0.1794	0.4655	0.0835	3.9175
86	772430	150958	0.1954	0.3820	0.0747	3.6647
87	611292	129140	0.2113	0.3073	0.0649	3.4335
88	473094	107609	0.2275	0.2424	0.0551	3.2192
89	355717	86624	0.2435	0.1873	0.0456	3.0198
90	262271	68231	0.2602	0.1417	0.0369	2.8309
91	187835	52498	0.2795	0.1048	0.0293	2.6506
92	130404	39128	0.3001	0.0755	0.0227	2.4848
93	87428	27897	0.3191	0.0529	0.0169	2.3356
94	56876	19202	0.3376	0.0360	0.0122	2.1958
95	35950	12868	0.3579	0.0238	0.0085	2.0601
96	22034	8369	0.3798	0.0153	0.0058	1.9298
97	13056	5242	0.4015	0.0095	0.0038	1.8055
98	7312	3128	0.4278	0.0057	0.0024	1.6813
99	3964	1969	0.4967	0.0033	0.0016	1.5644
100	1851	835	0.4511	0.0016	0.0007	1.6149
101	927	448	0.4833	0.0009	0.0004	1.5312
102	447	220	0.4922	0.0005	0.0002	1.4956
103	216	114	0.5278	0.0002	0.0001	1.4605
104	94	50	0.5319	0.0001	0.0001	1.5339
105	41	16	0.3902	0.0001	0.0000	1.7088
106	19	11	0.5789	0.0000	0.0000	1.4825
107	6	3	0.5000	0.0000	0.0000	1.8333
108	3	0	0.0000	0.0000	0.0000	2.1667
109	3	2	0.6667	0.0000	0.0000	1.1667

Female

x	N_x	D_x	q_x	l_x	d_x	e_x
80	3518883	322548	0.0917	1.0000	0.0917	6.3335
81	3109013	314113	0.1010	0.9083	0.0918	5.9222
82	2718885	305663	0.1124	0.8166	0.0918	5.5316
83	2345631	291402	0.1242	0.7248	0.0900	5.1689
84	1999530	273125	0.1366	0.6347	0.0867	4.8312
85	1678122	251163	0.1497	0.5480	0.0820	4.5164
86	1381416	227052	0.1644	0.4660	0.0766	4.2233
87	1113072	198342	0.1782	0.3894	0.0694	3.9557
88	879366	169497	0.1927	0.3200	0.0617	3.7050
89	679582	141327	0.2080	0.2583	0.0537	3.4702
90	515595	116060	0.2251	0.2046	0.0461	3.2501
91	381628	91619	0.2401	0.1586	0.0381	3.0490
92	276671	71789	0.2595	0.1205	0.0313	2.8543
93	194332	54063	0.2782	0.0892	0.0248	2.6792
94	132840	39470	0.2971	0.0644	0.0191	2.5191
95	88486	27887	0.3152	0.0453	0.0143	2.3726
96	57560	19411	0.3372	0.0310	0.0105	2.2344
97	36254	12781	0.3525	0.0205	0.0072	2.1169
98	22022	8378	0.3804	0.0133	0.0051	1.9973
99	12891	5166	0.4007	0.0082	0.0033	1.9167
100	7126	2875	0.4035	0.0049	0.0020	1.8641
101	3954	1651	0.4176	0.0029	0.0012	1.7866
102	2173	917	0.4220	0.0017	0.0007	1.7090
103	1148	521	0.4538	0.0010	0.0005	1.5917
104	581	274	0.4716	0.0005	0.0003	1.4989
105	291	151	0.5189	0.0003	0.0001	1.3903
106	127	61	0.4803	0.0001	0.0001	1.3506
107	55	33	0.6000	0.0001	0.0000	1.1368
108	19	10	0.5263	0.0000	0.0000	1.0921
109	8	7	0.8750	0.0000	0.0000	0.7500

Annex Table 3 (cont.).   Medium mortality countries   1970 - 1980

Male

x	N_x	D_x	q_x	l_x	d_x	e_x
80	2243584	263321	0.1174	1.0000	0.1174	5.5709
81	1939645	245321	0.1265	0.8826	0.1116	5.2452
82	1668175	228881	0.1372	0.7710	0.1058	4.9323
83	1422063	210850	0.1483	0.6652	0.0986	4.6371
84	1197093	192465	0.1608	0.5666	0.0911	4.3573
85	999592	172713	0.1728	0.4755	0.0822	4.0963
86	822744	152759	0.1857	0.3933	0.0730	3.8474
87	663560	133126	0.2006	0.3203	0.0643	3.6106
88	525018	112891	0.2150	0.2560	0.0551	3.3913
89	408196	93741	0.2296	0.2010	0.0462	3.1833
90	310188	77078	0.2485	0.1548	0.0385	2.9833
91	229560	61002	0.2657	0.1164	0.0309	2.8044
92	165617	47181	0.2849	0.0854	0.0243	2.6383
93	116082	35014	0.3016	0.0611	0.0184	2.4902
94	79581	25497	0.3204	0.0427	0.0137	2.3497
95	52738	17780	0.3371	0.0290	0.0098	2.2218
96	33706	11868	0.3521	0.0192	0.0068	2.0975
97	20906	7718	0.3692	0.0125	0.0046	1.9656
98	12677	4894	0.3861	0.0079	0.0030	1.8233
99	7359	3338	0.4536	0.0048	0.0022	1.6555
100	3775	1736	0.4599	0.0026	0.0012	1.6147
101	1937	926	0.4781	0.0014	0.0007	1.5637
102	962	440	0.4574	0.0007	0.0003	1.5380
103	488	250	0.5123	0.0004	0.0002	1.4129
104	209	102	0.4880	0.0002	0.0001	1.3718
105	100	61	0.6100	0.0001	0.0001	1.2029
106	38	21	0.5526	0.0000	0.0000	1.3024
107	18	8	0.4444	0.0000	0.0000	1.2937
108	7	4	0.5714	0.0000	0.0000	0.9286
109	3	3	1.0000	0.0000	0.0000	0.5000

Female

x	N_x	D_x	q_x	l_x	d_x	e_x
80	4551673	372736	0.0819	1.0000	0.0819	6.7682
81	4063566	369522	0.0909	0.9181	0.0835	6.3273
82	3589423	363638	0.1013	0.8346	0.0846	5.9103
83	3129628	352336	0.1126	0.7501	0.0844	5.5201
84	2684440	334147	0.1245	0.6656	0.0829	5.1570
85	2274605	310256	0.1364	0.5828	0.0795	4.8191
86	1898124	285583	0.1505	0.5033	0.0757	4.5013
87	1553649	253219	0.1630	0.4276	0.0697	4.2099
88	1253307	223164	0.1781	0.3579	0.0637	3.9323
89	990346	192141	0.1940	0.2942	0.0571	3.6759
90	767777	161344	0.2101	0.2371	0.0498	3.4404
91	581301	131658	0.2265	0.1873	0.0424	3.2226
92	429959	105173	0.2446	0.1448	0.0354	3.0198
93	310280	81531	0.2628	0.1094	0.0288	2.8358
94	218839	61159	0.2795	0.0807	0.0225	2.6684
95	149921	44745	0.2985	0.0581	0.0173	2.5094
96	99528	31660	0.3181	0.0408	0.0130	2.3643
97	64049	21400	0.3341	0.0278	0.0093	2.2339
98	40181	14118	0.3514	0.0185	0.0065	2.1040
99	24380	9305	0.3817	0.0120	0.0046	1.9729
100	14109	5628	0.3989	0.0074	0.0030	1.8820
101	7967	3331	0.4181	0.0045	0.0019	1.7990
102	4346	1863	0.4287	0.0026	0.0011	1.7324
103	2327	1004	0.4315	0.0015	0.0006	1.6571
104	1238	586	0.4733	0.0008	0.0004	1.5352
105	603	302	0.5008	0.0004	0.0002	1.4657
106	275	134	0.4873	0.0002	0.0001	1.4345
107	132	70	0.5303	0.0001	0.0001	1.3227
108	58	33	0.5690	0.0001	0.0000	1.2515
109	23	14	0.6087	0.0000	0.0000	1.2435

Annex Table 3 (cont.). Medium mortality countries 1980 - 1990

Male

x	N_x	D_x	q_x	l_x	d_x	e_x
80	3012217	317855	0.1055	1.0000	0.1055	6.0019
81	2612311	299323	0.1146	0.8945	0.1025	5.6509
82	2231173	277513	0.1244	0.7920	0.0985	5.3175
83	1876347	252910	0.1348	0.6935	0.0935	5.0018
84	1555516	226812	0.1458	0.6000	0.0875	4.7032
85	1267147	199664	0.1576	0.5125	0.0808	4.4207
86	1017671	173822	0.1708	0.4318	0.0737	4.1540
87	805197	147544	0.1832	0.3580	0.0656	3.9067
88	626908	123750	0.1974	0.2924	0.0577	3.6709
89	479627	101126	0.2108	0.2347	0.0495	3.4508
90	361508	82224	0.2274	0.1852	0.0421	3.2392
91	268920	65325	0.2429	0.1431	0.0348	3.0457
92	196094	51169	0.2609	0.1083	0.0283	2.8625
93	140159	39163	0.2794	0.0801	0.0224	2.6966
94	97465	29031	0.2979	0.0577	0.0172	2.5484
95	66307	20814	0.3139	0.0405	0.0127	2.4173
96	43969	14505	0.3299	0.0278	0.0092	2.2945
97	28371	9695	0.3417	0.0186	0.0064	2.1780
98	17914	6389	0.3566	0.0123	0.0044	2.0490
99	10994	4276	0.3889	0.0079	0.0031	1.9077
100	6362	2711	0.4261	0.0048	0.0021	1.8037
101	3429	1456	0.4246	0.0028	0.0012	1.7718
102	1823	800	0.4388	0.0016	0.0007	1.7104
103	947	446	0.4710	0.0009	0.0004	1.6569
104	473	211	0.4461	0.0005	0.0002	1.6867
105	237	101	0.4262	0.0003	0.0001	1.6425
106	121	57	0.4711	0.0002	0.0001	1.4910
107	51	24	0.4706	0.0001	0.0000	1.3735
108	26	13	0.5000	0.0000	0.0000	1.1500
109	10	9	0.9000	0.0000	0.0000	0.8000

Female

x	N_x	D_x	q_x	l_x	d_x	e_x
80	5814926	394228	0.0678	1.0000	0.0678	7.5390
81	5275154	400288	0.0759	0.9322	0.0707	7.0510
82	4727714	399902	0.0846	0.8615	0.0729	6.5889
83	4187458	395732	0.0945	0.7886	0.0745	6.1515
84	3663927	385277	0.1052	0.7141	0.0751	5.7413
85	3161058	368734	0.1166	0.6390	0.0745	5.3573
86	2685272	346282	0.1290	0.5644	0.0728	4.9987
87	2243243	318512	0.1420	0.4917	0.0698	4.6647
88	1836783	286205	0.1558	0.4218	0.0657	4.3539
89	1476710	252823	0.1712	0.3561	0.0610	4.0652
90	1162580	217308	0.1869	0.2951	0.0552	3.8017
91	898442	181389	0.2019	0.2400	0.0485	3.5607
92	678689	148659	0.2190	0.1915	0.0420	3.3350
93	501159	118603	0.2367	0.1496	0.0354	3.1301
94	360015	91225	0.2534	0.1142	0.0289	2.9456
95	252954	68269	0.2699	0.0852	0.0230	2.7756
96	172229	49455	0.2871	0.0622	0.0179	2.6167
97	114346	34611	0.3027	0.0444	0.0134	2.4694
98	73953	23345	0.3157	0.0309	0.0098	2.3242
99	46611	16147	0.3464	0.0212	0.0073	2.1657
100	28356	10403	0.3669	0.0138	0.0051	2.0486
101	16413	6330	0.3857	0.0088	0.0034	1.9460
102	9150	3686	0.4028	0.0054	0.0022	1.8538
103	4971	2051	0.4126	0.0032	0.0013	1.7671
104	2661	1162	0.4367	0.0019	0.0008	1.6571
105	1353	637	0.4708	0.0011	0.0005	1.5540
106	648	306	0.4722	0.0006	0.0003	1.4917
107	312	139	0.4455	0.0003	0.0001	1.3790
108	152	101	0.6645	0.0002	0.0001	1.0852
109	43	27	0.6279	0.0001	0.0000	1.2442

Annex Table 3 (cont.). High mortality countries 1950 - 1960

Male

x	N_x	D_x	q_x	l_x	d_x	e_x
80	354629	45706	0.1289	1.0000	0.1289	5.0326
81	302930	42312	0.1397	0.8711	0.1217	4.7032
82	255017	39265	0.1540	0.7494	0.1154	4.3856
83	207770	35191	0.1694	0.6341	0.1074	4.0928
84	166288	30579	0.1839	0.5267	0.0968	3.8254
85	130221	25912	0.1990	0.4298	0.0855	3.5747
86	99714	21438	0.2150	0.3443	0.0740	3.3385
87	74965	17654	0.2355	0.2703	0.0636	3.1159
88	54969	13795	0.2510	0.2066	0.0519	2.9217
89	39587	10753	0.2716	0.1548	0.0420	2.7331
90	27412	7966	0.2906	0.1127	0.0328	2.5659
91	18464	5674	0.3073	0.0800	0.0246	2.4121
92	12114	4099	0.3384	0.0554	0.0187	2.2604
93	7585	2629	0.3466	0.0367	0.0127	2.1607
94	4677	1759	0.3761	0.0239	0.0090	2.0416
95	2755	1041	0.3779	0.0149	0.0056	1.9709
96	1601	649	0.4054	0.0093	0.0038	1.8643
97	916	357	0.3897	0.0055	0.0022	1.7944
98	523	215	0.4111	0.0034	0.0014	1.6211
99	282	149	0.5284	0.0020	0.0010	1.4037
100	...	...	...	0.0009	...	1.4160

Female

x	N_x	D_x	q_x	l_x	d_x	e_x
80	494696	56157	0.1135	1.0000	0.1135	5.4848
81	423638	52756	0.1245	0.8865	0.1104	5.1231
82	358102	49444	0.1381	0.7761	0.1072	4.7807
83	293629	44364	0.1511	0.6689	0.1011	4.4665
84	238658	39531	0.1656	0.5679	0.0941	4.1724
85	189980	34109	0.1795	0.4738	0.0851	3.9015
86	148787	29117	0.1957	0.3887	0.0761	3.6458
87	114786	24104	0.2100	0.3127	0.0657	3.4112
88	87254	20016	0.2294	0.2470	0.0567	3.1850
89	64677	15813	0.2445	0.1903	0.0465	2.9843
90	46775	12436	0.2659	0.1438	0.0382	2.7883
91	32645	9317	0.2854	0.1056	0.0301	2.6170
92	22220	6632	0.2985	0.0754	0.0225	2.4625
93	14847	4827	0.3251	0.0529	0.0172	2.2974
94	9514	3156	0.3317	0.0357	0.0118	2.1633
95	5992	2238	0.3735	0.0239	0.0089	1.9890
96	3565	1424	0.3994	0.0150	0.0060	1.8767
97	1975	799	0.4046	0.0090	0.0036	1.7923
98	1136	480	0.4225	0.0053	0.0023	1.6703
99	621	294	0.4734	0.0031	0.0015	1.5267
100	...	...	...	0.0016	...	1.4497

Annex Table 3 (cont). High mortality countries 1960 - 1970

Male

x	N_x	D_x	q_x	l_x	d_x	e_x
80	492657	62828	0.1275	1.0000	0.1275	5.1018
81	428394	59449	0.1388	0.8725	0.1211	4.7744
82	366443	55805	0.1523	0.7514	0.1144	4.4632
83	308083	51025	0.1656	0.6370	0.1055	4.1751
84	255771	46008	0.1799	0.5315	0.0956	3.9046
85	208113	40759	0.1959	0.4359	0.0854	3.6514
86	165540	34986	0.2113	0.3505	0.0741	3.4189
87	128500	29025	0.2259	0.2764	0.0624	3.2011
88	97523	23904	0.2451	0.2140	0.0525	2.9892
89	71534	18734	0.2619	0.1615	0.0423	2.7975
90	51345	14677	0.2859	0.1192	0.0341	2.6127
91	35518	10830	0.3049	0.0852	0.0260	2.4583
92	23679	7521	0.3176	0.0592	0.0188	2.3174
93	15409	5256	0.3411	0.0404	0.0138	2.1633
94	9668	3531	0.3652	0.0266	0.0097	2.0244
95	5764	2257	0.3916	0.0169	0.0066	1.9015
96	3325	1348	0.4054	0.0103	0.0042	1.8034
97	1839	747	0.4062	0.0061	0.0025	1.6921
98	1049	479	0.4566	0.0036	0.0017	1.5076
99	555	300	0.5405	0.0020	0.0011	1.3544
100	...	...	...	0.0009		1.3596

Female

x	N_x	D_x	q_x	l_x	d_x	e_x
80	808052	85788	0.1062	1.0000	0.1062	5.6905
81	704543	82814	0.1175	0.8938	0.1051	5.3070
82	604512	78981	0.1307	0.7888	0.1031	4.9473
83	509760	73273	0.1437	0.6857	0.0986	4.6156
84	424183	67097	0.1582	0.5872	0.0929	4.3065
85	346970	60017	0.1730	0.4943	0.0855	4.0218
86	277533	52111	0.1878	0.4088	0.0768	3.7584
87	217792	44506	0.2044	0.3320	0.0678	3.5116
88	166500	36683	0.2203	0.2642	0.0582	3.2851
89	124016	29568	0.2384	0.2060	0.0491	3.0721
90	90647	23235	0.2563	0.1569	0.0402	2.8773
91	64515	17756	0.2752	0.1167	0.0321	2.6967
92	44411	13128	0.2956	0.0845	0.0250	2.5308
93	29594	9289	0.3139	0.0596	0.0187	2.3830
94	19193	6284	0.3274	0.0409	0.0134	2.2445
95	12225	4230	0.3460	0.0275	0.0095	2.0937
96	7500	2789	0.3719	0.0180	0.0067	1.9369
97	4435	1778	0.4009	0.0113	0.0045	1.7876
98	2493	1089	0.4368	0.0068	0.0030	1.6492
99	1341	636	0.4743	0.0038	0.0018	1.5405
100	...	...	...	0.0020		1.4792

Annex Table 3 (cont.). High mortality countries   1970 - 1980

	Male								Female						
x	N_x	D_x	q_x	l_x	d_x	e_x		x	N_x	D_x	q_x	l_x	d_x	e_x
80	534278	69936	0.1309	1.0000	0.1309	5.0746		80	1053716	106901	0.1015	1.0000	0.1015	5.8691
81	454767	64717	0.1423	0.8691	0.1237	4.7636		81	920224	102896	0.1118	0.8985	0.1005	5.4753
82	384289	59205	0.1541	0.7454	0.1148	4.4710		82	794673	98602	0.1241	0.7981	0.0990	5.1017
83	322125	53935	0.1674	0.6306	0.1056	4.1943		83	676383	93135	0.1377	0.6991	0.0963	4.7536
84	265927	48295	0.1816	0.5250	0.0953	3.9372		84	565675	85485	0.1511	0.6028	0.0911	4.4328
85	216230	41778	0.1932	0.4297	0.0830	3.7000		85	464686	76915	0.1655	0.5117	0.0847	4.1329
86	174006	36520	0.2099	0.3466	0.0728	3.4663		86	375701	68213	0.1816	0.4270	0.0775	3.8535
87	137059	30953	0.2258	0.2739	0.0619	3.2542		87	297246	59047	0.1986	0.3495	0.0694	3.5974
88	106123	25761	0.2427	0.2120	0.0515	3.0577		88	231368	49673	0.2147	0.2801	0.0601	3.3653
89	80152	20700	0.2583	0.1606	0.0415	2.8776		89	175793	41066	0.2336	0.2199	0.0514	3.1486
90	59324	16384	0.2762	0.1191	0.0329	2.7054		90	130851	32563	0.2489	0.1686	0.0419	2.9559
91	42697	12484	0.2924	0.0862	0.0252	2.5468		91	95200	25768	0.2707	0.1266	0.0343	2.7696
92	29968	9610	0.3207	0.0610	0.0196	2.3926		92	66938	19272	0.2879	0.0923	0.0266	2.6119
93	20140	6688	0.3321	0.0414	0.0138	2.2860		93	45963	13963	0.3038	0.0658	0.0200	2.4657
94	13331	4616	0.3463	0.0277	0.0096	2.1739		94	30847	10085	0.3269	0.0458	0.0150	2.3234
95	8608	3161	0.3672	0.0181	0.0066	2.0606		95	19945	6908	0.3464	0.0308	0.0107	2.2091
96	5362	2074	0.3868	0.0114	0.0044	1.9662		96	12562	4438	0.3533	0.0201	0.0071	2.1148
97	3180	1277	0.4016	0.0070	0.0028	1.8910		97	7797	2876	0.3689	0.0130	0.0048	1.9969
98	1850	775	0.4189	0.0042	0.0018	1.8245		98	4658	1894	0.4066	0.0082	0.0033	1.8717
99	1019	383	0.3759	0.0024	0.0009	1.7794		99	2594	998	0.3847	0.0049	0.0019	1.8117
100	...	...	...	0.0015	...	1.5498		100	...	...	...	0.0030	...	1.6319

Annex Table 3 (cont.). High mortality countries 1980 - 1990

Male

x	N_x	D_x	q_x	l_x	d_x	e_x
80	662767	85996	0.1298	1.0000	0.1298	5.1318
81	569141	80174	0.1409	0.8702	0.1226	4.8224
82	481109	73103	0.1519	0.7477	0.1136	4.5312
83	399914	66026	0.1651	0.6341	0.1047	4.2534
84	326532	58392	0.1788	0.5294	0.0947	3.9957
85	261911	50504	0.1928	0.4347	0.0838	3.7569
86	205578	42143	0.2050	0.3509	0.0719	3.5350
87	158770	35125	0.2212	0.2790	0.0617	3.3175
88	119402	28007	0.2346	0.2172	0.0510	3.1180
89	88355	22275	0.2521	0.1663	0.0419	2.9202
90	63669	17204	0.2702	0.1244	0.0336	2.7360
91	45017	13042	0.2897	0.0908	0.0263	2.5639
92	31342	9713	0.3099	0.0645	0.0200	2.4058
93	21243	7064	0.3325	0.0445	0.0148	2.2616
94	13875	4886	0.3521	0.0297	0.0105	2.1392
95	8854	3268	0.3691	0.0192	0.0071	2.0302
96	5501	2098	0.3814	0.0121	0.0046	1.9255
97	3434	1417	0.4126	0.0075	0.0031	1.8043
98	1992	837	0.4202	0.0044	0.0019	1.7207
99	1177	522	0.4435	0.0026	0.0011	1.6053
100	...	...	...	0.0014	...	1.4861

Female

x	N_x	D_x	q_x	l_x	d_x	e_x
80	1298797	122286	0.0942	1.0000	0.0942	6.1582
81	1154214	120440	0.1043	0.9058	0.0945	5.7464
82	1013520	117285	0.1157	0.8113	0.0939	5.3576
83	877748	112124	0.1277	0.7174	0.0916	4.9933
84	748244	106719	0.1426	0.6258	0.0893	4.6513
85	628160	97691	0.1555	0.5365	0.0834	4.3419
86	517161	88204	0.1706	0.4531	0.0773	4.0494
87	416490	77611	0.1863	0.3758	0.0700	3.7792
88	325892	66139	0.2029	0.3058	0.0621	3.5303
89	249754	54385	0.2178	0.2437	0.0531	3.3018
90	186480	43925	0.2355	0.1907	0.0449	3.0818
91	136392	34807	0.2552	0.1457	0.0372	2.8773
92	97317	26734	0.2747	0.1086	0.0298	2.6919
93	67377	20054	0.2976	0.0787	0.0234	2.5220
94	44904	14045	0.3128	0.0553	0.0173	2.3789
95	29147	9898	0.3396	0.0380	0.0129	2.2341
96	18249	6349	0.3479	0.0251	0.0087	2.1258
97	11329	4170	0.3681	0.0164	0.0060	1.9932
98	6844	2667	0.3897	0.0103	0.0040	1.8629
99	3990	1675	0.4198	0.0063	0.0026	1.7331
100	...	...	...	0.0037	...	1.6254

ANNEX TABLE 4. LIFE EXPECTANCY AT AGE 80 ACCORDING TO OFFICIAL LIFE TABLES
Single year or central year of life table.
Source: United Nations Demographic Yearbook, Several Issues

Year	M	F
Australia		
1954	5.47	6.30
1961	5.57	6.68
1966	5.51	6.72
1978	6.13	7.64
1979	6.27	7.83
1984	6.54	8.28
1985	6.32	8.07
1986	6.56	8.30
1989	6.51	8.36
1990	6.80	8.56
Austria		
1950	5.05	5.57
1960	5.24	5.98
1971	5.24	6.09
1977	5.65	6.64
1981	5.50	6.63
1983	5.63	6.77
1985	5.77	6.92
1987	6.23	7.26
1989	6.37	7.52
Belgium		
1961	5.29	6.07
1970	5.41	6.33
1974	5.53	6.54
1981	5.74	7.11
Czechoslovakia		
1955	5.79	6.16
1958	5.77	6.06
1960	5.25	5.78
1964	5.39	5.93
1969	5,38	6.06
1972	4.19	6.39
1977	5.47	6.36
1980	4.80	5.71
1983	5.37	6.31
1985	5.51	6.45
Denmark		
1953	5.80	6.01
1958	5.81	6.14
1963	5.70	6.30
Denmark (cont.)		
1968	5.99	6.77
1971	6.20	7.20
1974	6.20	7.50
1977	6.50	7.80
1982	6.30	7.90
1989	6.50	8.20
England & Wales		
1951	4.86	5.83
1954	5.17	5.25
1956	5.24	6.31
1959	5.30	6.40
1961	5.20	6.30
1964	5.30	6.70
1971	5.50	7.00
1977	5.60	7.20
1979	5.80	7.50
1984	6.10	8.00
Estonia		
1990	5.58	6.79
Finland		
1952	4.80	5.23
1958	5.04	5.46
1963	4.90	5.30
1968	4.86	5.42
1972	5.10	5.63
1977	5.24	6.37
1982	5.69	6.69
1986	6.11	7.47
1989	6.20	7.45
France		
1951	4.80	5.90
1954	4.90	5.59
1962	5.28	6.41
1965	5.50	6.70
1972	5.90	7.30
1978	6.09	7.64
1982	6.13	7.72
1985	6.32	8.01
1988	6.72	8.52
1990	6.85	8.68
Germany, East		
1952	5.03	5.48
1955	5.27	5.80
1961	5.21	5.73
1964	6.28	6.93
1967	5.96	6.62
1976	5.06	5.79
1977	5.01	6.00
1981	5.00	5.94
1984	5.15	6.10
1985	4.98	6.00
1988	5.34	6.40
Germany, West		
1958	5.19	5.71
1961	5.24	5.58
1964	5.43	6.17
1970	5.32	6.09
1972	5.36	6.23
1974	5.37	6.30
1977	5.57	6.63
1982	5.73	7.03
1984	5.87	7.26
1986	5.99	7.46
Hungary		
1954	4.62	5.03
1955	5.05	5.62
1959	4.86	5.40
1964	5.27	5.76
1972	5.23	6.05
1979	5.69	6.57
1983	5.53	6.49
1986	5.18	6.08
1988	5.39	6.36
1990	5.27	6.27
Iceland		
1955	6.20	7.10
1963	6.30	7.10
1968	6.00	6.50
1972	6.60	7.70
1975	7.40	8.40
1982	7.08	8.37

Year	M	F
Iceland (cont.)		
1986	7.47	8.89
1988	7.14	8.45
Ireland		
1951	4.98	5.64
1961	5.06	5.87
1966	5.23	6.06
1971	5.35	6.19
1981	5.36	6.65
1986	5.31	6.78
Italy		
1952	5.04	5.55
1956	5.17	5.75
1961	5.70	6.35
1971	5.82	6.7
1976	5.57	6.53
1981	5.84	7.28
1984	5.98	7.17
1985	6.21	7.48
1988	6.29	7.82
Japan		
1956	4.41	5.38
1963	4.98	6.04
1968	5.07	6.18
1972	5.49	6.64
1978	6.01	7.36
1982	6.45	7.73
1988	6.69	8.36
Luxembourg		
1986	5.32	6.75
Netherlands		
1953	5.80	6.10
1958	5.90	6.20
1963	6.00	6.60
1972	6.20	7.10
1975	6.10	7.20
1979	6.50	8.00
1982	6.39	8.13
1984	6.34	8.16
1986	6.51	8.40
1989	6.23	8.21
New Zealand		
1951	5.53	6.15
1956	5.70	6.46
1961	5.49	6.43
New Zealand (cont.)		
1971	5.52	6.75
1976	5.66	7.26
1981	5.89	7.70
1987	6.17	8.03
Norway		
1953	6.39	6.60
1958	6.28	6.64
1968	6.14	6.97
1972	6.16	7.03
1975	6.26	7.32
1979	6.43	7.68
1981	6.42	7.92
1985	6.47	8.01
1987	6.40	8.11
1989	6.46	8.12
Poland		
1952	5.40	6.10
1956	5.40	6.10
1958	6.00	7.30
1965	5.87	6.73
1980	5.69	7.20
1982	5.52	6.79
1985	5.15	6.46
1987	5.45	6.71
1988	5.71	6.99
1990	5.59	6.84
Portugal		
1951	4.97	5.65
1955	4.50	5.10
1961	5.07	5.85
1971	4.85	5.77
1981	5.31	6.31
1989	6.03	7.21
1990	5.65	6.73
Scotland		
1951	4.60	5.40
1954	4.97	5.68
1956	5.10	5.72
1959	5.18	5.74
1961	5.15	5.85
1964	5.14	6.30
1971	5.17	6.60
1977	5.31	6.90
1979	5.33	7.08
1983	5.86	7.63
Scotland (cont.)		
1985	5.83	7.46
Spain		
1950	4.81	5.24
1960	5.08	5.63
1970	5.99	6.80
1975	5.87	6.69
1980	7.07	7.88
1981	6.59	7.63
1985	6.66	7.73
Sweden		
1952	5.65	5.98
1958	5.74	6.20
1963	5.82	6.44
1969	6.00	6.78
1973	6.08	7.28
1976	6.07	7.40
1978	6.09	7.52
1983	6.30	7.97
1987	6.46	8.27
1990	6.56	8.29
Switzerland		
1951	5.24	5.74
1965	5.55	6.34
1977	6.40	7.60
1981	6.29	7.76
1984	6.70	7.90
1986	6.90	8.40
1988	6.80	8.60

Annex Table 5. MEAN VALUES OF q IN AGE GROUPS, PER 10.000

Country and period	MALE				FEMALE			
	80-84	85-89	90-94	95-99	80-84	85-89	90-94	95-99
Austria								
1960-70	1501	2194	3135	4000	1212	1903	2800	3693
1980-90	1287	1910	2727	3746	950	1618	2472	3453
Belgium								
1960-70	1416	2141	3023	3727	1169	1853	2725	3637
1980-90	1279	1862	2629	3485	866	1453	2225	3077
Czechoslovakia								
1960-70	1534	2269	3166	4338	1282	2000	2852	3766
1980-90	1557	2194	3103	4188	1182	1858	2762	3826
Denmark								
1960-70	1272	1959	2856	4010	1087	1736	2555	3582
1980-90	1158	1692	2478	3390	768	1302	2104	3043
England and Wales								
1960-70	1439	2110	2892	3805	1041	1638	2390	3256
1980-90	1270	1845	2563	3402	812	1332	2055	2900
Estonia								
1960-70	1418	2098	2937	3954	1105	1784	2561	3324
1980-90	1392	1998	2729	3413	1050	1637	2435	3210
Finland								
1960-70	1584	2333	3173	3903	1375	2125	2993	3861
1980-90	1249	1828	2621	3664	886	1451	2252	3050
France								
1960-70	1377	2068	2922	3571	1021	1664	2488	3280
1980-90	1124	1738	2571	3447	733	1300	2105	3021
Germany East								
1960-70	1531	2291	3276	4582	1332	2082	3022	4308
1980-90	1519	2247	3160	4150	1162	1891	2791	3746
Germany West								
1960-70	1447	2151	3025	4024	1213	1912	2766	3687
1980-90	1273	1872	2670	3473	883	1484	2273	3106
Hungary								
1960-70	1523	2283	3209	4271	1311	2038	2861	4082
1980-90	1536	2174	3042	3772	1176	1834	2677	3627
Iceland								
1961-70	1110	1807	2444	3536	980	1637	2430	3114
1980-89	930	1503	2281	2947	675	1159	1853	2359
Ireland								
1960-70	1413	2141	2875	4354	1171	1758	2401	3863
1980-89	1341	2004	2885	4439	962	1495	2259	3337
Italy								
1960-70	1345	2072	3042	4529	1124	1826	2731	4029
1980-89	1195	1790	2610	3512	848	1446	2269	3212

Annex Table 5. (cont.)

Country and period	MALE				FEMALE			
	80-84	85-89	90-94	95-99	80-84	85-89	90-94	95-99
Japan 1960-70 1980-90	1571 1063	2271 1661	3082 2413	3829 3233	1220 723	1909 1276	2759 2073	3736 2998
Latvia 1960-70 1980-90	1269 1346	1885 1928	2654 2519	3189 3077	1035 1025	1659 1632	2356 2343	3021 3023
Luxembourg 1960-70 1980-89	1513 1361	2153 1955	2837 2781	4443 4201	1288 935	1969 1541	2728 2253	4052 3052
Netherlands 1960-70 1980-90	1200 1148	1848 1687	2696 2373	3565 3150	1030 730	1664 1261	2465 2012	3421 2912
New Zealand 1960-70 1980-90	1314 1179	2006 1767	2698 2552	3650 3400	974 807	1608 1306	2336 2023	3392 2848
Norway 1960-70 1980-90	1204 1128	1838 1688	2717 2433	3588 3376	1024 758	1639 1311	2440 2082	3524 3006
Portugal 1960-70 1980-90	1514 1304	2249 1986	3090 2769	3912 3787	1170 988	1867 1605	2535 2328	3436 3212
Scotland 1960-70 1980-90	1509 1371	2210 1962	3135 2715	4014 3685	1143 901	1765 1434	2555 2186	3358 2775
Spain 1960-70 1980-86	1350 1104	1999 1653	2636 2221	3773 3094	1068 841	1657 1401	2262 2075	3302 3101
Sweden 1960-70 1980-90	1258 1130	1940 1744	2852 2557	3892 3519	1064 743	1722 1310	2508 2097	3390 3028
Switzerland 1960-70 1980-90	1360 1087	2073 1717	2958 2566	3947 3408	1116 730	1807 1290	2685 2139	3588 3135
Low mortality (8countries) 1960-70 1980-90	1403 1097	2075 1695	2910 2478	3666 3334	1096 731	1747 1289	2567 2087	3419 3008
Medium Mortality (5 countries) 1960-70 1980-90	1418 1251	2117 1842	3001 2622	4148 3472	1133 857	1788 1432	2603 2200	3591 3052
High Mortality (3 countries) 1960-70 1980-90	1530 1535	2284 2214	3234 3118	4430 4060	1314 1171	2051 1869	2941 2758	4078 3724
Thirteen countries (high & medium) 1960-70 1980-90	1411 1171	2100 1763	2964 2543	3947 3394	1117 797	1769 1362	2589 2144	3504 3032

ANNEX TABLE 6. AGE SHIFT OF MORTALITY FROM 1960-70 TO 1980-90.
Years of age by which the death rate moved up from age given at left.

MALE

Age in 1960-70	AUSTRIA	BELGIUM	CZECHOSLO-VAKIA	DENMARK	ENGLAND AND WALES	ESTONIA	FINLAND	FRANCE	GERMANY EAST
80	1,76	1,13	-0,47	0,76	1,47	-0,28	3,25	2,19	0,03
81	1,73	1,08	-0,33	0,98	1,47	0,07	3,15	2,24	0,05
82	1,86	1,27	-0,20	1,27	1,59	0,21	3,18	2,27	0,09
83	1,83	1,40	-0,09	1,44	1,60	0,22	3,10	2,26	0,13
84	1,87	1,53	0,01	1,73	1,75	0,40,	3,13	2,26	0,21
85	1,92	1,74	0,12	1,75	1,84	0,28	3,08	2,20	0,20
86	1,95	1,81	0,30	1,86	1,94	0,48	3,23	2,19	0,25
87	1,92	1,90	0,51	1,92	2,06	0,68	3,38	2,12	0,26
88	1,94	2,03	0,69	1,82	2,06	0,60	3,41	2,11	0,40
89	2,17	2,09	0,78	1,76	1,99	0,42	3,24	2,07	0,52
90	2,15	2,11	0,62	1,76	1,99	0,83	3,04	2,06	0,50
91	2,06	2,13	0,42	1,67	1,98	2,04	2,91	1,98	0,49
92	2,03	2,21	0,31	1,84	1,88	1,84	2,95	1,94	0,61
93	1,83	2,07	0,24	2,13	1,93	2,59	2,62	1,88	0,72
94	1,57	2,20	0,23	2,47	2,20	3,47	2,33	1,77	0,68
95	2,26	2,06	0,11	3,27	2,26	-	1,64	1,45	0,77
96	2,36	1,38	0,42	3,48	2,26	-	2,33	1,08	0,86
97	2,99	1,11	0,90	2,90	2,25	-	1,41	0,45	1,37
98	2,99	0,74	-	3,03	2,74	-	0,57	0,65	-
99	2,98	1,71	-	2,70	4,47	-	1,07	0,58	-
80-84	1,81	1,28	-0,22	1,24	1,58	0,72	3,16	2,24	0,10
85-89	1,98	1,91	0,48	1,82	1,82	0,49	3,27	2,14	0,33
90-94	1,93	2,14	0,36	1,97	2,00	2,15	2,77	1,93	0,60
80-94	1,91	1,78	0,24	1,65	1,80	0,92	3,07	2,10	0,34

ANNEX TABLE 6.   AGE SHIFT (cont.)

MALE

Age in 1960-70	GERMANY WEST	HUNGARY	ICELAND	IRELAND	ITALY	JAPAN	LUXEM-BURG	NETHER-LANDS	NEW ZEALAND
80	1,52	-0,28	2,80	1,76	1,12	4,41	1,64	-0,05	1,18
81	1,53	-0,20	2,17	0,43	1,28	4,37	1,58	0,27	1,08
82	1,61	-0,11	1,80	0,78	1,44	4,34	1,51	0,52	1,36
83	1,64	0,00	2,00	0,57	1,55	4,28	1,64	0,62	1,36
84	1,71	0,26	1,97	0,92	1,61	4,22	1,72	0,75	1,45
85	1,74	0,19	2,02	0,93	1,71	4,15	1,38	0,84	1,60
86	1,79	0,59	1,86	1,22	1,82	4,14	1,46	1,01	1,70
87	1,82	0,72	2,13	0,80	1,87	4,10	1,58	1,15	1,72
88	1,83	0,67	1,73	0,22	1,93	4,10	1,45	1,28	1,79
89	1,80	0,59	1,00	0,66	2,04	4,08	0,99	1,43	1,31
90	1,82	0,69	1,22	0,38	2,10	4,07	1,39	1,59	1,11
91	1,85	0,80	1,00	-0,04	2,25	4,04	0,39	1,67	0,89
92	2,05	0,95	1,14	-0,03	2,43	4,10	0,10	1,76	0,86
93	2,69	1,46	1,04	-0,65	2,60	4,00	-0,62	2,10	1,25
94	2,71	1,37	1,13	-0,08	2,71	4,13	-1,33	2,05	1,44
95	2,26	1,96	2,07	-0,38	2,92	3,97	-2,08	2,16	0,85
96	1,86	1,67	1,53	-0,16	3,40	4,00	0,67	1,85	1,13
97	2,09	-	0,89	-0,24	4,46	3,53	-	1,65	0,60
98	1,98	-	-	-0,40	-	3,38	-	2,68	-0,06
99	1,93	-	-	-1,61	-	1,99	-	4,22	-0,42
80-84	1,60	-0,07	2,15	0,89	1,40	4,32	1,62	0,42	1,29
85-89	1,80	0,55	1,75	0,77	1,87	4,11	1,37	1,14	1,62
90-94	2,22	1,05	1,11	-0,08	2,42	4,07	-0,01	1,83	1,13
80-94	1,87	0,51	1,67	0,53	1,90	4,17	0,66	1,13	1,35

ANNEX TABLE 6.   AGE SHIFT (cont.)

MALE

AGE IN 1960-70	NORWAY	PORTUGAL	SCOTLAND	SWEDEN	SWITZER-LAND	13	AGGREGATES LOW	AGGREGATES MEDIUM	AGGREGATES HIGH
80	0,65	1,79	1,17	1,18	2,27	2,11	2,39	1,37	-0,20
81	0,66	1,67	1,07	1,16	2,45	2,16	2,78	1,43	-0,13
82	0,82	1,66	1,26	1,20	2,44	2,22	2,75	1,55	-0,04
83	0,85	1,66	1,40	1,19	2,39	2,22	2,70	1,61	0,05
84	0,86	1,65	1,50	1,22	2,37	2,26	2,68	1,69	0,17
85	0,92	1,60	1,67	1,22	2,24	2,26	2,61	1,78	0,22
86	1,06	1,68	1,74	1,25	2,09	2,28	2,57	1,87	0,35
87	1,05	1,78	1,69	1,29	2,15	2,29	2,53	1,93	0,45
88	1,12	1,89	1,72	1,31	2,12	2,30	2,51	1,98	0,55
89	1,30	1,96	1,72	1,35	2,13	2,30	2,49	2,01	0,63
90	1,44	1,93	1,76	1,42	2,16	2,32	2,50	2,02	0,60
91	1,43	1,95	1,61	1,57	2,26	2,34	2,47	2,09	0,57
92	1,46	1,61	2,16	1,71	2,28	2,41	2,50	2,18	0,61
93	1,67	1,39	2,23	1,73	2,58	2,58	2,59	2,40	0,73
94	1,71	1,27	2,09	2,00	2,60	2,67	2,56	2,60	0,74
95	1,55	1,04	1,85	1,87	2,53	2,54	2,33	2,58	0,70
96	1,67	0,53	2,06	1,88	1,94	2,42	1,98	2,65	0,98
97	1,61	0,67	1,96	1,72	2,77	2,65	1,63	3,25	1,81
98	1,65	0,38	-	1,04	4,01	2,63	1,95	3,13	-
99	1,51	-	-	1,34	-	2,85	1,76	5,23	-
80-84	0,77	1,69	1,28	1,19	2,38	2,19	2,66	1,53	-0,03
85-89	1,09	1,78	1,71	1,28	2,15	2,29	2,54	1,91	0,44
90-94	1,54	1,63	1,97	1,69	2,38	2,46	2,52	2,26	0,65
80-94	1,13	1,70	1,65	1,39	2,30	2,31	2,57	1,90	0,35

ANNEX TABLE 6.   AGE SHIFT (CONT.)

FEMALE

Age in 1960-70	AUSTRIA	BELGIUM	CZECHO-SLOVAKIA	DENMARK	ENGLAND AND WALES	ESTONIA	FINLAND	FRANCE	GERMANY EAST
80	2,32	2,79	0,79	3,35	2,38	0,71	4,48	2,87	1,30
81	2,21	2,75	0,79	3,23	2,34	0,57	4,36	2,82	1,29
82	2,20	2,78	0,81	3,24	2,43	0,50	4,41	2,80	1,32
83	2,10	2,77	0,83	3,12	2,42	0,53	4,39	2,73	1,28
84	1,99	2,72	0,86	3,07	2,47	0,61	4,44	2,66	1,22
85	1,90	2,70	0,85	3,01	2,44	0,75	4,46	2,59	1,18
86	1,83	2,71	0,88	2,92	2,36	0,94	4,40	2,51	1,18
87	1,77	2,72	0,92	2,85	2,30	1,08	4,33	2,42	1,15
88	1,76	2,77	0,87	2,82	2,22	1,15	4,34	2,36	1,18
89	1,79	2,80	0,76	2,72	2,06	1,17	4,25	2,30	1,18
90	1,72	2,92	0,73	2,69	2,02	1,05	4,30	2,21	1,15
91	1,66	2,85	0,63	2,61	2,05	0,96	4,53	2,16	1,18
92	1,70	2,87	0,44	2,34	1,98	0,74	4,56	2,08	1,08
93	1,64	2,79	0,30	2,29	1,99	0,63	4,77	2,04	1,01
94	1,26	2,82	0,34	2,48	2,21	0,66	4,32	1,97	1,24
95	1,65	2,90	0,09	2,37	2,14	0,87	6,22	2,07	1,54
96	1,64	2,88	-0,14	2,28	2,08	1,00	5,62	1,76	2,05
97	1,49	3,06	-0,23	2,31	1,84	-	5,74	1,19	1,96
98	1,95	2,88	-0,52	2,23	1,79	-	4,92	1,71	-
99	1,77	3,29	-0,40	2,17	1,68	-	6,92	1,69	-
80-84	2,16	2,76	0,82	3,20	2,41	0,58	4,42	2,78	1,28
85-89	1,82	2,74	0,85	2,86	2,28	1,02	4,36	2,44	1,17
90-94	1,60	2,85	0,49	2,48	2,05	0,81	4,50	2,09	1,13
80-94	1,86	2,78	0,72	2,85	2,25	0,80	4,43	2,44	1,19

ANNEX TABLE 6. AGE SHIFT (cont.)

FEMALE

Age in 1960-70	GERMANY WEST	HUNGARY	ICELAND	IRELAND	ITALY	JAPAN	LUXEM-BURG	NETHER LANDS	NEW ZEALAND
80	2,89	1,04	2,11	3,68	2,46	4,71	2,81	2,96	2,29
81	2,85	1,03	2,73	1,99	2,53	4,62	3,21	2,88	1,52
82	2,86	1,16	3,33	1,97	2,56	4,57	3,13	2,84	1,86
83	2,81	1,22	3,36	1,67	2,56	4,45	3,26	2,83	1,89
84	2,77	1,24	3,49	2,19	2,53	4,34	3,00	2,78	2,22
85	2,73	1,25	3,95	2,28	2,51	4,24	2,64	2,78	2,29
86	2,69	1,26	4,13	2,37	2,47	4,13	2,37	2,71	2,23
87	2,69	1,26	3,66	2,07	2,45	4,05	2,65	2,69	2,24
88	2,69	1,22	4,12	2,08	2,43	3,94	2,32	2,66	2,17
89	2,71	1,20	3,85	1,37	2,39	3,83	2,25	2,63	1,95
90	2,77	1,16	3,81	1,23	2,38	3,81	2,95	2,58	1,99
91	2,84	1,10	3,55	0,85	2,36	3,75	2,99	2,59	2,16
92	2,94	0,94	5,19	0,88	2,46	3,68	2,84	2,40	1,99
93	3,08	1,11	4,34	0,45	2,60	3,61	2,90	2,21	1,72
94	2,99	0,87	4,53	1,07	2,71	3,80	3,76	2,26	1,93
95	2,79	1,02	3,99	0,97	2,87	3,78	-	2,22	2,42
96	2,76	1,17	3,41	-	3,14	3,91	-	2,40	2,44
97	2,61	1,84	3,03	-	3,64	4,13	-	2,36	2,93
98	3,29	-	2,22	-	3,08	4,38	-	2,42	2,70
99	3,49	-	1,52	-	2,96	4,36	-	2,34	-
80-84	2,84	1,14	3,00	2,30	2,53	4,54	3,08	2,86	1,96
85-89	2,70	1,24	3,94	2,03	2,45	4,04	2,45	2,69	2,18
90-94	2,92	1,03	4,28	0,90	2,50	3,73	3,09	2,41	1,96
80-94	2,82	1,14	3,74	1,74	2,49	4,10	2,87	2,65	2,03

ANNEX TABLE 6. AGE SHIFT (cont.)

FEMALE

Age in 1960-70	NORWAY	PORTUGAL	SCOTLAND	SWEDEN	SWITZER-LAND	13	AGGREGATES LOW	MEDIUM	HIGH
80	2,53	1,85	2,37	2,97	3,62	3,11	3,60	2,62	1,12
81	2,56	1,55	2,46	3,07	3,70	3,06	3,54	2,59	1,10
82	2,65	1,55	2,54	3,10	3,66	3,07	3,50	2,63	1,16
83	2,66	1,52	2,53	3,02	3,58	3,01	3,40	2,60	1,15
84	2,58	1,65	2,52	3,00	3,50	2,96	3,32	2,59	1,14
85	2,44	1,65	2,42	2,94	3,31	2,90	3,23	2,55	1,12
86	2,31	1,76	2,39	2,86	3,24	2,83	3,12	2,50	1,13
87	2,26	1,89	2,32	2,76	3,21	2,75	3,03	2,45	1,13
88	2,21	1,81	2,25	2,66	3,12	2,70	2,95	2,42	1,10
89	2,19	1,64	2,15	2,56	2,96	2,61	2,85	2,35	1,09
90	2,15	1,68	2,11	2,53	2,86	2,57	2,77	2,33	1,05
91	2,14	1,44	2,16	2,34	2,89	2,54	2,70	2,35	1,03
92	2,00	1,24	2,60	2,15	3,01	2,52	2,60	2,40	0,89
93	1,99	1,28	3,19	2,10	2,98	2,53	2,52	2,51	0,84
94	2,12	1,29	-	2,07	2,72	2,59	2,52	2,62	0,88
95	2,28	1,20	-	2,08	2,43	2,55	2,46	2,60	1,02
96	2,94	1,54	-	2,02	2,23	2,56	2,35	2,64	1,18
97	3,57	1,18	-	1,81	2,10	2,46	2,10	2,68	1,49
98	3,65	0,71	-	1,98	2,72	2,53	2,43	2,59	-
99	3,56	-	-	1,48	3,50	2,41	2,32	2,44	-
80-84	2,59	1,62	2,48	3,03	3,61	3,04	3,47	2,61	1,13
85-89	2,28	1,75	2,31	2,76	3,17	2,76	3,04	2,45	1,11
90-94	2,08	1,39	2,51	2,24	2,89	2,55	2,62	2,44	0,94
80-94	2,32	1,59	2,43	2,68	3,22	2,78	3,04	2,50	1,06

ANNEX TABLE 7. SURVIVORS FROM AGE 80 TO 100 IN ACTUAL COHORTS

Country and cohort	Male			Female		
	Age 80	Reach age 100		Age 80	Reach age 100	
		Number	per 1000		Number	per 1000
Austria						
1870-79	84 504	138	1.63	129 766	424	3.27
1880-89	94 322	203	2.15	174 348	793	4.55
Belgium						
1870-79	125 439	230	1.83	168 000	610	3.63
1880-89	138 591	422	3.04	205 481	1 419	6.91
Czechoslovakia						
1870-79	114 108	200	1.75	164 487	510	3.10
1880-89	126 513	172	1.36	216 099	611	2.83
Denmark						
1870-79	56 666	194	3.43	64 220	454	7.07
1880-89	69 366	373	5.38	88 145	1 022	11.59
England & Wales						
1870-70	564 291	1 297	2.30	939 363	7 782	8.28
1880-89	594 491	2 073	3.49	1 170 719	14 105	12.05
Finland						
1870-79	25 763	34	1.32	50 418	142	2.82
1880-89	30 820	74	2.40	63 245	463	7.32
France						
1870-79	563 986	1 547	2.74	960 617	6 870	7.15
1880-89	605 130	2 426	4.01	1 198 632	13 425	11.20
Germany, East						
1874-79	154 946	204	1.32	215 776	476	2.21
1880-79	259 216	339	1.31	425 695	1 095	2.57
Germany, West						
1871-79	587 408	983	1.67	761 758	2 550	3.35
1880-89	731 801	2 075	2.84	1 186 680	7 317	6.17
Hungary						
1870-79	85 565	86	1.01	114 433	301	2.63
1880-89	106 928	174	1.63	166 258	551	3.31
Italy						
1872-79	468 233	1 082	2.31	579 386	2 573	4.44
1880-89	637 935	2 197	3.44	923 891	6 607	7.15
Japan						
1870-79	410 725	741	1.80	697 333	2 902	4.16
1880-89	592 706	2 223	3.75	966 093	7 877	8.15
Netherlands						
1880-89	154 084	1 087	7.05	187 232	2 412	12.98

ANNEX TABLE 7. (cont.)

Country and cohort	Male			Female		
	Age 80	Reach age 100		Age 80	Reach age 100	
		Number	per 1000		Number	per 1000
Norway						
1870-79	46 241	228	4.93	59 766	499	8.35
1880-89	53 570	323	6.03	73 447	891	12.13
Scotland						
1870-79	61 221	107	1.75	92 018	542	5.89
1880-89	59 111	145	2.45	108 649	1 255	11.55
Sweden						
1870-79	103 578	382	3.69	123 117	872	7.08
1880-89	125 663	553	4.40	162 604	1 995	12.27
Switzerland						
1870-79	54 605	128	2.34	82 217	400	4.86
1880-89	67 734	294	4.34	107 604	1 031	9.58
Total						
1870-79	3 507 189	7 581	2.16	5 021 469	27 877	5.55
1880-89	4 447 981	15 153	3.41	7 424 822	62 819	8.46

ANNEX TABLE 8. PROBABILITY OF DYING AT AGES 100 AND OVER.
Pooled data for 14 countries[1]

Age x	Males			Females		
	Reached age x	Died before age x+1	1000q	Reached age x	Died before age x+1	1000q
1950-60						
100	1643	820	499	5933	2632	444
101	771	336	436	3072	1343	437
102	402	190	473	1592	711	447
103	190	93	489	793	383	483
104	93	45	484	376	174	463
105	45	24	533	173	82	474
106	22	12	545	79	34	430
107	9	2	222	47	30	638
108	7	5	714	16	10	625
109	2	2	1000	5	5	
1960-70						
100	3623	1663	459	13134	5476	417
101	1773	831	469	7166	3000	419
102	880	412	468	3907	1661	425
103	442	219	495	2059	940	457
104	197	110	558	1032	486	471
105	82	41	500	513	254	495
106	38	23	605	237	118	498
107	13	6	462	105	62	590
108	6	2	333	38	21	553
109	5	4	800	16	12	750
110	1	0		4	2	500
111	1	1		2	1	500

[1] To the group of thirteen countries is added Belgium beginning with 1974.

ANNEX TABLE 8. (cont.)

	Males			Females		
Age x	Reached age x	Died before age x+1	1000q	Reached age x	Died before age x+1	1000q
1970-80						
100	7612	3449	453	27520	10881	395
101	3912	1796	459	15435	6310	409
102	1993	914	459	8448	3587	425
103	1002	495	494	4452	1943	436
104	473	234	495	2310	1082	468
105	229	126	550	1118	558	499
106	98	49	500	516	260	504
107	45	23	511	243	126	519
108	18	11		112	68	607
109	7	6		37	24	649
110	1	1		11	3	273
111	0	0		7	4	571
112	0	0		3	2	667
113	0	0		1	1	
1980-90						
100	13433	5658	421	56926	20927	368
101	7293	3097	425	33003	12646	383
102	3856	1657	430	18547	7363	397
103	2032	942	464	10249	4308	420
104	1007	445	442	5382	2332	433
105	495	223	451	2759	1267	459
106	243	110	453	1342	610	455
107	109	53	486	644	307	477
108	53	29		297	167	562
109	19	15		116	70	603
110	5	2		40	21	
111	2	1		14	5	
112				6	2	
113				4	1	
114				3	1	

ANNEX TABLE 9.　　GENDER INDICATORS OF MORTALITY.
Thirteen countries with good data.　　　　　　1950 - 1960

x	$q_x \; 10^4$				$p_x \; 10^4$			Female age delay
	M	F	M/F	M-F	M	F	F/M	
80	1237	1000	1.238	238	8763	9000	1.027	2.15
81	1350	1101	1.227	249	8650	8899	1.029	2.11
82	1477	1219	1.212	258	8523	8781	1.030	2.08
83	1606	1336	1.202	270	8394	8664	1.032	2.05
84	1747	1466	1.192	282	8253	8534	1.034	2.06
85	1894	1600	1.184	295	8106	8400	1.036	2.07
86	2048	1738	1.178	310	7952	8262	1.039	2.09
87	2206	1883	1.171	323	7794	8117	1.041	2.13
88	2367	2035	1.164	333	7633	7965	1.044	2.11
89	2532	2184	1.159	348	7468	7816	1.047	2.11
90	2701	2348	1.151	354	7299	7652	1.048	2.10
91	2875	2514	1.144	362	7125	7486	1.051	2.07
92	3049	2684	1.136	366	6951	7316	1.053	1.99
93	3239	2862	1.132	377	6761	7138	1.056	1.97
94	3417	3051	1.120	365	6583	6949	1.055	1.85
95	3602	3245	1.110	357	6398	6755	1.056	1.72
96	3796	3448	1.101	349	6204	6552	1.056	1.56
97	4054	3662	1.107	392	5946	6338	1.066	1.81
98	4324	3902	1.108	422	5676	6098	1.074	2.39
99	4445	4090	1.087	355	5555	5910	1.064	1.98
100	4594	4249	1.081	345	5406	5751	1.064	2.77
101	4731	4442	1.065	289	5269	5558	1.055	3.36
102	4762	4546	1.047	215	5238	5454	1.041	2.44
103	4830	4607	1.048	223	5170	5393	1.043	
104	5050	4593	1.099	456	4950	5407	1.092	
105	4549	4977	0.914	-428	5451	5023	0.921	
106	4998	5261	0.950	-263	5002	4739	0.948	
98-100	4454	4080	1.092	374	5546	5920	1.067	
101-103	4774	4532	1.054	243	5226	5468	1.046	
104-106	4866	4944	0.988	-78	5134	5056	0.987	

ANNEX TABLE 9. (cont.) 1960 - 1970

x	$q_x \, 10^4$				$p_x \, 10^4$			Female age delay
	M	F	M/F	M-F	M	F	F/M	
80	1181	902	1.309	279	8819	9098	1.032	2.44
81	1291	1002	1.288	289	8709	8998	1.033	2.49
82	1410	1115	1.264	294	8590	8885	1.034	2.42
83	1530	1230	1.244	301	8470	8770	1.035	2.32
84	1662	1355	1.227	307	8338	8645	1.037	2.27
85	1798	1486	1.210	312	8202	8514	1.038	2.20
86	1945	1623	1.198	322	8055	8377	1.040	2.16
87	2096	1767	1.186	329	7904	8233	1.042	2.13
88	2255	1920	1.175	335	7745	8080	1.043	2.10
89	2421	2074	1.167	347	7579	7926	1.046	2.07
90	2596	2238	1.160	359	7404	7762	1.048	2.07
91	2773	2409	1.151	364	7227	7591	1.050	2.06
92	2957	2584	1.145	374	7043	7416	1.053	2.03
93	3147	2761	1.140	385	6853	7239	1.056	2.06
94	3333	2951	1.129	382	6667	7049	1.057	2.03
95	3515	3135	1.121	380	6485	6865	1.059	2.04
96	3702	3328	1.112	374	6298	6672	1.059	1.94
97	3938	3506	1.123	432	6062	6494	1.071	2.36
98	4151	3715	1.117	436	5849	6285	1.075	2.70
99	4348	3883	1.120	464	5652	6117	1.082	2.84
100	4508	4034	1.118	475	5492	5966	1.086	2.84
101	4685	4201	1.115	484	5315	5799	1.091	2.96
102	4899	4376	1.120	523	5101	5624	1.103	2.63
103	4981	4533	1.099	449	5019	5467	1.089	
104	5255	4691	1.120	563	4745	5309	1.119	
105	5241	5022	1.044	219	4759	4978	1.046	
106	4917	5214	0.943	-297	5083	4786	0.942	
98-100	4336	3877	1.118	458	5664	6123	1.081	
101-103	4855	4370	1.111	485	5145	5630	1.094	
104-106	5138	4976	1.036	162	4862	5024	1.035	

ANNEX TABLE 9. (cont.) 1970 - 1980

x	$q_x \; 10^4$				$p_x \; 10^4$			Female age delay
	M	F	M/F	M-F	M	F	F/M	
80	1113	777	1.434	337	8887	9223	1.038	3.26
81	1210	869	1.392	341	8790	9131	1.039	3.09
82	1319	976	1.352	343	8681	9024	1.040	2.98
83	1430	1083	1.321	347	8570	8917	1.041	2.83
84	1550	1199	1.293	351	8450	8801	1.042	2.71
85	1677	1322	1.268	355	8323	8678	1.043	2.58
86	1810	1452	1.247	358	8190	8548	1.044	2.46
87	1949	1591	1.225	358	8051	8409	1.044	2.35
88	2099	1739	1.207	360	7901	8261	1.046	2.25
89	2257	1892	1.192	364	7743	8108	1.047	2.18
90	2421	2057	1.177	365	7579	7943	1.048	2.13
91	2594	2226	1.166	369	7406	7774	1.050	2.09
92	2769	2398	1.155	371	7231	7602	1.051	2.04
93	2947	2577	1.144	371	7053	7423	1.053	2.03
94	3121	2761	1.130	360	6879	7239	1.052	2.00
95	3294	2941	1.120	353	6706	7059	1.053	1.89
96	3460	3121	1.109	339	6540	6879	1.052	1.72
97	3693	3315	1.114	378	6307	6685	1.060	1.93
98	3939	3517	1.120	421	6061	6483	1.070	2.26
99	4164	3706	1.124	458	5836	6294	1.079	2.49
100	4356	3893	1.119	463	5644	6107	1.082	2.45
101	4588	4071	1.127	517	5412	5929	1.095	2.61
102	4726	4262	1.109	464	5274	5738	1.088	2.33
103	4935	4472	1.104	463	5065	5528	1.091	2.34
104	4996	4661	1.072	334	5004	5339	1.067	1.42
105	5123	4856	1.055	267	4877	5144	1.055	
106	5428	5190	1.046	238	4572	4810	1.052	
98-100	4153	3705	1.121	447	5847	6295	1.077	
101-103	4750	4268	1.113	481	5250	5732	1.092	
104-106	5182	4902	1.057	280	4818	5098	1.058	

For 1980-1990, see Table 25 in text.

ANNEX TABLE 10. STATIONARY OLDEST-OLD POPULATION BY COUNTRY IN 1980-90
Based on 10.000 persons (3500 male and 6500 female) annually reaching the age of 80 years.

Country and age	Number			Percent		
	Male	Female	Total	Male	Female	Total
Australia						
80-84	13427	27538	40965	17.61	36.12	53.72
85-89	6446	16712	23158	8.45	21.92	30.37
90-94	2128	7322	9450	2.79	9.60	12.39
95-99	413	1963	2376	0.54	2.57	3.12
100-	39	264	302	0.05	0.35	0.40
Total	22452	53799	76251	29.44	70.56	100.00
Austria						
80-84	12984	26210	39194	19.69	39.75	59.45
85-89	5624	13636	19261	8.53	20.68	29.21
90-94	1616	4611	6227	2.45	6.99	9.45
95-99	260	876	1136	0.39	1.33	1.72
100-	24	88	112	0.04	0.13	0.17
Total	20508	45422	65930	31.11	68.89	100.00
Belgium						
80-84	12992	26706	39697	18.74	38.53	57.27
85-89	5701	14801	20502	8.22	21.35	29.58
90-94	1696	5623	7319	2.45	8.11	10.56
95-99	298	1296	1594	0.43	1.87	2.30
100-	28	173	201	0.04	0.25	0.29
Total	20715	48598	69312	29.89	70.11	100.00
Czechoslovakia						
80-84	12153	24798	36951	21.07	42.99	64.06
85-89	4464	11254	15718	7.74	19.51	27.25
90-94	1067	3269	4337	1.85	5.67	7.52
95-99	126	505	631	0.22	0.88	1.09
100-	6	36	42	0.01	0.06	0.07
Total	17817	39862	57679	30.89	69.11	100.00

ANNEX TABLE 10. (cont.) STATIONARY OLDEST-OLD POPULATION BY COUNTRY IN 1980-90

Country and age	Number			Percent		
	Male	Female	Total	Male	Female	Total
Denmark						
80-84	13331	27294	40626	17.95	36.76	54.71
85-89	6384	16192	22576	8.60	21.81	30.41
90-94	2102	6677	8779	2.83	8.99	11.82
95-99	398	1625	2023	0.54	2.19	2.72
100-	40	208	248	0.05	0.28	0.33
Total	22256	51996	74252	29.97	70.03	100.00
England & Wales						
80-84	13015	26996	40011	18.09	37.53	55.62
85-89	5752	15670	21422	8.00	21.78	29.78
90-94	1759	6467	8226	2.44	8.99	11.43
95-99	325	1666	1991	0.45	2.32	2.77
100-	35	253	288	0.05	0.35	0.40
Total	20886	51052	71938	29.03	70.97	100.00
Estonia						
80-84	12673	25566	38239	20.07	40.49	60.57
85-89	5162	12720	17883	8.18	20.15	28.32
90-94	1416	4349	5765	2.24	6.89	9.13
95-99	251	868	1119	0.40	1.37	1.77
100-	25	105	130	0.04	0.17	0.21
Total	19527	43608	63136	30.93	69.07	100.00
Finland						
80-84	13039	26567	39605	18.83	38.37	57.21
85-89	5868	14640	20508	8.48	21.15	29.62
90-94	1780	5555	7335	2.57	8.02	10.60
95-99	305	1267	1572	0.44	1.83	2.27
100-	24	187	212	0.04	0.27	0.31
Total	21016	48216	69232	30.36	69.64	100.00
France						
80-84	13504	27572	41076	17.95	36.65	54.60
85-89	6446	16543	22989	8.57	21.99	30.56
90-94	2042	6820	8862	2.71	9.07	11.78
95-99	372	1670	2042	0.49	2.22	2.71
100-	34	231	265	0.05	0.31	0.35
Total	22398	52837	75235	29.77	70.23	100.00

ANNEX TABLE 10. (cont.) STATIONARY OLDEST-OLD POPULATION BY COUNTRY IN 1980-90

Country and age	Number			Percent		
	Male	Female	Total	Male	Female	Total
Germany, East						
80-84	12310	24962	37272	21.20	42.99	64.18
85-89	4550	11340	15890	7.83	19.53	27.36
90-94	1030	3219	4249	1.77	5.54	7.32
95-99	123	494	617	0.21	0.85	1.06
100-	6	37	43	0.01	0.06	0.07
Total	18018	40053	58071	31.03	68.97	100.00
Germany, West						
80-84	13016	26609	39626	18.95	38.74	57.69
85-89	5716	14567	20283	8.32	21.21	29.53
90-94	1682	5401	7083	2.45	7.86	10.31
95-99	293	1221	1514	0.43	1.78	2.20
100-	27	158	185	0.04	0.23	0.27
Total	20735	47956	68692	30.19	69.81	100.00
Hungary						
80-84	12241	24841	37082	21.01	42.64	63.65
85-89	4557	11382	15939	7.82	19.54	27.36
90-94	1090	3375	4465	1.87	5.79	7.66
95-99	147	567	714	0.25	0.97	1.23
100-	11	47	58	0.02	0.08	0.10
Total	18045	40212	58258	30.98	69.02	100.00
Iceland						
80-84	14133	27947	42080	17.27	34.16	51.43
85-89	7611	17554	25165	9.30	21.45	30.76
90-94	2799	8175	10974	3.42	9.99	13.41
95-99	625	2436	3061	0.76	2.98	3.74
100-	80	463	543	0.10	0.57	0.66
Total	25248	56575	81823	30.86	69.14	100.00
Ireland						
80-84	12857	26079	38936	19.43	39.42	58.85
85-89	5360	13807	19167	8.10	20.87	28.97
90-94	1438	5163	6601	2.17	7.80	9.98
95-99	195	1138	1333	0.29	1.72	2.01
100-	9	118	126	0.01	0.18	0.19
Total	19858	46305	66163	30.01	69.99	100.00

ANNEX TABLE 10. (cont.) STATIONARY OLDEST-OLD POPULATION BY COUNTRIES IN 1980-90.

Country and age	Number			Percent		
	Male	Female	Total	Male	Female	Total
Italy						
80-84	13251	26822	40073	18.80	38.06	56.86
85-89	6112	15004	21116	8.67	21.29	29.96
90-94	1880	5654	7535	2.67	8.02	10.69
95-99	333	1243	1577	0.47	1.76	2.24
100-	31	146	177	0.04	0.21	0.25
Total	21608	48869	70476	30.66	69.34	100.00
Japan						
80-84	13701	27627	41329	17.87	36.04	53.91
85-89	6792	16710	23503	8.86	21.80	30.66
90-94	2284	7012	9296	2.98	9.15	12.13
95-99	470	1749	2219	0.61	2.28	2.89
100-	58	256	314	0.08	0.33	0.41
Total	23305	53355	76660	30.40	69.60	100.00
Latvia						
80-84	12769	25696	38465	19.83	39.90	59.73
85-89	5377	12994	18371	8.35	20.18	28.53
90-94	1597	4473	6070	2.48	6.95	9.43
95-99	320	990	1310	0.50	1.54	2.03
100-	44	138	182	0.07	0.21	0.28
Total	20107	44291	64399	31.22	68.78	100.00
Luxembourg						
80-84	12705	26232	38937	19.21	39.66	58.87
85-89	5355	13964	19319	8.10	21.11	29.21
90-94	1513	4928	6441	2.29	7.45	9.74
95-99	182	1099	1280	0.27	1.66	1.94
100-	10	152	163	0.02	0.23	0.25
Total	19766	46375	66140	29.88	70.12	100.00
Netherlands						
80-84	13363	27459	40822	17.76	36.50	54.26
85-89	6370	16436	22806	8.47	21.85	30.31
90-94	2134	6931	9064	2.84	9.21	12.05
95-99	441	1781	2222	0.59	2.37	2.95
100-	54	263	317	0.07	0.35	0.42
Total	22362	52869	75231	29.72	70.28	100.00

ANNEX TABLE 10. (cont.) STATIONARY OLDEST-OLD POPULATION BY COUNTRY IN 1980-90.

Country and age	Number			Percent		
	Male	Female	Total	Male	Female	Total
New Zealand						
80-84	13240	27054	40293	18.08	36.94	55.02
85-89	6166	15797	21963	8.42	21.57	29.99
90-94	1955	6610	8565	2.67	9.03	11.69
95-99	366	1740	2106	0.50	2.38	2.88
100-	30	284	314	0.04	0.39	0.43
Total	21757	51484	73241	29.71	70.29	100.00
Norway						
80-84	13480	27385	40865	18.00	36.57	54.57
85-89	6508	16269	22777	8.69	21.72	30.41
90-94	2156	6700	8856	2.88	8.95	11.83
95-99	425	1670	2095	0.57	2.23	2.80
100-	48	249	298	0.06	0.33	0.40
Total	22617	52273	74891	30.20	69.80	100.00
Poland						
80-84	12560	25517	38077	20.30	41.23	61.53
85-89	5019	12374	17392	8.11	20.00	28.10
90-94	1346	3911	5257	2.17	6.32	8.49
95-99	245	772	1017	0.40	1.25	1.64
100-	33	107	140	0.05	0.17	0.23
Total	19203	42681	61884	31.03	68.97	100.00
Portugal						
80-84	12956	25984	38940	19.85	39.82	59.67
85-89	5478	13303	18781	8.40	20.39	28.78
90-94	1502	4656	6158	2.30	7.14	9.44
95-99	232	1004	1237	0.36	1.54	1.90
100-	19	120	139	0.03	0.18	0.21
Total	20188	45068	65256	30.94	69.06	100.00
Scotland						
80-84	12708	26415	39123	18.70	38.87	57.57
85-89	5277	14581	19858	7.76	21.46	29.22
90-94	1474	5623	7097	2.17	8.27	10.44
95-99	239	1382	1621	0.35	2.03	2.39
100-	19	240	259	0.03	0.35	0.38
Total	19717	48241	67958	29.01	70.99	100.00

ANNEX TABLE 10. (cont.) STATIONARY OLDEST-OLD POPULATION BY COUNTRY IN 1980-90.

Country and age	Number			Percent		
	Male	Female	Total	Male	Female	Total
Singapore-Chinese						
80-84	13529	26789	40317	17.82	35.29	53.12
85-89	6818	15745	22562	8.98	20.74	29.73
90-94	2629	6952	9581	3.46	9.16	12.62
95-99	708	2152	2861	0.93	2.84	3.77
100-	83	498	581	0.11	0.66	0.77
Total	23767	52136	75902	31.31	68.69	100.00
Spain						
80-84	13547	26883	40430	18.69	37.09	55.79
85-89	6613	15165	21778	9.12	20.93	30.05
90-94	2318	6067	8385	3.20	8.37	11.57
95-99	501	1378	1879	0.69	1.90	2.59
Total	22979	49493	72472	31.71	68.29	100.00
Sweden						
80-84	13499	27484	40983	18.04	36.72	54.76
85-89	6426	16383	22808	8.59	21.89	30.47
90-94	2029	6744	8772	2.71	9.01	11.72
95-99	372	1652	2024	0.50	2.21	2.70
100-	34	223	258	0.05	0.30	0.34
Total	22359	52486	74845	29.87	70.13	100.00
Switzerland						
80-84	13610	27611	41220	17.99	36.49	54.48
85-89	6628	16621	23250	8.76	21.97	30.73
90-94	2100	6826	8926	2.78	9.02	11.80
95-99	389	1629	2017	0.51	2.15	2.67
100-	39	204	243	0.05	0.27	0.32
Total	22766	52891	75657	30.09	69.91	100.00

ANNEX TABLE 11. YEARS LIVED AT SPECIFIED AGE INTERVALS PER EACH PERSON REACHING AGE 80.
(For exceptions from full decades, see footnote).

Country and age interval	Male				Female			
	1950-60	1960-70	1970-80	1980-90	1950-60	1960-70	1970-80	1980-90
Australia[1]								
80 - 85	...	...	3.71	3.84	...	...	4.10	4.24
85 - 90	...	...	1.62	1.84	...	...	2.27	2.57
90 - 95	...	...	0.48	0.61	...	...	0.90	1.13
95 - 100	...	...	0.09	0.12	...	...	0.22	0.30
100 -105	...	...	0.01	0.01	...	...	0.03	0.04
Total	...	...	5.91	6.41	...	...	7.52	8.28
Austria								
80 - 85	3.50	3.53	3.55	3.71	3.70	3.79	3.87	4.03
85 - 90	1.26	1.33	1.37	1.61	1.54	1.69	1.81	2.10
90 - 95	0.27	0.31	0.33	0.46	0.40	0.48	0.54	0.71
95 - 100	0.03	0.04	0.04	0.07	0.06	0.07	0.09	0.13
100 -105	0.00	0.00	0.00	0.01	0.00	0.01	0.01	0.01
Total	5.07	5.21	5.29	5.86	5.70	6.03	6.31	6.99
Belgium								
80 - 85	3.54	3.60	3.62	3.71	3.75	3.83	3.93	4.11
85 - 90	1.32	1.42	1.49	1.63	1.62	1.75	1.94	2.28
90 - 95	0.29	0.34	0.39	0.48	0.44	0.51	0.62	0.87
95 - 100	0.04	0.05	0.06	0.09	0.07	0.08	0.11	0.20
100 -105	0.00	0.00	0.00	0.01	0.01	0.01	0.01	0.03
Total	5.19	5.42	5.55	5.92	5.88	6.18	6.61	7.48
Czechoslovakia								
80 - 85	3.47	3.50	3.45	3.47	3.63	3.73	3.75	3.82
85 - 90	1.22	1.28	1.23	1.28	1.45	1.58	1.63	1.73
90 - 95	0.25	0.29	0.27	0.30	0.35	0.42	0.44	0.50
95 - 100	0.03	0.03	0.03	0.04	0.05	0.06	0.07	0.08
100 -	0.00	0.00	0.00	0.00	0.00	0.00	0.01	0.01
Total	4.97	5.10	4.99	5.09	5.48	5.80	5.89	6.13
Denmark								
80 - 85	3.71	3.73	3.81	3.81	3.79	3.90	4.12	4.20
85 - 90	1.56	1.61	1.79	1.82	1.69	1.89	2.31	2.49
90 - 95	0.41	0.44	0.56	0.60	0.48	0.59	0.87	1.03
95 - 100	0.06	0.06	0.10	0.11	0.07	0.11	0.20	0.25
100 -	0.00	0.00	0.01	0.01	0.00	0.01	0.03	0.03
Total	5.74	5.84	6.27	6.36	6.04	6.50	7.52	8.00

[1] The following life tables were exceptions to full decades: Australia 1980-85; Germany (East) 1954-60; Germany (West) 1956-60; Iceland 1961-70 and 1980-89; Ireland 1980-89: Italy 1952-60 and 1980-89; Luxembourg 1953-60 and 1980-89; Netherlands 1980-89; Poland 1971-70; Singapore 1982-90; Spain 1980-86.

ANNEX TABLE 11. (cont.)

Country and age interval	Male				Female			
	1950-60	1960-70	1970-80	1980-90	1950-60	1960-70	1970-80	1980-90
England & Wales								
80 - 85	3.52	3.58	3.62	3.72	3.84	3.94	4.03	4.15
85 - 90	1.28	1.41	1.48	1.64	1.77	1.97	2.14	2.41
90 - 95	0.29	0.36	0.41	0.50	0.55	0.68	0.79	1.00
95 - 100	0.03	0.05	0.06	0.09	0.10	0.14	0.17	0.26
100 -105	0.00	0.00	0.00	0.01	0.01	0.02	0.02	0.04
Total	5.12	5.40	5.57	5.96	6.27	6.75	7.15	7.86
Estonia								
80 - 85	3.48	3.61	3.57	3.62	3.78	3.87	3.89	3.93
85 - 90	1.28	1.43	1.44	1.47	1.67	1.84	1.91	1.96
90 - 95	0.30	0.37	0.38	0.40	0.47	0.57	0.63	0.67
95 - 100	0.04	0.05	0.06	0.07	0.08	0.11	0.13	0.13
100 -105	0.00	0.00	0.01	0.01	0.01	0.01	0.02	0.02
Total	5.10	5.46	5.46	5.58	6.01	6.40	6.58	6.71
Finland								
80 - 85	3.44	3.45	3.59	3.73	3.62	3.64	3.91	4.09
85 - 90	1.20	1.23	1.43	1.66	1.42	1.46	1.89	2.25
90 - 95	0.26	0.27	0.38	0.51	0.34	0.36	0.61	0.86
95 - 100	0.03	0.03	0.06	0.09	0.05	0.05	0.11	0.19
100 -105	0.00	0.00	0.00	0.01	0.00	0.00	0.02	0.03
Total	4.93	4.98	5.46	6.00	5.43	5.51	6.54	7.42
France								
80 - 85	3.52	3.64	3.73	3.86	3.82	3.96	4.09	4.24
85 - 90	1.28	1.47	1.63	1.84	1.73	1.99	2.24	2.55
90 - 95	0.28	0.38	0.47	0.58	0.50	0.66	0.82	1.05
95 - 100	0.04	0.06	0.07	0.11	0.08	0.13	0.18	0.25
100 -	0.00	0.00	0.01	0.01	0.01	0.01	0.02	0.04
Total	5.12	5.55	5.91	6.40	6.14	6.75	7.36	8.13
Germany, East								
80 - 85	3.54	3.52	3.50	3.52	3.67	3.69	3.74	3.84
85 - 90	1.30	1.27	1.29	1.30	1.49	1.51	1.59	1.74
90 - 95	0.28	0.28	0.28	0.29	0.38	0.38	0.42	0.50
95 - 100	0.03	0.03	0.04	0.04	0.05	0.05	0.06	0.07
100 -	0.00	0.00	0.00	0.00	0.00	0.00	0.00	0.01
Total	5.15	5.10	5.11	5.15	5.59	5.63	5.81	6.16

ANNEX TABLE 11. (cont.)

Country and age interval	Male				Female			
	1950-60	1960-70	1970-80	1980-90	1950-60	1960-70	1970-80	1980-90
Germany. West								
80 - 85	3.55	3.57	3.59	3.72	3.72	3.79	3.90	4.10
85 - 90	1.34	1.39	1.42	1.63	1.56	1.68	1.89	2.24
90 - 95	0.30	0.33	0.37	0.48	0.42	0.48	0.58	0.83
95 - 100	0.04	0.05	0.06	0.08	0.06	0.07	0.10	0.19
100 -105	0.00	0.00	0.00	0.01	0.00	0.01	0.01	0.02
Total	5.23	5.34	5.44	5.92	5.76	6.03	6.48	7.38
Hungary								
80 - 85	3.46	3.52	3.50	3.50	3.58	3.71	3.78	3.83
85 - 90	1.19	1.28	1.28	1.30	1.37	1.54	1.66	1.75
90 - 95	0.24	0.29	0.30	0.32	0.32	0.41	0.46	0.52
95 - 100	0.03	0.03	0.04	0.04	0.04	0.06	0.07	0.08
100 -105	0.00	0.00	0.00	0.00	0.00	0.00	0.01	0.01
Total	4.92	5.12	5.12	5.16	5.31	5.72	5.98	6.19
Iceland								
80 - 85	...	3.84	4.01	4.04	...	4.02	4.21	4.30
85 - 90	...	1.80	2.09	2.17	...	2.06	2.47	2.70
90 - 95	...	0.58	0.73	0.80	...	0.68	1.06	1.25
95 - 100	...	0.11	0.20	0.18	...	0.14	0.29	0.38
100 -105	...	0.01	0.01	0.02	...	0.02	0.05	0.07
Total	...	6.34	7.04	7.21	...	6.92	8.08	8.70
Ireland								
80 - 85	3.57	3.62	3.61	3.67	3.73	3.82	3.89	4.01
85 - 90	1.34	1.41	1.42	1.53	1.63	1.76	1.88	2.12
90 - 95	0.33	0.35	0.38	0.41	0.52	0.58	0.64	0.80
95 - 100	0.06	0.05	0.06	0.06	0.10	0.11	0.13	0.17
100 -	0.00	0.00	0.00	0.00	0.01	0.01	0.01	0.02
Total	5.30	5.43	5.47	5.67	5.99	6.28	6.55	7.12
Italy								
80 - 85	3.69	3.66	3.69	3.78	3.83	3.87	3.97	4.13
85 - 90	1.56	1.51	1.57	1.75	1.81	1.81	2.01	2.31
90 - 95	0.43	0.37	0.43	0.54	0.58	0.53	0.66	0.87
95 - 100	0.07	0.05	0.06	0.09	0.10	0.08	0.13	0.19
100 -	0.00	0.00	0.01	0.01	0.01	0.01	0.01	0.02
Total	5.75	5.59	5.76	6.17	6.33	6.30	6.78	7.52

ANNEX TABLE 11. (cont.)

Country and age interval	Male				Female			
	1950-60	1960-70	1970-80	1980-90	1950-60	1960-70	1970-80	1980-90
Japan								
80 - 85	3.42	3.47	3.70	3.92	3.70	3.78	4.00	4.25
85 - 90	1.19	1.25	1.58	1.94	1.57	1.68	2.05	2.57
90 - 95	0.26	0.28	0.43	0.65	0.42	0.48	0.68	1.08
95 - 100	0.03	0.04	0.07	0.13	0.07	0.07	0.13	0.27
100 -105	0.00	0.00	0.01	0.02	0.00	0.01	0.01	0.04
Total	4.90	5.04	5.79	6.66	5.76	6.02	6.87	8.21
Latvia								
80 - 85	3.64	3.72	3.66	3.64	3.89	3.95	3.94	3.95
85 - 90	1.51	1.63	1.59	1.54	1.88	1.97	2.00	2.00
90 - 95	0.40	0.48	0.47	0.46	0.64	0.67	0.69	0.69
95 - 100	0.07	0.09	0.10	0.09	0.16	0.15	0.16	0.15
100 -105	0.01	0.01	0.01	0.01	0.02	0.02	0.02	0.02
Total	5.63	5.93	5.83	5.74	6.59	6.76	6.81	6.81
Luxembourg								
80 - 85	3.50	3.50	3.53	3.63	3.71	3.72	3.88	4.03
85 - 90	1.28	1.32	1.43	1.53	1.52	1.59	1.84	2.15
90 - 95	0.25	0.33	0.33	0.44	0.41	0.44	0.55	0.76
95 - 100	0.02	0.05	0.06	0.05	0.07	0.08	0.09	0.17
100 -105	0.00	0.00	0.00	0.00	0.00	0.00	0.01	0.02
Total	5.05	5.20	5.26	5.65	5.71	5.83	6.37	7.13
Netherlands								
80 - 85	...	3.79	3.80	3.83	...	3.95	4.10	4.24
85 - 90	...	1.72	1.79	1.82	...	1.97	2.25	2.57
90 - 95	...	0.51	0.58	0.62	...	0.66	0.85	1.10
95 - 100	...	0.08	0.11	0.13	...	0.13	0.20	0.29
100 -	...	0.01	0.01	0.02	...	0.01	0.02	0.04
Total	...	6.11	6.29	6.42	...	6.72	7.42	8.24
New Zealand								
80 - 85	3.73	3.69	3.71	3.79	3.96	4.01	4.09	4.16
85 - 90	1.59	1.55	1.60	1.76	1.97	2.07	2.26	2.43
90 - 95	0.46	0.43	0.47	0.56	0.67	0.72	0.88	1.02
95 - 100	0.08	0.07	0.08	0.10	0.14	0.15	0.21	0.27
100 -	0.01	0.01	0.01	0.01	0.01	0.02	0.03	0.04
Total	5.87	5.57	5.87	6.22	6.75	6.97	7.47	7.92

ANNEX TABLE 11. (cont.)

Country and age interval	Male				Female			
	1950-60	1960-70	1970-80	1980-90	1950-60	1960-70	1970-80	1980-90
Norway								
80 - 85	3.86	3.79	3.81	3.85	3.94	3.97	4.08	4.21
85 - 90	1.81	1.72	1.79	1.86	1.97	2.00	2.22	2.50
90 - 95	0.55	0.51	0.56	0.61	0.66	0.67	0.82	1.03
95 - 100	0.09	0.08	0.10	0.13	0.12	0.13	0.18	0.26
100 -105	0.01	0.01	0.01	0.01	0.01	0.01	0.02	0.04
Total	6.32	6.11	6.27	6.46	6.70	6.78	7.32	8.04
Poland								
80 - 85	...	...	3.59	3.59	...	...	3.88	3.93
85 - 90	...	...	1.47	1.44	...	...	1.89	1.90
90 - 95	...	...	0.40	0.38	...	...	0.62	0.60
95 - 100	...	...	0.07	0.07	...	...	0.12	0.12
100 -105	...	...	0.01	0.01	...	...	0.02	0.02
Total	...	...	5.54	5.49	...	...	6.53	6.57
Portugal								
80 - 85	3.51	3.52	3.58	3.70	3.78	3.82	3.88	3.99
85 - 90	1.25	1.30	1.40	1.57	1.68	1.75	1.85	2.05
90 - 95	0.28	0.30	0.34	0.43	0.51	0.52	0.57	0.72
95 - 100	0.04	0.04	0.05	0.06	0.10	0.10	0.11	0.15
100 -105	0.00	0.00	0.00	0.01	0.01	0.01	0.01	0.02
Total	5.08	5.16	5.37	5.77	6.08	6.20	6.42	6.93
Scotland								
80 - 85	3.45	3.52	3.54	3.63	3.71	3.84	3.97	4.06
85 - 90	1.18	1.31	1.38	1.51	1.57	1.81	2.04	2.25
90 - 95	0.25	0.31	0.35	0.42	0.43	0.57	0.71	0.86
95 - 100	0.03	0.04	0.06	0.06	0.07	0.11	0.15	0.21
100 -	0.00	0.00	0.00	0.01	0.00	0.01	0.02	0.04
Total	4.91	5.18	5.33	5.63	5.78	6.34	6.89	7.42
Singapore								
80 - 85	...	...	...	3.86	...	...	...	4.12
85 - 90	...	...	...	1.95	...	...	...	2.42
90 - 95	...	...	...	0.75	...	...	...	1.07
95 - 100	...	...	...	0.21	...	...	...	0.33
100 -	...	...	...	0.02	...	...	...	0.08
Total	...	...	...	6.79	...	...	...	8.02

ANNEX TABLE 11. (cont.)

Country and age interval	Male				Female			
	1950-60	1960-70	1970-80	1980-90	1950-60	1960-70	1970-80	1980-90
Spain								
80 - 85	3.58	3.67	3.74	3.87	3.82	3.92	4.00	4.13
85 - 90	1.38	1.52	1.66	1.89	1.77	1.93	2.09	2.34
90 - 95	0.37	0.42	0.50	0.66	0.61	0.68	0.75	0.93
95 - 100	0.07	0.08	0.09	0.16	0.14	0.15	0.16	0.23
100 -105	0.00	0.00	0.00	0.00	0.00	0.00	0.00	0.00
Total	5.40	5.69	5.99	6.58	6.34	6.68	7.00	7.63
Sweden								
80 - 85	3.70	3.74	3.78	3.86	3.79	3.92	4.10	4.22
85 - 90	1.54	1.63	1.72	1.83	1.71	1.92	2.26	2.52
90 - 95	0.39	0.45	0.52	0.58	0.49	0.61	0.86	1.04
95 - 100	0.05	0.07	0.09	0.11	0.07	0.12	0.20	0.26
100 -105	0.00	0.00	0.01	0.01	0.01	0.01	0.02	0.03
Total	5.68	5.89	6.12	6.39	6.07	6.58	7.44	8.07
Switzerland								
80 - 85	3.57	3.66	3.77	3.88	3.76	3.88	4.09	4.25
85 - 90	1.36	1.49	1.69	1.90	1.63	1.83	2.20	2.56
90 - 95	0.30	0.37	0.50	0.60	0.46	0.55	0.80	1.05
95 - 100	0.05	0.06	0.08	0.11	0.07	0.09	0.16	0.25
100 -105	0.00	0.00	0.01	0.01	0.00	0.01	0.02	0.03
Total	5.28	5.58	6.05	6.50	5.92	6.36	7.27	8.14

ANNEX TABLE 12. YEARS LIVED AT SPECIFIED AGE INTERVALS PER EACH PERSON REACHING THE INTERVAL.
(for exceptions from full decades, see footnote).

Country and age interval	Male				Female			
	1950-60	1960-70	1970-80	1980-90	1950-60	1960-70	1970-80	1980-90
Australia[1]								
80 - 85	...	...	3.71	3.84	...	...	4.10	4.24
85 - 90	...	...	3.22	3.38	...	...	3.59	3.76
90 - 95	...	...	2.74	2.81	...	...	30.7	3.20
95 - 100	...	...	2.23	2.26	...	...	2.43	2.53
100 - 105	...	...	2.14	1.84	...	...	2.14	2.03
Austria								
80 - 85	3.50	3.53	3.55	3.71	3.70	3.79	3.87	4.03
85 - 90	2.93	3.00	3.03	3.20	3.11	3 22	3.29	3.46
90 - 95	2.34	2.41	2.44	2.65	2.53	2 61	2.65	2.83
95 - 100	1.90	1.97	2.01	2.10	2.01	2 09	2.11	2.22
100 - 105	1.28	1.64	1.68	1.76	1.67	1 67	1.71	1.85
Belgium								
80 - 85	3.54	3.60	3.62	3.71	3.75	3.83	3.93	4.11
85 - 90	2.97	3.04	3.12	3.23	3.17	3.26	3.26	3.58
90 - 95	2.38	2.47	2.54	2.69	2.58	2.64	2.64	2.98
95 - 100	1.98	2.06	2.01	2.17	2.07	2.16	2.16	2.42
100 - 105	1.67	1.63	1.52	1.73	1.63	1.67	1.67	2.03
Czechoslovakia								
80 - 85	3.47	3.50	3.45	3.47	3.63	3.73	3.75	3.82
85 - 90	2.88	2.95	2.92	2.97	3.05	3.14	3.17	3.25
90 - 95	2.31	2.38	2.39	2.45	2.46	2.56	2.57	2.64
95 - 100	1.88	1.82	2.00	1.86	1.93	2.05	2.07	2.05
100 - 105	1.41	1.39	1.69	1.44	1.53	1.61	1.68	1.59
Denmark								
80 - 85	3.71	3.73	3.81	3.81	3.79	3.90	4.12	4.20
85 - 90	3.15	3.17	3.31	3.37	3.22	3.36	3.60	3.71
90 - 95	2.51	2.59	2.75	2.81	2.61	2.74	2.96	3.08
95 - 100	2.02	1.94	2.18	2.21	2.07	2.17	2.38	2.44
100 - 105	1.25	1.44	1.65	1.77	1.31	1.77	1.99	1.92

[1] The following life tables were exceptions to full decades: Australia 1980-98; Germany(East) 1956-60; Germany(West) 1956-60; Iceland 1961-70 and 1980-89; Ireland 1980-89; Italy 1952-60 and 1980-89; Luxembourg 1963-60 and 1980-89; Netherlands 1980-89; Poland 1971-70; Singapore 1982-90; Spain 1980-86.

ANNEX TABLE 12. (cont.)

Country and age interval	Male				Female			
	1950-60	1960-70	1970-80	1980-90	1950-60	1960-70	1970-80	1980-90
England & Wales								
80 - 85	3.52	3.58	3.62	3.72	3.84	3.94	4.03	4.15
85 - 90	2.93	3.06	3.13	3.24	3.28	3.42	3.52	3.68
90 - 95	2.41	2.54	2.60	2.75	2.75	2.87	2.94	3.11
95 - 100	1.86	2.03	2.07	2.23	2.20	2.31	2.37	2.53
100 -	1.66	1.57	1.68	1.92	1.81	1.93	2.00	2.12
Estonia								
80 - 85	3.48	3.61	3.57	3.62	3.78	3.87	3.89	3.93
85 - 90	2.95	3.08	3.09	3.12	3.22	3.31	3.40	3.41
90 - 95	2.51	2.56	2.61	2.61	2.66	2.73	2.82	2.85
95 - 100	1.77	1.94	2.13	2.28	2.23	2.21	2.38	2.29
100 -	1.64	1.53	1.91	1.80	1.67	1.85	1.99	1.92
Finland								
80 - 85	3.43	3.45	3.59	3.73	3.62	3.64	3.91	4.09
85 - 90	2.90	2.91	3.10	3.27	3.03	3.05	3.36	3.58
90 - 95	2.37	2.37	2.55	2.72	2.44	2.47	2.80	2.98
95 - 100	1.89	1.94	1.94	2.13	1.95	2.00	2.31	2.43
100 -	1.12	1.43	1.42	1.67	1.76	1.80	2.01	2.22
France								
80 - 85	3.52	3.64	3.73	3.86	3.82	3.96	4.09	4.24
85 - 90	2.93	3.09	3.21	3.34	3.34	3.41	3.56	3.72
90 - 95	2.36	2.51	2.64	2.75	2.75	2.80	2.93	3.08
95 - 100	1.95	2.11	2.15	2.22	2.22	2.25	2.34	2.46
100 -	1.38	1.56	1.57	1.68	1.68	1.79	1.93	2.05
Germany-East								
80 - 85	3.53	3.51	3.50	3.52	3.67	3.69	3.75	3.84
85 - 90	2.95	2.93	2.95	2.96	3.08	3.09	3.13	3.24
90 - 95	2.32	2.32	2.37	2.39	2.49	2.47	2.52	2.62
95 - 100	1.88	1.81	1.92	1.90	1.87	1.93	2.03	2.07
100 -	1.44	1.32	1.54	1.45	1.45	1.40	1.59	1.62
Germany-West								
80 - 85	3.55	3.57	3.58	3.72	3.71	3.80	3.91	4.09
85 - 90	2.98	3.03	3.08	3.23	3.12	3.23	3.34	3.56
90 - 95	2.37	2.48	2.52	2.68	2.56	2.63	2.72	2.95
95 - 100	1.95	1.99	2.06	2.20	2.01	2.12	2.16	2.42
100 -	1.46	1.50	1.52	1.71	1.51	1.59	1.59	2.02

ANNEX TABLE 12. (cont.)

Country and age interval	Male				Female			
	1950-60	1960-70	1970-80	1980-90	1950-60	1960-70	1970-80	1980-90
Hungary								
80 - 85	3.46	3.52	3.49	3.50	3.58	3.70	3.78	3.82
85 - 90	2.86	2.93	2.97	3.00	3.01	3.12	3.20	3.27
90 - 95	2.28	2.38	2.44	2.44	2.41	2.55	2.60	2.67
95 - 100	1.89	1.89	1.87	2.02	1.87	2.03	2.07	2.13
100 -	1.41	1.41	1.39	1.61	1.34	1.48	1.65	1.68
Iceland								
80 - 85	...	3.83	4.01	4.04	...	4.03	4.21	4.30
85 - 90	...	3.25	3.45	3.54	...	3.45	3.71	3.83
90 - 95	...	2.84	2.94	2.94	...	2.77	3.21	3.30
95 - 100	...	2.21	2.80	2.40	...	2.36	2.43	2.74
100 -	...	1.17	0.79	1.77	...	1.76	1.92	2.00
Ireland								
80 - 85	3.56	3.62	3.61	3.67	3.73	3.82	3.89	4.01
85 - 90	2.97	3.01	3.06	3.15	3.21	3.29	3.37	3.52
90 - 95	2.55	2.52	2.60	2.58	2.80	2.82	2.88	2.96
95 - 100	2.06	1.95	1.97	1.92	2.27	2.16	2.23	2.35
100 -	1.32	2.18	1.74	1.64	1.54	1.61	1.92	1.84
Italy								
80 - 85	3.69	3.67	3.69	3.79	3.84	3.87	3.97	4.13
85 - 90	3.15	3.10	3.18	3.30	3.33	3.28	3.42	3.59
90 - 95	2.60	2.47	2.59	2.72	2.78	2.66	2.79	2.96
95 - 100	1.97	1.88	2.11	2.19	2.14	2.04	2.22	2.35
100 -	1.68	1.74	1.62	1.79	1.93	1.90	1.85	1.92
Japan								
80 - 85	3.42	3.47	3.71	3.91	3.70	3.78	4.00	4.25
85 - 90	2.89	2.93	3.16	3.40	3.16	3.22	3.44	3.74
90 - 95	2.34	2.41	2.60	2.84	2.57	2.63	2.80	3.11
95 - 100	1.96	1.98	2.10	2.32	2.06	2.10	2.25	2.48
100 -	1.94	1.79	1.84	2.02	1.85	1.83	1.93	2.16
Latvia								
80 - 85	3.64	3.72	3.66	3.65	3.88	3.95	3.94	3.95
85 - 90	3.12	3.21	3.22	3.22	3.37	3.40	3.44	3.43
90 - 95	2.57	2.68	2.72	2.72	2.88	2.87	2.88	2.88
95 - 100	2.31	2.37	2.41	2.41	2.60	2.43	2.44	2.42
100 -	2.01	1.94	2.10	2.10	2.16	2.06	2.04	2.05

ANNEX TABLE 12.   (cont.)

Country and age interval	Male				Female			
	1950-60	1960-70	1970-80	1980-90	1950-60	1960-70	1970-80	1980-90
Luxembourg								
80 - 85	3.50	3.50	3.53	3.63	3.70	3.72	3.88	4.04
85 - 90	2.95	3.00	3.01	3.18	3.02	3.16	3.31	3.51
90 - 95	2.25	2.53	2.53	2.66	2.63	2.64	2.71	2.86
95 - 100	1.71	1.92	2.14	1.63	2.20	2.12	2.13	2.38
100 -	...	1.36	1.69	1.43	1.39	1.49	1.69	2.04
Netherlands								
80 - 85	...	3.79	3.81	3.82	...	3.95	4.09	4.24
85 - 90	...	3.26	3.33	3.36	...	3.40	3.58	3.75
90 - 95	...	2.68	2.80	2.87	...	2.81	2.98	3.14
95 - 100	...	2.12	2.19	2.35	...	2.26	2.38	2.52
100 -	...	.158	1.84	1.97	...	1.79	2.05	2.14
New Zealand								
80 - 85	3.73	3.70	3.71	3.78	3.96	4.01	4.09	4.16
85 - 90	3.17	3.14	3.21	3.30	3.40	3.45	3.60	3.70
90 - 95	2.74	2.68	2.71	2.76	2.89	2.90	3.03	3.12
95 - 100	2.11	2.10	2.15	2.26	2.24	2.31	2.46	2.54
100 -	2.44	1.65	1.45	1.48	1.58	2.10	1.93	2.21
Norway								
80 - 85	3.86	3.79	3.81	3.85	3.95	3.97	4.08	4.21
85 - 90	3.30	3.27	3.33	3.38	3.41	3.43	3.55	3.71
90 - 95	2.69	2.66	2.75	2.83	2.80	2.83	2.95	3.09
95 - 100	2.06	2.11	2.17	2.24	2.21	2.21	2.37	2.47
100 -	1.97	1.69	1.89	2.00	1.97	1.78	1.93	2.20
Poland								
80 - 85	...	...	3.59	3.59	...	...	3.89	3.93
85 - 90	...	...	3.12	3.09	...	...	3.37	3.34
90 - 95	...	...	2.64	2.63	...	...	2.80	2.77
95 - 100	...	...	2.30	2.29	...	...	2.35	2.32
100 -	...	...	2.00	1.99	...	...	2.04	2.02
Portugal								
80 - 85	3.50	3.52	3.58	3.70	3.78	3.83	3.88	4.00
85 - 90	2.90	2.96	3.04	3.15	3.21	3.25	3.32	3.44
90 - 95	2.45	2.40	2.50	2.61	2.73	2.75	2.75	2.89
95 - 100	2.04	1.96	2.01	2.05	2.18	2.21	2.22	2.34
100 -	1.46	1.55	1.67	1.82	1.68	1.79	2.04	1.95

ANNEX TABLE 12. (cont.)

Country and age interval	Male				Female			
	1950-60	1960-70	1970-80	1980-90	1950-60	1960-70	1970-80	1980-90
Scotland								
80 - 85	3.45	3.52	3.54	3.63	3.70	3.84	3.97	4.06
85 - 90	2.86	2.97	3.06	3.15	3.16	3.32	3.46	3.60
90 - 95	2.34	2.45	2.54	2.63	2.61	2.77	2.89	3.01
95 - 100	1.93	1.96	2.02	2.08	2.06	2.21	2.32	2.54
100 -	1.36	1.50	1.59	1.65	1.61	1.83	1.91	2.25
Singapore-Chinese								
80 - 85	...	...	...	3.87	...	...	...	4.12
85 - 90	...	...	...	3.49	...	...	...	3.74
90 - 95	...	...	...	3.07	...	...	...	
95 - 100	...	...	...	2.63	...	...	...	3.20
100 -	...	...	...	1.99	...	...	...	2.76
								2.57
Spain								
80 - 85	3.58	3.67	3.74	3.87	3.82	3.92	4.01	4.14
85 - 90	3.02	3.14	3.25	3.39	3.30	3.40	3.48	3.62
90 - 95	2.69	2.69	2.70	2.93	2.93	2.93	2.90	3.08
95 - 100	2.08	2.04	2.05	2.11	2.14	2.17	2.10	2.13
100 -	1.60	1.61	1.86	2.00	1.80	1.86	1.96	2.00
Sweden								
80 - 85	3.70	3.74	3.78	3.86	3.79	3.93	4.10	4.23
85 - 90	3.10	3.20	3.27	3.34	3.24	3.36	3.57	3.71
90 - 95	2.49	2.58	2.71	2.75	2.64	2.78	2.99	3.08
95 - 100	1.94	2.01	2.13	2.21	2.05	2.23	2.38	2.45
100 -	1.51	1.72	1.68	1.76	1.71	1.84	1.98	2.01
Switzerland								
80 - 85	3.57	3.65	3.77	3.89	3.76	3.88	4.09	4.25
85 - 90	2.97	3.09	3.25	3.37	3.18	3.31	3.52	3.74
90 - 95	2.43	2.50	2.65	2.74	2.62	2.69	2.90	3.06
95 - 100	2.00	1.98	2.16	2.23	2.04	2.14	2.29	2.43
100 -	1.75	1.80	1.73	1.82	1.58	1.69	1.60	2.00

ANNEX Table 13. ANNUAL POPULATION GROWTH (%) IN COUNTRIES INVOLVED AND NOT INVOLVED IN WORLD WAR I.

Age	Involved in war[1]						Not involved in war[2]					
	Male			Female			Male			Female		
	1960 to 1970	1970 to 1980	1980 to 1990	1960 to 1970	1970 to 1980	1980 to 1990	1960 to 1970	1970 to 1980	1980 to 1990	1960 to 1970	1970 to 1980	1980 to 1990
80	0.47	2.20	2.72	2.53	2.60	2.39	1.35	2.00	2.53	2.65	3.61	2.83
81	0.46	1.67	3.33	2.58	2.61	2.74	1.82	1.87	2.35	3.06	3.71	2.99
82	0.49	1.33	3.60	2.67	2.78	2.79	1.78	1.70	2.39	3.08	3.80	3.14
83	0.27	1.33	3.96	2.58	3.16	2.98	2.02	2.09	2.10	3.32	4.11	3.26
84	0.59	0.49	4.64	2.78	2.94	3.27	2.21	1.94	2.30	3.43	4.22	3.62
85	1.02	0.50	4.72	3.20	3.14	3.56	2.71	1.98	2.57	4.04	4.30	4.04
86	1.66	0.90	4.35	3.61	3.46	3.64	2.67	2.67	2.26	4.04	4.94	4.04
87	1.84	0.81	4.80	3.87	3.28	4.45	3.04	2.33	2.88	4.21	4.75	4.99
88	3.08	0.90	4.49	4.91	3.55	4.53	3.61	2.99	2.61	.462	5.30	5.04
89	2.83	1.20	4.52	4.48	3.64	4.88	4.19	2.60	2.82	.463	5.38	5.35
90	3.48	1.47	3.74	4.79	3.97	4.67	4.97	2.60	2.65	5.00	5.27	5.63
91	4.04	1.71	3.46	5.10	4.36	4.82	5.40	3.28	2.57	5.38	5.94	5.73
92	4.75	1.83	3.39	5.65	4.29	5.21	5.68	3.38	2.35	5.49	5.90	5.84
93	4.58	1.96	3.60	5.53	4.37	5.75	4.42	4.26	3.01	4.90	6.19	6.47
94	5.24	2.46	2.58	5.66	4.94	5.55	5.03	4.22	3.25	4.82	7.02	6.42
95	5.71	3.46	2.87	5.58	5.40	6.18	5.66	5.01	2.99	5.48	7.22	6.67
96	5.27	4.53	2.98	5.64	5.77	6.50	5.00	4.81	4.73	4.91	7.80	7.15
97	5.70	4.30	3.33	6.39	5.90	6.39	5.54	5.47	4.88	6.79	7.49	6.87
98	5.69	5.76	3.60	5.84	7.29	6.77	2.57	7.89	5.20	4.03	7.67	8.27
99	6.34	5.82	3.88	7.21	6.37	6.99	4.56	7.39	4.45	7.18	7.83	7.97
100	7.74	6.09	5.52	7.43	7.17	8.20	6.35	8.22	-0.44	5.57	9.73	4.09
101	7.83	5.49	7.56	7.40	7.61	9.24	4.67	11.61	-1.30	5.79	10.53	4.56
102	4.22	7.43	7.71	7.85	8.99	8.01	8.31	9.37	2.21	8.39	10.54	2.94
103	15.67	8.84	5.54	10.29	7.50	8.88	4.81	12.07	-1.27	5.62	12.73	4.19
104	9.15	9.60	8.69	10.26	8.66	8.87	0.00	-6.70	28.21	1.06	13.98	3.85

[1]Austria, Czechoslovakia, England & Wales, France, Germany (East and West), Hungary, Italy, New Zealand, Scotland.
[2]Denmark, Netherlands, Norway, Sweden, Switzerland.

ANNEX TABLE 14.   OLDEST-OLD POPULATION ON 1 JANUARY, 1960-1990

Date	80-84	85-89	90-94	95-99	100-	Total
Western Europe (13 countries)						
Male						
1960	1 143 569	392 811	75 910	7 995	324	1 620 609
1970	1 220 552	478 847	115 792	13 701	660	1 829 552
1980	1 439 430	538 481	143 302	21 268	1 346	2 143 827
1990	2 031 058	832 096	204 537	30 315	2 279	3 100 285
Female						
1960	1 784 305	677 152	161 331	22 190	1 253	12 646 231
1970	2 312 400	984 330	266 399	38 173	2 590	3 603 892
1980	3 095 178	1 402 492	414 789	70 007	5 727	4 988 193
1990	4 140 168	2 137 588	699 849	135 417	12 430	7 125 452
Eastern Europe (3 countries)						
Male						
1960	165 895	52 116	8 866	747	...	227 624
1970	176 106	62 414	13 283	1 273	...	253 076
1980	200 823	64 175	14 410	1 760	...	281 168
1990	238 694	85 777	17 534	1 753	...	343 758
Female						
1960	247 042	80 616	15 891	1 624	...	345 173
1970	324 710	118 197	26 299	2 912	...	472 118
1980	432 721	161 206	37 406	4 653	...	635 986
1990	524 973	221 556	56 995	7 213	...	810 737
Japan						
Male						
1960	164 655	44 392	7 112	538	32	216 729
1970	233 934	68 817	13 242	1 352	82	317 427
1980	401 590	129 656	27 342	2 942	171	561 701
1990	650 315	268 508	67 071	8 941	666	995 501
Female						
1960	301 953	98 438	20 116	2 050	123	422 680
1970	399 819	155 357	38 540	4 579	263	598 558
1980	648 769	252 137	69 193	9 742	747	980 588
1990	1 098 745	535 616	165 128	25 937	2 460	1 827 886

ANNEX TABLE 15.   PERSONS AGED 80 AND OVER, 1960-1990. BOTH SEXES.

	Country	1.1.1960	1.1.1970	1.1.1980	1.1.1990
	Australia	...	186876	243379	362115
*	Austria	121225	155642	197719	277808
	Belgium	169173	201557	257070	347150
	Canada	224085	329793	426319	589457 1)
**	Czechoslovakia	149761	193807	260721	353912
*	Denmark	74432	101086	144296	198458
*	England & Wales	895107	1117200	1344324	1852018
**	Estonia	19227	26137	32247	40387
*	Finland	40594	51153	81948	138281
*	France	909205	1154926	1494182	2084462
**	Germany, East	314798	378751	448644	541034
*	Germany, west	836638	1121126	1556512	2394224
**	Hungary	108238	152636	207789	259632
*	Iceland	2526 2)	2980	5009	6321
	Ireland	58266	60218	65044	77235
*	Italy	777347	935286	1211292	1745513
*	Japan	639409	915985	1542289	2823387
**	Latvia	37293	48973	57472	72125
	Luxembourg	4683	5761	7769	11338
*	Netherlands	155340	222736	309963	427146
	New Zealand	35276	45185	51687	72092
*	Norway	70138	84154	117358	156279
	Poland	...	321895 3)	491462	733676
	Portugal	107575	136730	172120	247547
	Scotland	84939	100354	123439	166308
	Spain	368107	505937	689205	960691 4)
*	Sweden	137957	183736	254389	358935
*	Switzerland	80707	107459	160907	243975
*	13 countries of low or medium mortality	4740625	6153469	8420188	12706807
**	5 countries of high mortality	629317	800304	1006873	1267090

1) 1989;   2) 1961;   3) 1971;   4) 1987

ANNEX TABLE 16. POPULATION GROWTH FACTOR FROM 1960 TO 1990

P = projected at constant mortality
A = actually observed

MALE

Country	80-84		85-89		90-94		95-99		100-		Total	
	P	A	P	A	P	A	P	A	P	A	P	A
Austria	1.56	1.69	1.63	2.13	1.61	2.51	1.69	3.08	2.44	8.80	1.58	1.83
Belgium	1.32	1.40	1.35	1.67	1.61	2.64	1.62	3.46	...	...	1.34	1.53
Czechoslovakia	1.88	1.90	1.73	1.83	1.70	2.10	1.62	1.79	...	...	1.83	1.89
Denmark	1.62	1.67	1.77	2.09	2.01	2.94	2.09	4.24	2.88	9.11	1.68	1.86
England & Wales	1.63	1.74	1.50	1.94	1.42	2.42	1.56	3.95	1.64	6.51	1.59	1.83
Estonia	1.78	1.86	1.74	2.02	1.73	2.24	1.69	2.59	...	...	1.77	1.93
Finland	2.55	2.78	2.25	3.11	2.46	4.72	1.70	4.15	2.14	11.00	2.47	2.94
France	1.73	1.93	1.70	2.47	1.67	3.28	1.62	4.48	1.98	6.96	1.72	2.13
Germany. East	1.11	1.12	1.41	1.42	1.70	1.77	2.40	2.72	...	...	1.20	1.21
Germany. West	1.66	1.76	1.87	2.30	2.01	3.06	2.46	5.02	...	11.00	1.72	1.94
Hungary	1.73	1.78	1.87	2.07	1.82	2.30	1.56	2.43	...	...	1.77	1.86
Iceland	1.61	1.68	2.09	2.56	1.78	2.57	1.75	2.83	1.00	1.00	1.73	1.97
Ireland	0.97	1.01	0.98	1.18	1.06	1.26	1.39	1.19	1.68	0.86	0.98	1.06
Italy	1.63	1.69	1.53	1.76	1.62	1.96	1.90	2.50	2.83	7.05	1.60	1.73
Japan	3.44	3.95	3.70	6.05	3.88	9.43	4.57	16.62	5.31	21.48	3.51	4.59
Latvia	1.66	1.66	1.65	1.70	1.89	1.97	1.76	2.47	...	...	1.67	1.69
Luxembourg	1.46	1.53	1.56	1.90	1.92	3.34	2.72	5.00	...	...	1.50	1.68
Netherlands	1.31	1.31	1.36	1.44	1.38	1.66	1.66	2.56	...	...	1.33	1.38
New Zealand	1.54	1.58	1.57	1.74	1.61	1.81	2.08	2.47	...	...	1.56	1.64
Norway	1.67	1.67	1.79	1.84	2.00	2.26	1.98	2.62	2.31	3.70	1.73	1.77
Portugal	2.18	2.32	2.09	2.59	2.08	3.11	2.32	3.66	...	...	2.15	2.42
Scotland	1.37	1.45	1.27	1.61	1.18	1.85	1.55	3.34	...	...	1.34	1.52
Sweden	1.83	1.92	1.87	2.24	1.96	2.81	1.70	3.31	1.79	4.96	1.84	2.05
Switzerland	2.07	2.28	2.16	3.05	2.30	4.32	2.49	6.07	3.37	8.50	2.10	2.56

ANNEX TABLE 16. (cont.)

FEMALE

Country	80-84		85-89		90-94		95-99		100-		Total	
	P	A	P	A	P	A	P	A	P	A	P	A
Austria	2.00	2.21	2.25	3.15	2.52	4.25	2.93	5.99	3.63	9.40	2.09	2.55
Belgium	1.87	2.07	1.97	2.81	2.05	3.84	2.13	5.64	...	...	1.91	2.40
Czechoslovakia	2.34	2.47	2.42	2.93	2.63	3.72	2.46	3.82	...	...	2.37	2.65
Denmark	2.38	2.64	2.56	3.79	2.58	5.44	2.71	8.68	4.18	24.30	2.44	3.16
England & Wales	1.72	1.87	1.84	2.52	1.97	3.48	2.18	4.99	2.54	7.78	1.77	2.19
Estonia	1.89	1.98	1.98	2.33	2.33	3.23	1.99	2.94	...	...	1.94	2.16
Finland	2.88	3.26	2.54	4.00	2.76	6.60	1.81	7.02	2.49	13.22	2.78	3.63
France	1.76	1.97	1.89	2.83	2.02	4.11	2.12	5.95	2.74	11.14	1.81	2.37
Germany. East	1.74	1.84	2.08	2.46	2.52	3.28	3.26	4.54	...	...	1.86	2.06
Germany. West	2.66	2.97	3.03	4.41	3.44	6.56	4.08	11.25	...	21.40	2.79	3.51
Hungary	2.30	2.49	2.55	3.31	2.70	4.24	2.44	5.13	...	...	2.38	2.77
Iceland	1.74	1.86	1.97	2.63	1.83	3.17	1.73	4.47	2.35	7.50	1.81	2.23
Ireland	1.24	1.34	1.33	1.76	1.53	2.28	1.79	2.65	1.87	3.38	1.29	1.54
Italy	2.20	2.40	2.19	2.89	2.43	3.57	2.71	4.29	3.72	7.94	2.22	2.63
Japan	3.16	3.64	3.28	5.44	3.42	8.21	3.84	12.65	4.58	20.00	3.20	4.32
Latvia	1.88	1.93	2.04	2.19	2.39	2.45	2.25	2.13	...	...	1.97	2.04
Luxembourg	2.31	2.56	2.50	3.61	2.59	4.84	3.05	6.71	...	...	2.37	2.95
Netherlands	1.91	2.06	1.99	2.60	2.05	3.31	2.15	4.24	...	...	1.94	2.32
New Zealand	1.97	2.08	2.10	2.58	2.28	3.23	3.08	6.01	...	...	2.04	2.33
Norway	2.13	2.28	2.28	2.90	2.23	3.39	2.04	3.96	1.90	4.26	2.18	2.57
Portugal	2.01	2.15	1.93	2.31	2.02	2.82	2.05	3.06	...	2.57	1.98	2.25
Scotland	1.73	1.90	1.80	2.58	1.84	3.56	1.90	5.44	...	...	1.75	2.21
Sweden	2.32	2.60	2.42	3.60	2.37	4.84	2.08	6.13	2.14	9.30	2.34	3.03
Switzerland	2.38	2.72	2.59	4.14	2.76	6.12	2.70	8.42	2.57	12.86	2.45	3.30